Antiarrhythmic Therapy: A Pathophysiologic Approach

by
Members of the Sicilian Gambit Who Coauthored
the Volume:

Günter Breithardt, M.D.
A. John Camm, M.D.
Ronald W. F. Campbell, M.D.
Harry A. Fozzard, M.D.
Brian F. Hoffman, M.D.
Michiel J. Janse, M.D.
Ralph Lazzara, M.D.
Samuel Lévy, M.D.
Robert J. Myerburg, M.D.
Dan M. Roden, M.D., C.M.
Michael R. Rosen, M.D.
Peter J. Schwartz, M.D.
Harold C. Strauss, M.D.
Albert L. Waldo, M.D.
Andrew L. Wit, Ph.D.
Raymond L. Woosley, M.D., Ph.D.
Antonio Zaza, M.D.
Douglas P. Zipes, M.D.

Futura Publishing Company, Inc.
Armonk, NY
1994

Library of Congress Cataloging-in-Publication Data

Members of the Sicilian Gambit.
   Antiarrhythmic therapy : a pathophysiologic approach.
      p. cm.
   Developed by the Members of the Sicilian Gambit at the Harriman
meeting.
   Includes bibliographical references and index.
   ISBN 0-87993-596-0
   1. Arrhythmia—Treatment. 2. Arrhythmia—Pathophysiology.
I. Title.
   [DNLM: 1. Arrhythmia—drug therapy. 2. Arrhythmia—
physiopathology. 3. Anti-Arrhythmia Agents—pharmacology. WG 330
1994]
RC685.A65M45   1994
616.1'28—dc20
DNLM/DLC
for Library of Congress   94-13905
                                                                       CIP

Published by
Futura Publishing Company, Inc.
135 Bedford Road
Armonk, New York 10504-0418

LC#: 94-13905
ISBN #: 0-87993-596-0

Every effort has been made to ensure that the information in this book
is as up to date and as accurate at the time of publication. However,
due to the constant developments in medicine, neither the authors,
nor the editor, nor the publisher can accept any legal or any other
responsibility for any errors or omissions that may occur.

Printed in the United States of America

This book is printed on acid-free paper.

Contributors

Günter Breithardt, M.D.   Medizinische Klinik und Poliklinik, Innere Medizin C—Kardiologie, Westfalische Wilhelms, Universitat Münster, Münster, Germany

A. John Camm, M.D.   Professor of Clinical Cardiology, Department of Cardiological Sciences, St. George's Hospital Medical School, London, United Kingdom

Ronald W. F. Campbell, M.D.   Professor of Cardiology, University of Newcastle upon Tyne, Freeman Hospital, Newcastle upon Tyne, United Kingdom

Harry A. Fozzard, M.D.   The Otho S. A. Sprague Distinguished Service Professor of Medical Sciences, Chairman, Departments of Pharmacological and Physiological Sciences and Medicine, University of Chicago, Chicago, Illinois

Brian F. Hoffman, M.D.   David Hosack Professor of Pharmacology, and Chairman, Department of Pharmacology, Columbia University, New York, New York

Michiel J. Janse, M.D.   Professor, Klinische en Experimentele Cardiologie, Academisch Ziekenhuis Bij de Universiteit van Amsterdam, Academisch Medisch Centrum, Amsterdam, The Netherlands

Ralph Lazzara, M.D.   Professor of Medicine, Department of Medicine, Chief, Cardiovascular Section, The University of Oklahoma Health Sciences Center, Oklahoma City, Oklahoma

Samuel Lévy, M.D.   Professor of Medicine, Chief, Division of Cardiology, Hopital Nord, University of Marseille, Marseille, France

Robert J. Myerburg, M.D. Professor of Medicine, Chairman, Division of Cardiology, University of Miami Medical Center, Miami, Florida

Dan M. Roden, M.D., C.M. Professor of Medicine, Division of Clinical Pharmacology, School of Medicine, Vanderbilt University, Nashville, Tennesee

Michael R. Rosen, M.D. Gustavus A. Pfeiffer Professor of Pharmacology, Professor of Pediatrics, Columbia University, New York, New York

Peter J. Schwartz, M.D. Professor of Medicine, Instituto di Clinica Medica Generale e Terapia Medica, Università di Milano, Milano, Italy

Harold C. Strauss, M.D. The Edward S. Orgain Professor of Cardiology, Professor of Medicine and Pharmacology, Department of Medicine, Cardiovascular Division, Duke University Medical Center, Durham, North Carolina

Albert L. Waldo, M.D. Professor of Medicine, Department of Medicine, Case Western Reserve University, University Hospitals of Cleveland, Cleveland, Ohio

Andrew L. Wit, Ph.D. Professor of Pharmacology, Department of Pharmacology, Columbia University, New York, New York

Raymond L. Woosley, M.D., Ph.D. Professor of Pharmacology, Chairman, Department of Pharmacology, Georgetown University Medical Center, Washington, DC

Antonio Zaza, M.D. Assistant Professor of Physiology, Dipartimento di Fisiologia e Biochimica Generali, Università Degli Studi di Milano, Sezione di Fisiologia Generale, Laboratorio di Electrofisiologia, Milano, Italy

Douglas P. Zipes, M.D. Distinguished Professor of Medicine, Indiana University School of Medicine, Krannert Institute of Cardiology, Indianapolis, Indiana

Foreword

Cardiac arrhythmias associated with ischemia, infarction, and sudden death represent the final common pathway of many, if not most, cardiac-related deaths. Recent estimates indicate loss of life from malignant disturbances of cardiac rhythm approaches 300,000 each year in the United States alone. Despite the magnitude of this threat, and unlike impressive results achieved with many other aspects of cardiac disease, progress in developing effective therapeutic strategies for rhythm disorders has been slow, complicated, and difficult to realize. Notable improvements have occurred in the areas of ablation and defibrillator technologies; however, these invasive approaches seem unlikely to be useful in many cases, and both involve increased cost and surgical risk.

The original Sicilian Gambit paper published at the end of 1991 helped initiate a reevaluation of pharmacologic antiarrhythmic options, directing attention and emphasis towards specific molecular targets, ion currents, and vulnerable parameters. It encouraged a search for better drugs for treating arrhythmias and urged departure from restrictive monolithic associations between arrhythmia causes and cures to focus attention back to mechanisms of both. This emphasis was particularly timely given the disarray in drug discovery spawned by the Cardiac Arrhythmia Suppression Trial (CAST). CAST delivered the sobering message that "rational" design of better drugs through the 1980s had seemingly failed. This was because CAST showed, convincingly, that three new Na channel blocking compounds that were effective in suppressing premature ventricular depolarizations did not increase life expectancy but, in fact, increased mortality in a selected population of patients.

Much of the original Sicilian Gambit paper was directed at a basic assessment of different targets in cardiac cells, focusing attention on potassium channels. This reflected an ongoing shift in thinking that important targets were likely to emerge in the control of cell repolarization rather than, or in addition to, depolarization. Subsequent experience has confirmed the value of this approach, and of the initial paper's other emphasis, that attention should be given to the emerging issues of how different transport proteins function in an integrated manner, their molecular diversity, regulation, and influence on disease.

That emphasis is continued in the present volume, further developing the idea of an integrated basic pharmacologic approach to address vulnerable targets, while complementing this with an equally rigorous emphasis on a rational empirical standard of clinical outcome. Its intent, as indicated in Ch. 1, seems to be to move closer to a pathophysiologic approach and a clinical test of mechanistic appreciation and eventual prediction. This recognition seems to reflect in part the field's awareness that the earlier paradigm—that arrhythmias might likely be controlled readily by a better, more sharply focused targeting of aberrations in individual currents—has been, perhaps, too simplistic. The recognition that some of our most promising drugs, such as amiodarone and sotalol, show multifunctional activity against a variety of different currents, targets, and pathways argues strongly in a new direction. This enhances, rather than diminishes, the argument that a great deal more basic research needs to be done to relate how state-of-the-art findings, as elaborated here, can be used to achieve a better understanding of real-time propagation of cardiac action potentials in three-dimensional, anisotropic tissue. It also emphasizes the need to look more deeply into other aspects of cell function and excitability, into different components of seemingly unrelated pathways of signalling, contraction, and communication, into ways of manipulating receptor subtypes or altering their expression and intercellular interactions at a more basic, even genetic level, and into improving outcomes in the search for better cardiac rhythm control.

The urgency of that need is further emphasized by one recent estimation: that despite the advances made with newly developed drugs, even preliminary evaluations suggest these will, at best, prove efficacious in less than a third of patient cases. With its emphasis on clinical relevance and arrhythmo-pathophysiologic mechanisms, this volume, like the original Sicilian Gambit paper, should help direct both new research and its understanding and application in productive new directions.

Peter M. Spooner, Ph.D.
Chief, Cardiac Functions Branch
Division of Heart and Vascular Diseases
National Heart, Lung and Blood Institute
Bethesda, Maryland

Preface

The contributors to the Sicilian Gambit constitute a loosely organized group of basic and clinical investigators who have met, both formally and informally since 1990, to discuss and pool their ideas about cardiac arrhythmias and their therapy and to share this information with the community. The membership of the group is in constant flux, and the intent of the Gambit is to have individual names and egos subserve the deliberations of the group. Hence, the content of this book reflects the combined efforts of the following individuals: Günter Breithardt, A. John Camm, Ronald W. F. Campbell, Harry A. Fozzard, Brian F. Hoffman, Michiel J. Janse, Ralph Lazzara, Samuel Lévy, Robert J. Myerburg, Dan M. Roden, Michael R. Rosen, Peter J. Schwartz, Harold C. Strauss, Albert L. Waldo, Andrew L. Wit, Raymond L. Woosley, Antonio Zaza, and Douglas P. Zipes. Each contributed in equal fashion to the volume and most engaged, as well, in three exhaustive and exhausting days of group meetings, breakout workshops, and writing sessions at Arden House, in Harriman, New York, from October 17–21, 1993. All came to the conference with outlines on preassigned topics and all summarized and prepared rough drafts of the group's deliberations of their subject areas during the actual course of the meeting. The group followed a pattern set in the original Sicilian Gambit meeting in 1990; that is, whereas organizers (Drs. Lévy, Rosen, and Schwartz), a meeting chair (Dr. Rosen), and breakout session chairs (Drs. Lazzara, Schwartz, and Strauss) were administrative necessities, the product of the meeting and the credit for authorship of the volume goes to all participants equally. All have read and edited the entire volume and contributed to each of its chapters. Hence, the chapters, while prepared by one to three participants, have no individual authorships listed.

ix

Several additional individuals deserve recognition for their roles in the meeting and in the preparation of the volume. First is Eric Prystowsky who was asked to provide a critique of the volume and whose efforts led to reconsideration of several areas; second are the underwriters of the Sicilian Gambit, Dr. Horst Mertens and Roberto Gradnik and Mr. Ernst Schneider and Mrs. Karen Camping-Van Etten from Knoll AG; and third are the original "angels" behind the Gambit, although no longer at Knoll AG, Drs. Siegfried Rhein and Bernard Ayton. It should be mentioned that all aid provided by Knoll AG was via educational grants, and there was no attempt to influence the meeting or the contents of the resulting volume.

Two individuals provided assistance of inestimable value in preparing and overseeing the operation of the meeting and in preparing the volume, and so we thank both Alla Kuznetsova and Eileen Franey, who elegantly and unobtrusively saw to the myriad details required. Finally, our sincere thanks to Jan Plotczyk and his staff at Arden House, who provided the setting and the conference support that eased our way through this project; to our publishers, Steven Korn and Jacques Strauss, at Futura Publishing Company, who offered encouragement and professionalism throughout; and to our Production Editor, Janet Foltin, who tirelessly reviewed every word written, and ensured that what we meant to say was communicated accurately.

Members of the Sicilian Gambit

Contents

SECTION I

The Sicilian Gambit:
General Introduction

Chapter 1

The Sicilian Gambit:
Overview and Intent

This book reflects the deliberations of a group of basic and clinical scientists who met for three days in a secluded location to discuss the status of cardiac antiarrhythmic therapy. The framework for our discussion was provided by The Sicilian Gambit (1991), which proposed a break from traditional methods of drug classification to a system wherein one might better than previously meld the knowledge and needs of the diverse community engaged in antiarrhythmic drug research, development, and therapy. The name "Sicilian Gambit" was chosen for several reasons: to reflect the site of the initial meeting in Taormina, Sicily; to reflect the fact that this was viewed as not only a new opening to the classification of antiarrhythmic drugs but to the entire way in which we think about them; and, equally importantly, to indicate that the contributors to the group, all of whom had individual views and prejudices that were often disparate, had argued their points of view and agreed on a synthesis.

As originally published, the Sicilian Gambit (1991) stated the following: that any drug may act on one or several "targets" including channels, pumps, receptors, and/or other cardiac or extracardiac loci (Fig. 1). These targets are not only acted on by drugs but may be affected by other endogenous and exogenous substances. The importance of the targets is seen in their involvement in normal rhythm and in either the initiation or the perpetuation of an arrhythmia. Moreover, they are potentially amenable to study at the clinical or the experimental level.

From *Antiarrhythmic Therapy: A Pathophysiologic Approach* edited by Members of the Sicilian Gambit © 1994, Futura Publishing Co., Inc., Armonk, NY.

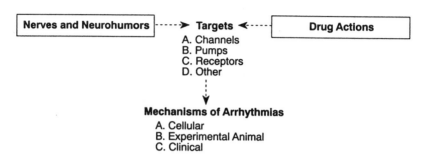

Figure 1. *Elements for a classification system. See text for discussion. Reproduced with permission from The Sicilian Gambit: A new approach to the classification of antiarrhythmic drugs based on their actions on arrhythmogenic mechanisms. Circulation 1991; 84:1831–1851. Copyright 1991 American Heart Association.*

Contributing to and complicating the Gambit approach is the understanding that very few, if any, drugs manifest a single targeted effect; in fact, most drugs act at several sites, sharing a spectrum of actions with other drugs. This factor leads us to reject classifications that reduce drug actions to rigid or simplistic schemes. As stated originally in the Sicilian Gambit (1991), "for two decades, the approach to antiarrhythmic drug development and administration has focused on the Vaughan Williams classification (e.g., Vaughan Williams, 1971, 1984; Harrison et al, 1981). This classification, presented in Table 1, has been useful in teaching students and physicians because it is physiologically based, can be learned quickly, and facilitates discussion of the potentially beneficial or deleterious actions of drugs. The Vaughan Williams classification originated at a time when our knowledge of electrophysiological mechanisms (including the roles of receptors and channels) was less extensive than now and relatively few antiarrhythmic agents were available. In the ensuing years there has been a continuing attempt to fit new concepts about arrhythmias and about the actions of new agents into its general framework."

A major criticism of the Vaughan Williams system arose from the extent to which the categorization of drugs in Classes I to IV led to oversimplified views of their common and dissimilar actions. This had reached a point at which the classification was not readily usable to either the basic scientist or the clinician without a great deal of additional explanation. Indeed, the stratification of Class I drugs into three subclasses and, more recently, the beginnings of stratification of Class

Table 1
Vaughan Williams Classification of Antiarrhythmic Drugs*

	Class I	Class II	Class III	Class IV
	Drugs with direct membrane action (Na channel blockade)	Sympatholytic drugs	Drugs that prolong repolarization	Calcium channel blocking drugs
IA	Depress phase 0 Slow conduction Prolong repolarization			
IB	Little effect on phase 0 in normal tissue Depress phase 0 in abnormal fibers Shorten repolarization			
IC	Markedly depress phase 0 Markedly slow conduction Slight effect on repolarization			

* This is the classification as modified by Harrison et al (1981)

III, are symptomatic of the extent to which the complex realities of drug properties and physiologic systems have rendered what was a simple classification system at best unwieldy and, at worst, misleading. Hence, while the Vaughan Williams system has offered an admirable shorthand that has been especially useful for teaching, its usefulness is ever more limited beyond that point.

It was the belief of the original Gambit authors (1991) that no structured "class" approach should be applied to any group of antiarrhythmics; that is, drugs that modify a sodium channel in various fashions may, at the same time, differently affect potassium and/or calcium channels as well as other targets in ways that must be given recognizance by the physician if he/she is to understand the patient-drug interaction and accurately interpret the outcome of drug administration. The Gambit group, during its meeting in October, 1993, still does not propose a new drug classification system. What it does offer is the challenge to clinicians and scientists alike to explore the common ground between their various disciplines in synthesizing an approach to arrhythmias. The means for doing this is exemplified by Figure 2, which considers the pathophysiologic or "rational" approach proposed by the Gambit and the empiric approach used by physicians. This in no way implies that empiricism does not have a rational basis. Rather, it emphasizes that many of the steps that appear superficially ignored and/or taken for granted by the empiric approach do, in fact, have ready scientific explanations. Moreover, it emphasizes that—to the extent that a clinician is availed of this information—he/she may better understand the vagaries of arrhythmogenesis and treatment in a particular patient as well as contribute to a more rational approach to therapy.

Let us now consider Figure 2 in detail. Panel A shows, on the left, the Sicilian Gambit approach and, on the right, the usual empiric approach. The Gambit approach is pathophysiologic and starts with the assumption that a physician will make a diagnosis of an arrhythmia as, for example, atrioventricular nodal reentrant tachycardia (depicted in Fig. 2, Panel B). For any arrhythmia, the mechanism may be either suspected or known. For this tachycardia, it is known to be reentrant, involving the atrioventricular node. A set of critical components contributes to the arrhythmia. Critical components may be considered as individual factors, all of which are essential to the expression of the arrhythmia. They may participate in the maintenance of the arrhythmia or contribute solely to its initiation. In the case of atrioventricular nodal reentry, slow conduction in the node and a pathway of rapid or slow conduction in the atrium would be considered critical components.

Among the critical components contributing to any arrhythmia may be a vulnerable parameter or parameters. The vulnerable parameter is the factor or factors (structurally or functionally) particularly amenable to a therapeutic approach. In the case of atrioventricular nodal reentry, one vulnerable parameter amenable to pharmacologic therapy is the atrioventricular nodal action potential, which is generated by a particular subcellular target, the L-type calcium channel. Interventions such as calcium channel blockade or β-blockade have a reasonably predictable clinical outcome in this setting. Moreover, the response to this or any intervention can have further impact on both the ability to diagnose and to select a therapy. It is to be stressed that

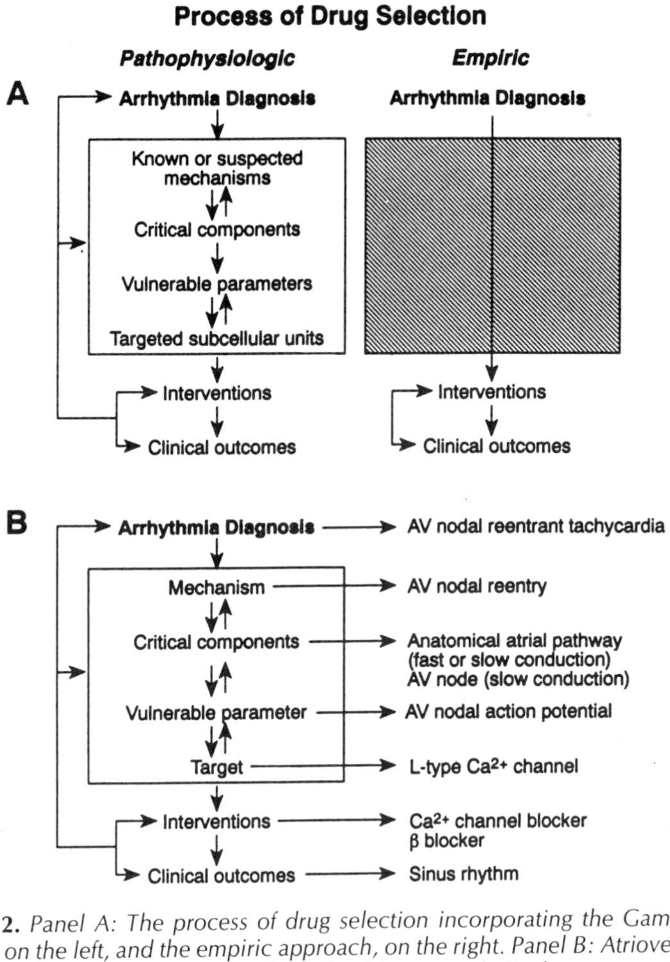

Process of Drug Selection

Pathophysiologic   *Empiric*

A   Arrhythmia Diagnosis   Arrhythmia Diagnosis

Known or suspected mechanisms

Critical components

Vulnerable parameters

Targeted subcellular units

Interventions   Interventions

Clinical outcomes   Clinical outcomes

B   Arrhythmia Diagnosis ⟶ AV nodal reentrant tachycardia

Mechanism ⟶ AV nodal reentry

Critical components ⟶ Anatomical atrial pathway (fast or slow conduction) AV node (slow conduction)

Vulnerable parameter ⟶ AV nodal action potential

Target ⟶ L-type Ca^{2+} channel

Interventions ⟶ Ca^{2+} channel blocker β blocker

Clinical outcomes ⟶ Sinus rhythm

Figure 2. *Panel A: The process of drug selection incorporating the Gambit approach on the left, and the empiric approach, on the right. Panel B: Atrioventricular nodal reentry as an example of the Gambit approach. Each component in the pathophysiologic Gambit approach is matched with its counterpart that contributes to the pathophysiology and therapy of atrioventricular nodal reentry. See text for discussion. Reproduced with permission from The Sicilian Gambit: A new approach to the classification of antiarrhythmic drugs based on their actions on arrhythmogenic mechanisms. Circulation 1991; 84:1831–1851. Copyright 1991 American Heart Association.*

application of other techniques can identify other vulnerable parameters among the critical components of an arrhythmia. For example, catheter techniques have identified anatomic loci in the atria as essential to atrioventricular nodal reentry, rendering them vulnerable parameters to radiofrequency ablation. Hence, using the example of a single arrhythmia, we can see that the framework within which the Gambit operates does provide a wedding between pathophysiology and therapy, and a rationale for drug selection and prioritization.

That the Gambit approach represents nothing more than an expansion of the traditional empiric approach to arrhythmias is emphasized in Figure 2, Panel A, right panel. Here, diagnosis is followed by a decision on intervention and observation of outcome. The cross-hatched area is literally a "black box" incorporating, unconsciously, all the information that is, in fact, made available by the Gambit approach.

If for a specific arrhythmia the Gambit provides a rational approach and this, in fact, reflects and complements the empiric approach used by many physicians in treating this arrhythmia, what are the problems with the Gambit method? One is the identification of "vulnerable parameters," which are no more or less than descriptors of what might be viewed as "Achilles heels," contributing to an arrhythmia and susceptible to therapeutic intervention. It is imperative to understand that a site that currently is identified as vulnerable to drugs may not be the sole contributor to an arrhythmia that one might attack, either with future drugs or with alternative therapies. As mentioned above, the advent of catheter ablation has made it possible to cure atrioventricular nodal reentrant tachycardias by interrupting a site in the reentrant circuit that is not in the atrioventricular node and that is not uniquely accessible to any drug or drugs. Hence, the recognition must exist that, as ideas and technologies advance, any of several critical components contributing to an arrhythmia can be identified as potentially vulnerable parameters to therapy, and as certain components become accessible to therapy and, therefore, vulnerable, others may no longer be desirable targets because of associated side effects of the therapy and/or lesser efficacy of the intervention.

A second and more global problem of the original Gambit publication (1991) was that it was heavily oriented to the basic sciences. Hence, it dealt in detail with targets and arrhythmogenic mechanisms considered at the cellular and experimental levels, but less so at the clinical level. Clinicians were justifiably concerned about the extent to which the Gambit could be used in support of their daily thinking about arrhythmias and their therapy. They also were concerned that although the Gambit exposed a number of flaws in existing drug classification systems, it offered no classification to replace these systems. Rather, it expressed the view that while one could categorize arrhythmias by their mechanisms and vulnerable parameters, this represented only a first step towards a new classification rather than the replacement of the old. This conclusion left many clinicians perplexed. It is for this reason that in this book we pay particular attention to the arrhythmias that confront clinicians, in addition to expanding on the scientific basis for the Gambit. With this in mind, the volume is organized as follows: Section I reviews the basic molecular, electrophysiologic, and pharmacologic principles underlying the Gambit approach, thereby providing a basis for the clinical interpretations that follow. In Section II, the focus is on the clinical electrophysiologic identification of arrhythmia mechanisms and an exploration of the clinical application of the vulnerable parameter concept. Section III systematically explores a series of clinically occurring arrhythmias in light of the pathophysiologic approach recommended by the Gambit. Finally, Section IV considers the future of antiarrhythmic drug development.

The last point to be emphasized in these introductory remarks is that in considering arrhythmias, we are dealing with highly complex and dynamic processes. This statement can best be understood if we remember that arrhythmias are conditioned not only by pathophysiologic events in the heart but by the multiple modifiers of cardiac action, including the central nervous system, autonomic nerves, neurohumors, and a host of others. Normal rhythm and arrhythmias are conditioned as well by the normal physiologic processes of development, maturation, and aging. Hence, the substrate on which any pathophysiologic event is superimposed is conditioned by age and by environment. Additionally, these same modifying factors apply to drugs and their metabolism and interaction with the body. Finally, many pathophysiologic processes are themselves dynamic. The net result is that, for most arrhythmias, the application of antiarrhythmic therapy is not akin to an expert shooting at a bull's-eye with a bow and arrow. Rather, it resembles the attempt to hit an elusive target with a changing array of weapons, with which we have uneven skills and whose capabilities we only partially understand. At one extreme, the bull's-eye philosophy may be applied well, as with the atrioventricular nodal reentrant tachycardia treated with a calcium channel blocker or with ablation. But at the other extreme, in the setting of coronary artery disease or cardiomyopathy of various etiologies, we are dealing with high levels of complexity that we can only partially comprehend.

And so, to the clinician or scientist approaching this book, we state the following: if you are looking for simple answers, you will not find them here. The field of cardiac arrhythmias and their therapy is no simpler than that of cancer in its multiple forms and therapies. To think of antiarrhythmic treatment in one-dimensional paradigms involving pure empiricism (e.g., for this arrhythmia on electrocardiogram, give "drug X") is to do justice neither to the patient's well-being nor to the physician's intellect. With this in mind, it will be apparent in reading the clinical sections of this book that, for some clinical arrhythmias, the Gambit approach works well, and for others, there is not sufficient understanding of pathophysiology and therapy to adequately apply the Gambit philosophy. It is in these areas that we believe we face our greatest challenges.

Hence, if you are looking for a summary of what we think we do and do not know, and for a framework within which to consider your therapeutic successes and failures in a way that directs you to different therapeutic modalities and research opportunities, we believe this book will be helpful. In fact, one way to use it practically is to apply the approach to arrhythmias outlined in Figure 2 to each of the clinical arrhythmias discussed in Sections II and III of the book. In conclusion, we offer the Gambit as a basis for a continuing learning process, with the hope that as our knowledge evolves, so will the application of this knowledge to patient benefit.

Chapter 2

Molecular Targets for Drug Action

Our ability to identify drug targets and the nature of drug-target interactions has increased dramatically with the availability of a variety of molecular techniques. We now know the primary molecular structures of many ion channels, pumps, and receptors, and this provides the opportunity to determine drug-binding sites. This understanding has greatly increased our insight into the complex interplay of ionic currents that underlies cardiac electrical behavior. This chapter identifies the molecular targets for drug action on electrophysiologic function and provides a functional definition of the characteristics of drug action on these targets.

Channels

Channels are large glycoproteins that span the membrane bilayer and, under an appropriate stimulus, form pores that permit ions to cross the membrane rapidly, thereby creating ion currents. A channel is often selective for certain ions (e.g., sodium channels or potassium channels), although different channels can incorporate regions in which the amino acid sequences are quite similar (homologous).

The sections entitled "Channels" and "Pumps/Carriers" are reproduced and updated with permission from the American Heart Association, Inc., from The Sicilian Gambit: A new approach to the classification of antiarrhythmic drugs based on their actions on arrhythmogenic mechanisms. Task force of the working group on arrhythmias of the European Society of Cardiology. Circulation 84:1831–1851, 1991.

From *Antiarrhythmic Therapy: A Pathophysiologic Approach* edited by Members of the Sicilian Gambit © 1994, Futura Publishing Co., Inc., Armonk, NY.

Channel proteins that have similar sequences and physiologic properties are termed "isoforms." Some channels only open after a delay following the stimulus, and some channels rectify; that is, they conduct ions more effectively in one direction across the membrane than the other. Stimuli for channel opening include a change in membrane voltage; chemical signals, which may act directly or by occupying an adjacent receptor; or mechanical deformation. It appears likely that these stimuli act by inducing conformational changes in the channel proteins.

The process whereby an ion channel protein responds to an external stimulus to change conformation is termed "gating." Channel activation is similar to (but may not be synonymous with) channel opening. The rate of change of channel conformation (gating kinetics) can be very rapid, with major changes in channel function occurring in less than one millisecond, or quite slow, with changes occurring over seconds. Gating kinetics should not be confused with the kinetics of antiarrhythmic drug binding to or dissociation from channels, which occur at different rates for different drugs. Once open, channel proteins may stay open until closed by another signal, or they may inactivate, that is, close even in the face of a maintained stimulus. Inactivated channels generally do not reopen when restimulated until they have recovered from inactivation, a time- (and often voltage-) dependent process.

Channels can be classified according to the mechanisms that govern their opening: voltage-gated or ligand-gated. A number of channel types have been purified, cloned, and sequenced from heart and from other excitable cells (Catterall, 1992; Pongs, 1992). They share considerable homology, especially in the intramembranous segments, such that it is not surprising that some channel-active drugs interact with more than one channel type. In addition, channels of one type (e.g., the sodium channels) are even more homologous among tissues, so that drugs that interact with one channel type in the heart may also interact with that channel type in the nervous system. The progress in determining channel structure encourages us to believe that it will soon be possible to determine key structural differences and drug-binding sites and to tailor drugs that are tissue- and channel-specific. A schematic representation of the role of channels and pumps/carriers in generating the normal transmembrane resting and action potentials is illustrated in Figure 1. Knowledge of the structure and function of

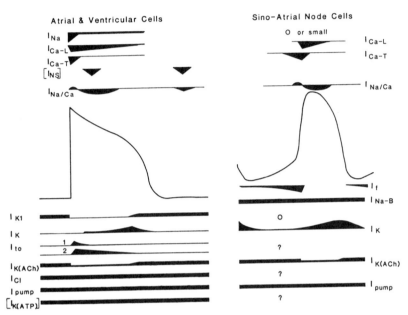

Atrial & Ventricular Cells

Sino-Atrial Node Cells

Figure 1. *Currents and channels involved in generating the resting and action potential. The time course of a stylized action potential of atrial and ventricular cells is shown on the left and of sinoatrial node cells on the right. Above and below are the various channels and pumps that contribute the currents underlying the electrical events. See text for identification of the symbols and description of the channels or currents. Where possible, the approximate time courses of the currents associated with the channels or pumps are shown symbolically without effort to represent their magnitudes relative to each other. I_K incorporates at least two currents, I_{Kr} and I_{Ks}. There appears to be an ultrarapid component, as well, designated I_{Kur}. The heavy bars for I_{Cl}, I_{pump}, and $I_{K(ATP)}$ only indicate the presence of these channels or pump, without implying magnitude of currents, since that would vary with physiologic and pathophysiologic conditions. The channels identified by brackets (I_{NS} and $I_{K(ATP)}$) imply that they are active only under pathologic conditions. For the sinoatrial node cells, I_{Na} and I_{K1} are small or absent. Question marks indicate that experimental evidence is not yet available to determine the presence of these channels in sinoatrial cell membranes. Although it is likely that other ionic current mechanisms exist, they are not shown here because their roles in electrogenesis are not sufficiently well defined.*

channels and pumps/carriers is increasing rapidly, and the following tabulation will thus require a regular update.

Channels That Carry Inward Currents

Sodium Channels

These channels represent a family of large proteins with multiple subunits (Catterall, 1992). The main (α-) subunit contains about 2000 amino acids and includes four major repeated internal sequences that represent internal subunits. Presently, 10 members of this family have been cloned and expressed, including two from heart muscle. In brain and skeletal muscle, the α-subunit is normally accompanied by other subunits, but it is functional even when alone. The α-subunit in the heart is also functional alone (Satin et al, 1992), although some evidence suggests that there may be an additional subunit. Functional evidence points to at least two isoforms of the cardiac sodium channel.

I_{Na} is the inward excitatory current carried by Na^+ through a voltage-activated sodium channel. The current is activated at threshold to produce rapid depolarization and to provide the current to drive action potential or impulse propagation in atrial, His-Purkinje, and ventricular cells. These Na^+ channels are sparse or absent in sinoatrial and atrioventricular nodal cells (Brown, 1982).

I_{Na-B} is a proposed background Na^+ current through a voltage-independent channel in sinoatrial nodal cells (Hagiwara et al, 1992). It is offset by an outward K^+ current at the beginning of phase 4, but as the K^+ current decays, it contributes to pacemaker behavior.

Ca^{2+} Channels

These channels also represent a family of proteins with multiple subunits. Some of the subunits from various tissues, including a cardiac subunit of the L-type, have been cloned and sequenced, and they show extensive homology. There are at least two types of calcium channels in the heart (Pelzer et al, 1990). The L-type (I_{Ca-L}), which is blocked by verapamil, diltiazem, and the dihydropyridines, predominates in all cardiac tissues studied. The T-type (I_{Ca-T}) is prominent in pacemaker tissues. Ca^{2+} channels are also found in high density in vascular smooth muscle, endocrine cells, and the brain.

I_{Ca-L} is the calcium current that is activated regeneratively from a relatively depolarized threshold potential to produce depolarization and propagation in sinoatrial and atrioventricular nodal cells. It is also present in atrial, His-Purkinje, and ventricular cells, where it contributes to the plateau and triggers calcium release from the sarcoplasmic reticulum. It can be the source of repolarizing current in the early afterdepolarization phenomenon that contributes to torsades de pointes (see Ch. 4). I_{Ca-L} is inactivated by both depolarization and $[Ca^{2+}]_i$, but it usually lasts long enough to contribute to the overall plateau currents. It is the target for the clinically useful calcium channel blockers, and it is strongly modulated by neurotransmitters (Pelzer et al, 1990).

I_{Ca-T} is a calcium current through a different voltage-gated channel that is activated at potentials intermediate between thresholds for I_{Na} and I_{Ca-L}. It probably contributes inward current to the later stages of phase 4 depolarization in sinoatrial node and His-Purkinje cells, and it may also play a role in abnormal automaticity in atria (Hagiwara et al, 1992). It is almost absent from ventricular cells.

Other Inward Current Channels

There are two cationic nonselective channels that, under normal physiologic conditions, allow current to be carried by Na^+. They are not well characterized, and no structural information is available yet.

I_f is an inward current carried by Na^+ through a relatively nonselective cationic channel that is activated by polarization to high membrane potentials in sinoatrial and atrioventricular nodal cells and His-Purkinje cells (DiFrancesco et al, 1986). This current generates phase 4 depolarization and contributes to pacemaker function. Its kinetics are fairly slow, and it is strongly modulated by neurotransmitters.

I_{NS} is a channel that is gated by $[Ca^{2+}]_i$ (Ehara et al, 1988). It is a cationic nonselective channel that, if activated at the resting potential, produces an inward current carried by Na^+. Under some conditions, it is activated by Ca^{2+} release from the sarcoplasmic reticulum during $[Ca^{2+}]_i$ overload and contributes to delayed afterdepolarizations (see Ch. 4).

Channels That Carry Outward Currents

Many functionally different types of potassium channels have been identified in heart and other tissues. Indeed, almost all cells have some type of potassium channel. The voltage-gated potassium channels are composed of four subunits, each about one quarter the size of the sodium channel subunit (Pongs, 1992). It seems likely that naturally occurring potassium channels are composed of a mix of different subunit types. Some of the cloned channels have been matched with the functional currents. Other potassium channels are quite different, with either one or two transmembrane segments.

I_{K1} is the K^+ current responsible for maintaining the resting potential near the K^+ equilibrium potential in atrial, atrioventricular nodal, His-Purkinje, and ventricular cells (Giles and Imaizumi, 1988). This current, which is also called the inward rectifier, shuts off during depolarization (inward rectification). It has recently been cloned and found to have only two transmembrane segments, in contrast to the voltage-gated potassium channels (Ishii et al, 1994). Its absence from sinoatrial node cells is important in letting small currents control the pacemaker rate.

I_K is a K^+ current carried through voltage-gated channels with slow activation kinetics, giving it the name delayed rectifier. I_K turns on slowly during the action potential plateau and is the major current causing repolarization. After repolarization, it turns off slowly enough in the sinoatrial node to contribute to phase 4 depolarization. I_K can be modulated by neurotransmitters (Sanguinetti and Jurkiewicz, 1990; Walsh and Kass, 1988). There are at least two distinct components to I_K, a rapidly activating current called I_{Kr} and a slowly activating one called I_{Ks}. There are probably separate gene products, as well (Roberds et al, 1993). Recent studies have indicated there is an additional, ultrarapid component to I_K, designated I_{Kur} (Backx and Marban, 1993; Wang et al, 1993b).

I_{to} is a K^+ current that turns on rapidly after depolarization and then inactivates. One type of I_{to} is activated by $[Ca^{2+}]_i$, and the other is voltage activated and modulated by neurotransmitters (Coraboeuf and Carmeliet, 1982). I_{to} can play an important role in modifying action potential duration and in contributing to the heterogeneity of repolarization because of its nonuniform distribution (it is present in subepicardial but not subendocardial muscle). Similar currents, called I_A, are found in nerve and skeletal muscle cells.

$I_{K(ACh)}$ is a K^+ current whose channel is activated by the muscarinic (M_2) receptor via guanosine triphosphate regulatory (G-) protein signal transduction (Sakmann et al, 1983). This channel has recently been cloned (Kubo et al, 1993b). It shuts down somewhat during depolarization (inward rectification), but it contributes outward current both at rest and during the action potential. It is particularly important in the sinoatrial and atrioventricular nodes and in atrial cells, where it can produce substantial hyperpolarization, and in atrium, where it produces marked acceleration of repolarization. This channel is also opened by activation of the purinergic (adenosine) receptor, and so the current is also designated $I_{K(Ado)}$.

$I_{K(ATP)}$ is a K^+ current carried through a metabolically-regulated channel (Carmeliet et al, 1990). This channel is blocked by adenosine triphosphate and is strongly activated during hypoxia. The channel has been present in all cardiac cells studied, but it has not been identified in the sinoatrial node. It may contribute to shortening of the action potential during ischemia. Experimentally available antiarrhythmic drugs can either increase or decrease this K^+ current, thereby accelerating or prolonging repolarization.

I_{Cl} is a Cl^- current, usually quite small, but which can be greatly increased by adrenergic receptor activation, favoring repolarization (Harvey et al, 1990). Because the Cl^- concentration is sometimes above what is expected for equilibrium, the Cl^- channel could, under those circumstances, generate inward current. Because the channel rectifies, the inward current could be quite small, but it might contribute to pacemaker depolarization.

$I_{K(Ca)}$ is a K^+ current carried through a channel that is activated by $[Ca^{2+}]_i$. It appears to require very high levels of $[Ca^{2+}]_i$ for activation. Its presence in cardiac cells has been hard to establish, and its physiologic role is not yet clear (Giles and Imaizumi, 1988).

Some Other Important Channels

Cardiac cells are coupled electrically and chemically to one another by large channels called gap junctions or connexons (Page and Manjunath, 1986). These junctions are composed of two multimeric complexes, one set for each cell. The two sets align themselves to form a large pore between the cells that permits passage of ions and small molecules. The conductance of gap junctions is regulated by $[Ca^{2+}]_i$ and pH_i and perhaps by phosphorylation via activation of the β-adrenergic receptor system. They play a major role in isolating cells damaged by ischemic injury or trauma from adjacent, more normal cells.

A calcium channel in the sarcoplasmic reticulum can be triggered to release Ca^{2+} by calcium entry through I_{Ca-L}. Because it also can be modulated by the drug ryanodine, it is often called the ryanodine receptor (Nakai et al, 1990).

Pumps/Carriers

Active Transport

At least two adenosine triphosphate-dependent pumps in the sarcolemma generate ionic current, the Na/K pump (which is blocked by digitalis) and the calcium pump. Several isoforms of the Na/K pump have been identified by differing affinities for digitalis. A different adenosine triphosphate-dependent calcium pump is found in the sarcoplasmic reticulum. Both sarcolemmal pumps have been cloned and sequenced, and several isoforms of the Na/K pump are present. Some evidence suggests that they are modulated by phosphorylation through the adrenergic-receptor system. $I_{Na/K\ pump}$ is the current generated by the Na/K pump. Because each cycle transports three Na^+ out and two K^+ into the cell, it generates a small outward current that is relatively constant during the cardiac cycle (Gadsby, 1984).

Carriers

This group of membrane proteins facilitates exchange of ions or substrates, or pumps them using energy. It includes the Na/Ca countertransport system in the sarcolemma and in the mitochondria, the Na/H exchanger, the Na/K/Cl cotransporter, and the Cl/HCO_3 exchanger. The cardiac Na/Ca exchanger has recently been cloned, but no selective blocking or activating drugs are presently known. Amiloride blocks the Na/K/Cl cotransporter and the Na/H exchanger, as well as several types of channels.

$I_{Na/Ca}$ is the current generated by the Na/Ca countertransport system, which exchanges one Ca^{2+} for three Na^+ (Sheu and Blaustein,

1992). It is the chief means of Ca^{2+} efflux through the sarcolemma. The direction of the current depends on the relation between the Na^+ and Ca^{2+} gradients and the membrane potential. At the resting potential, the exchanger generates a small inward current, but upon depolarization, the current may show a brief outward phase and then become inward as $[Ca^{2+}]_i$ rises. During $[Ca^{2+}]_i$ overload, the sarcoplasmic reticulum may release Ca^{2+} spontaneously during diastole, causing the Na/Ca exchanger to generate a larger inward current, and thereby contributing to the generation of delayed afterdepolarizations (see Ch. 4).

Receptors

The autonomic nervous system is an important modulator of cardiac rhythms. α- and β-Adrenergic, muscarinic, and purinergic receptors influence various channels and pumps, which, in turn, influence the initiation and propagation of normal and abnormal cardiac impulses. The receptor systems in the heart are coupled by G-proteins to their effector systems (Gilman, 1987). These G-proteins translate the results of an external stimulus, such as receptor occupancy, into a physiologic response, such as activation of a kinase and subsequent phosphorylation of target proteins (e.g., ion channels). Alternatively, they may link receptors to second messenger systems and pumps.

The β-Adrenergic Receptor-Effector Coupling System

β_1- and β_2-Adrenoceptors have been demonstrated in the hearts of various species, including man, using radioligand binding, autoradiographic, and functional techniques (Brodde, 1991; Jones et al, 1989; Masini et al, 1991). β_2/β_1 Ratios vary depending on cardiac tissue, species, and technique, from 0/100 or 11/89 in guinea pig ventricle (Engle et al, 1981; Molenaar et al, 1990) to about 30/70 in human atrium (Brodde, 1991) or rat atrium (Juberg et al, 1985), and about 40/60 in guinea pig His bundle (Molenaar et al, 1990). In dogs, β_1-adrenergic receptor-effector coupling is the major sympathetic modulator of cardiac electrical activity. However, β_2-adrenergic stimulation has been reported to increase heart rate, atrioventricular conduction velocity, and atrial contractility, and to decrease atrial refractory periods

(Akahane et al, 1989; Motomura and Hashimoto, 1992; Takei et al, 1992a; Takei et al, 1992b). β_1- and β_2-Receptor subtypes are coupled to adenylate cyclase via the G-protein, G_s. β-Adrenergic-receptor stimulation modulates L-type calcium channels, the I_f channel, various K channels, I_{Cl}, and, under certain conditions, Na channels.

The binding of agonist to β-adrenergic receptor in cardiac myocytes increases intracellular cyclic AMP levels, activating the cyclic AMP-dependent protein kinase and phosphorylating a peptide associated with the L-type Ca^{2+} channel, increasing Ca^{2+} current and contractility (Hescheler and Trautwein, 1989). The chronotropic effect of β-adrenergic stimulation is also mediated by an increase in cyclic AMP that appears to shift the activation curve of the pacemaker current I_f towards more positive potentials (DiFrancesco, 1985). β-Adrenergic stimulation also enhances Na/K pump function (Désilets and Baumgarten, 1986; Wasserstrom et al, 1982), which would tend to hyperpolarize cardiac fibers, especially those that are partially depolarized, as in the setting of acute ischemia.

A direct G-protein (G_s) coupling between β-adrenoceptors and Ca, I_f, and Na channels has been documented (Yatani et al, 1990). The delayed rectifier K current, I_K, and a component of the transient outward current, I_{to}, are enhanced by β-adrenergic stimulation (Yazawa and Kameyama, 1990), while the inward rectifier, I_{K1}, does not appear to be affected (Ehara et al, 1988). β-Adrenergic stimulation enhances voltage-dependent K^+ and voltage-independent Cl^- currents (Harvey and Hume, 1989).

These actions appear to have physiologic and pathophysiologic importance, as follows: the effect on the L-type Ca^{2+} channel could, in its own right, induce early afterdepolarizations and triggered activity, as well as increase free intracellular Ca^{2+} concentrations that, in turn, would potentiate delayed afterdepolarizations and resultant triggered activity. The effect on I_f can increase the rate of impulse initiation of the sinus node pacemaker, as well as of latent atrial and ventricular pacemakers. The potassium channel effects tend to accelerate repolarization and shorten refractoriness, and both the Ca^{2+} and K^+ channel effects may combine to accelerate atrioventricular nodal conduction and shorten atrioventricular nodal refractoriness. These ion channel effects can account for the tachycardias and QT interval shortening associated with sympathetic stimulation of the intact heart.

Clinically, β-adrenergic blocking agents have well-established effects on those arrhythmias that require the participation of the atrioventricular node. The β-adrenergic blocking effects result largely from drug-induced decreases in conduction velocity and prolongation of refractoriness in the atrioventricular node, actions reflecting block of catecholamine effects on Ca^{2+} and K^+ channels. Limited subsets of patients with various ventricular arrhythmias, e.g., some ventricular premature depolarizations, exercise-induced ventricular tachycardias, some ventricular tachycardias inducible by programmed stimulation, and adenosine-sensitive ventricular tachycardias also may respond to β-adrenergic blockade. β-Adrenergic blocking drugs also reduce the risk of sudden cardiac death in selected population subgroups (e.g., postmyocardial infarction, long QT syndrome) (Schwartz and Locati, 1985). In postmyocardial infarction patients, the mechanisms of protection are not yet fully understood.

The α-Adrenergic Receptor-Effector Coupling System

There are two, and possibly three, α_1-adrenergic-receptor subtypes in the heart (del Balzo et al, 1990), linked via G-proteins to a series of effector processes (Na/K pump) (Shah et al, 1988), K channels (Apkon and Nerbonne, 1988), and phospholipase C (del Balzo et al, 1990), that modulate impulse initiation and repolarization. Information on second messenger involvement in these processes is incomplete. The Na/K pump-stimulating effect is responsible for a decrease in the rate of impulse initiation by automatic fibers outside the sinus node, and the decreases induced in I_K, I_{K1}, and/or I_{to} result in prolongation of repolarization (Shah et al, 1988; Fedida et al, 1989; Lee and Rosen, 1994).

Studies in isolated tissues suggest that α_1-adrenergic-receptor subtype stimulation also can be arrhythmogenic. α_1-Agonists induce triggered rhythms via delayed or early afterdepolarizations and abnormal automatic rhythms (Kimura et al, 1984; Lee and Rosen, 1993; Anyukhovsky et al, 1992) studied in settings where $[Ca^{2+}]_o$ is elevated, repolarization is prolonged, ischemia and reperfusion are simulated, or infarction is induced. In intact cats after coronary occlusion and reperfusion, there is an increase in α_1-adrenergic-receptor number and affinity (Sheridan et al, 1980). This is associated with ventricular tachycardia and fibrillation that start occasionally during ischemia and invariably within one to three minutes of reperfusion.

For humans, only limited data are available concerning α-adrenergic involvement in cardiac arrhythmias. The efficacy of phentolamine against arrhythmias in a small group of patients in the immediate postmyocardial infarction period has been reported. Patients with the congenital long QT syndrome, a subset whose arrhythmias are not blocked by propranolol, do respond to left thoracic sympathectomy, leading to the speculation that α-adrenergic mechanisms may be involved (Malfatto et al, 1992). In sum, the clinical antiarrhythmic potential of α-adrenergic blockade remains largely untested.

The Muscarinic Receptor-Effector Coupling System

The M_2 receptor has been identified pharmacologically as the dominant cardiac muscarinic receptor (Peralta et al, 1987). Its density is two to five times higher in the atria than in the ventricles (Fields et al, 1978). The M_2 receptor is coupled directly to the ligand-operated K channel ($I_{K(ACh)}$) by the G-protein, G_K (Yatani et al, 1987). The M_2 receptor also inhibits adenylate cyclase via G_i and, in this way, affects currents that are modulated by the cyclic AMP dependent protein kinase, including I_{Ca-L}, I_f, and, presumably, I_K (Lindemann and Watanabe, 1989).

A major aspect of muscarinic action on the heart is the antagonism of adrenergic effects at the level of the adenylate cyclase-cyclic AMP system (Lindemann and Watanabe, 1989). Whereas β-adrenergic agonists stimulate the cyclic AMP second messenger system via the G-protein, G_s, muscarinic agonists such as acetylcholine inhibit this same system via G_i (Yatani et al, 1987). The effects of muscarinic activation on Ca^{2+} and K^+ currents contribute to the depression of conduction in the atrioventricular node. The effects of M_2 agonists to decrease I_f and to increase conductance of the muscarinic K^+ channel suppress the sinus node pacemaker (DiFrancesco et al, 1989). M_2-receptor activation leads to an increase in $I_{K(ACh)}$, which hyperpolarizes and shortens the action potential in atrial tissues (DiFrancesco et al, 1989).

Increased vagal activity (whether due to direct electrical stimulation or to pharmacologic activation) reduces the incidence of ventricular fibrillation during acute myocardial ischemia in intact animals

(Vanoli et al, 1991). This effect is only in part dependent on heart rate reduction; it also depends on the antiadrenergic action of muscarinic activation. Muscarinic blockade with atropine sometimes increases the incidence of ventricular fibrillation during ischemia.

Clinically, vagal activation is effective against arrhythmias involving the atrium and atrioventricular node, but there is no direct evidence for an antiarrhythmic effect of vagal activation at the ventricular level in human subjects. There is indirect evidence that impairments of or decreases in either vagal tone (heart rate variability) (Kleiger et al, 1987) or reflexes (baroreflex sensitivity) (LaRovere et al, 1988) are associated with increased mortality and incidence of sudden death among postmyocardial infarction patients. Hence, an antiarrhythmic action of muscarinic agonists occurs at the supraventricular level, and an important role may be played in ventricular arrhythmias and sudden death.

The Purinergic Receptor-Effector Coupling System

The cardiac purinergic receptor population is designated as A_1. It is coupled presumably by G_K to the ligand-operated K channel ($I_{K(Ado)}$) (Kirsch et al, 1990). As such, its actions are thought to reflect operation at the same effector coupling pathway as that described for the M_2 muscarinic receptor, resulting in hyperpolarization and acceleration of repolarization of cells in the atrium and atrioventricular junction. Like acetylcholine, adenosine reduces calcium current (Cerbai et al, 1988; Visentin et al, 1990) and reduces catecholamine effects as a result of accentuated antagonism. Via these mechanisms, adenosine suppresses both automatic rhythms and triggered rhythms in supraventricular tissues.

Clinically, a subset of benign ventricular tachycardias is terminated by the A_1 agonist, adenosine. Of greater importance, reentrant tachycardias involving the atrioventricular node are consistently terminated by adenosine (Belhassen et al, 1983). Other mechanisms effectively treated are nonreentrant ventricular and supraventricular tachycardias presumed due to triggered activity (Lerman et al, 1986; Lerman, 1993; DiMarco et al, 1985). Hence, this receptor-effector system offers an attractive target for therapeutic interventions.

Cytoplasmic Regulators of Second Messengers

We are becoming increasingly aware of the roles a variety of molecules may play in the regulation of second messengers. The latter, in turn, exert important influences on ionic currents. For example, agents that block cyclic AMP-phosphodiesterase may increase cyclic adenosine monophosphate and affect target channels such as the L-type Ca channel. Receptors for angiotensin and α_1 adrenoreceptors activate phospholipase C which, in turn, activates protein kinase C via diacylglycerol and releases inositol trisphosphate. The diacylglycerol-protein kinase C pathway results in phosphorylation of transsarcolemmal Ca^{2+} channels, and the inositol trisphosphate pathway induces sarcoplasmic reticulum release of Ca^{2+}. Both events would increase free intracellular Ca^{2+}. Other examples of regulators are: phospholipase A_2, which may stimulate the ligand-activated $K_{(ACh)}$ channel via arachidonic acid metabolic pathways; long chain fatty acids, which are reported to activate delayed rectifier K currents; and, finally, dephosphorylation, which is promoted by phosphatases and a specific muscle phosphatase inhibitor, okadaic acid, that is known to increase cardiac Ca currents.

Chapter 3

How Specific Targets Can Be Identified and Attacked

Considerations in the Development of Targets

The numerous, significant advances made in our understanding of the basic mechanisms underlying arrhythmias, of the function of the ion channels that contribute to the action potentials throughout the heart, and in the determination of amino acid sequences and related functional information about many different ion channel proteins raise the prospect of identifying highly specific targets for the development of new antiarrhythmic drugs. Ultimately, knowledge of the roles played by individual proteins in the generation of cardiac arrhythmias should enable us to design and develop compounds whose action should be well circumscribed, i.e., drugs that produce specific desired effects and avoid undesirable effects (see also Ch. 16). Moreover, as our basic understanding of the cellular and molecular determinants of processes governing cardiac electrophysiologic properties and their response to pharmacologic agents increases, novel targets for drug action will continue to be identified.

As examples, the concept of blocking Ca^{2+} channels to suppress arrhythmias was not envisioned until I_{Ca} was described, nor was the prospect of using adenosine in patients to terminate paroxysmal su-

From *Antiarrhythmic Therapy: A Pathophysiologic Approach* edited by Members of the Sicilian Gambit © 1994, Futura Publishing Co., Inc., Armonk, NY.

praventricular tachycardia considered until its effects on atrioventricular nodal function were systematically evaluated. Similarly, the identification of different K^+ channel clones and dissection of the role played by different K^+ channels in the repolarization process has led to the prospect of identifying drugs that effect an increase in action potential duration with minimal undesirable effects. Thus, detailed characterization of arrhythmia mechanisms and cellular regulatory pathways as well as identification of ion channel proteins and regulatory subunits are essential for development of new approaches to arrhythmia suppression. It is the philosophy of the participants of the Sicilian Gambit that further understanding of these basic mechanisms, from the molecule to the integrated behavior of the whole heart, may lead to identification of novel targets for antiarrhythmic drug action, which will lead to safer and more effective therapies. It is important to point out that a number of serious obstacles must be overcome if a strategy targeted at a highly specific molecular site is to be successfully implemented.

As addressed in the Sicilian Gambit (1991), specific target(s) or vulnerable parameters for certain arrhythmias can be modified in a reproducible and predictable fashion by specific antiarrhythmic drugs, resulting in arrhythmia termination. Characterization of an arrhythmia may permit one to identify integrated measures of function such as conduction, refractoriness, automaticity, or triggered activity as the parameter vulnerable to an antiarrhythmic drug. But, in fact, it is current flow through specific ion channels or the conformational state in which the channel finds itself that generates or is responsible for the particular parameter of interest. Thus, the channels are prime molecular targets of drug action. Hence, one conclusion that can be derived is that knowledge of the ionic mechanism(s) underlying each vulnerable parameter and availability of specific ion channel blockers would allow one to target therapy more specifically, and potentially to identify which ion channel type(s) represent the vulnerable molecular target or parameter for a given arrhythmia type. A detailed consideration of targets is presented in Ch. 2. For the reader's convenience, a glossary of abbreviations for those targets to be considered in this chapter is provided in Table 1.

We can begin our consideration of strategic considerations using reentry as an example. In the case of paroxysmal atrioventricular nodal reentrant tachycardia, atrioventricular nodal conduction is the vulnerable parameter. In contrast to adjacent cell types, propagation

Table 1
Glossary of Abbreviations

I_{to1}	Voltage-activated Ca^{2+} insensitive transient outward current (Campbell et al, 1993a and 1993b).
I_{to2}	Ca^{2+}-activated transient outward current (Callewaert et al, 1986).
I_{Kr}	Rapid component of delayed rectifier current (Sanguinetti and Jurkiewicz, 1990)
I_{Kur}	Ultrarapid component of delayed rectifier current (Backx and Marban, 1993; Wang et al, 1993b).
I_{Ks}	Slow component of delayed rectifier current (Sanguinetti and Jurkiewicz, 1990).
I_{K1}	Inward rectifier current (Rasmusson et al, 1990; Luo and Rudy, 1994).
$I_{Na/Ca}$	Na/Ca exchanger current (Sheu and Blaustein, 1992).
$I_{Na/K}$	Na/K pump current (Eisner and Smith, 1992).
I_{Na}	Sodium current (Fozzard, 1992).
I_{Ca}	Calcium current (Catterall, 1992).

through a selected part of the atrioventricular node that is obligatorily part of the reentry circuit is primarily Ca^{2+} channel dependent. As a result, the Ca^{2+} channel represents the appropriate molecular target of drug action, which can be realized through use of Ca^{2+} channel blocking drugs, β-adrenergic blockers, or adenosine. However, propagation in other parts of the reentrant circuit is Na^+ current dependent and, as a result, Na^+ channel blockers may also be effective in terminating this arrhythmia.

On the other hand, if refractoriness is identified as the vulnerable parameter in a given arrhythmia, then the problem becomes much more complicated. One can increase refractoriness by increasing repolarization or by delaying the recovery of available Na^+ channels (Hondeghem and Snyders, 1990; Snyders et al, 1992a and 1992b; Hille, 1992). However, which molecular target is the optimal one, where the goal is to increase action potential duration, is currently little understood. The reason for this ambiguity is due to the presence of at least eight outward currents (I_{to1}, I_{to2}, I_{Kr}, I_{Kur}, I_{Ks}, I_{K1}, $I_{Na/Ca}$, $I_{Na/K}$) and two inward currents (I_{Na}, I_{Ca}) that contribute to repolarization in ventricular myocytes (Colatsky et al, 1990; Rasmusson et al, 1994; Eisner and Smith, 1992; Sheu and Blaustein, 1992; Sanguinetti and Jurkiewicz, 1990; Backx and Marban, 1993; Campbell et al, 1993a and 1993b; Luo and Rudy, in press). Thus, we have the dilemma of identifying which current to target to effect an increase in repolarization. In part, the answer to this dilemma reflects the relative contribution of a particular current to repolarization at the heart rate of interest, for differences in channel-gating properties allow the current contribution to repolarization to vary as a function of heart rate. Some have proposed that I_{Kr} is the ideal target to achieve an increase in action potential duration (Colatsky et al, 1990). However, at fast heart rates, the contribution to repolarization by incomplete I_{Ks} deactivation, and enhanced $I_{Na/Ca}$ and $I_{Na/K}$ due to increased Na^+ and Ca^{2+} influx is substantially larger than at slow rates. Thus, I_{Kr} block may exert little effect on repolarization at fast rates. Conversely, the relative contribution of I_{Kr} is larger at slow rates than at fast rates and, as a result, I_{Kr} block at slow rates causes a larger effect on repolarization. Other potential targets include I_{to}, I_{Ks} and I_{Kp}. However, other variables that need to be taken into account when considering the relative contribution of the different currents to repolarization are cell type and location in the myocardium (e.g., epicardium versus endocardium) (Litovsky and Antzelevitch, 1988; Antzelevitch et al, 1991; Furukawa et al, 1992; Wang et al, 1993b). Another variable, temperature, has largely been ignored in the extrapolation of myocyte data to the in situ heart (Campbell et al, 1993a, 1993b, and 1994). For example, information concerning the rate dependence of I_{to} and its contribution to repolarization is difficult to evaluate at this time because of the high Q_{10} of gating kinetics and the fact that much of the data on I_{to} is available from studies carried out at 22°C.

Ionic currents are a reflection of both the permeation and gating properties of ion channels. Many gating transitions in most cardiac ion channels are voltage dependent. In addition to transmembrane voltage, a variety of intracellular enzymes and second messengers such as G-proteins, kinases and phosphatases, inositol trisphosphate, diacylglycerol, arachidonic acid, and cyclic GMP are now widely recognized to also modulate ion channel gating, thereby affecting current magnitude and time course in these cells (Hille, 1992). In addition, it is now recognized that associated subunits can substantially modify the functional properties of ion channels and may account for differences in functional properties of ionic currents between different tissues (Isom et al, 1992; Catterall, 1992; Collin et al, 1993; Makita et al, 1993). On the other hand, current density in myocardial cells can also be affected by factors regulating gene expression such as transcriptional control and posttranslational control mechanisms. Hence, antiarrhythmic drug blockade of ion channels designed to reduce a particular current through direct action on the channel is but one of many approaches that can result in a reduction of a particular ionic current in myocardial cells. Conversely, many antiarrhythmic drug effects can or could be substantially modified by changes in any of the factors that modulate ion channel function or expression of the gene that encodes the channel (Sherman and Catterall, 1984; Offord and Catterall, 1989; Pragnell et al, 1991; Levitan et al, 1991; Sanguinetti et al, 1991; Duff et al, 1992; Lee et al, 1993; Matsubara et al, 1993). What has received scant attention is the fact that these modulators of ion channel function could also serve as molecular targets of drug action. In essence, this approach is successful and is used in some cases to treat patients with the coadministration of a β-adrenergic blocking agent with an antiarrhythmic drug. This combination represents a direct approach to action on two molecular targets, the ion channel and the receptor and, as a result of action on the receptor, an indirect approach to action on the channel via a G-protein and protein kinase A.

Drug-Channel Interactions

The mechanism of antiarrhythmic drug interaction with ion channels has been studied in detail during the past three decades, but only during the past decade in a manner designed to analyze the biophysical basis of drug interaction with ion channels. Interpretation of these studies is based on the analysis of patterns of current reduction at the single channel and macroscopic current level that reflect intermittent drug binding to a certain type of ion channel (Snyders et al, 1992a; Rasmussen et al, 1994). This cycle of association and dissociation means that antiarrhythmic drugs that block the Na^+ and Ca^{2+} channel typically display use dependence (Fig. 1, upper panel). This term indicates that the greater the frequency of channel activation, the greater the fraction of blocked channels. K^+ channel blockers also display use-dependent blocking characteristics. However, for many of these compounds, the fraction of K^+ channels blocked decreases with increasing frequency of channel activation, and is referred to as reverse use dependence (Fig. 1, lower panel) (Hondeghem and Snyders, 1990; Colatsky et al, 1990; Roden, 1993). The pattern of blockade is also dependent on the conformational state of the channel to which binding occurs (Rasmusson et al, 1994).

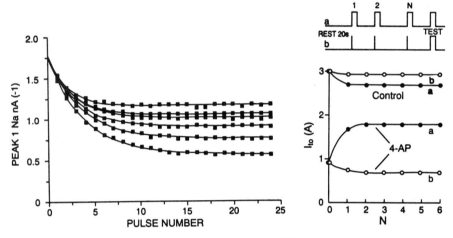

Figure 1. *Examples of two prototypic ion channel blockers, a Na^+ and a K^+ channel blocker interacting with their respective ion channels in a frequency-dependent manner. Lidocaine represents the prototypic Na^+ channel blocker and 4-aminopyridine (4-AP) represents a blocker of the transient outward current, I_{to1}. Lidocaine (80 μm) interacts with the sodium channel in a frequency-dependent manner (Left Panel), demonstrating an exponential decline in sodium current during different pulse trains (interstimulus interval of each pulse train was constant and the interstimulus interval of different pulse trains ranged between 150 [bottom curve] and 650 [top curve] ms). The sequence of the pulse within the train is plotted on the abscissa and demonstrates the shorter the interval between pulses (the faster the rate), the greater the degree of steady-state block observed. 4-aminopyridine also interacts with the transient outward current channel in a more complicated manner, demonstrating under different experimental conditions either reverse use dependence or use dependence (Right Panel). The change in I_{to} following an abrupt transition from a 20-s rest period to a pulse train with a 2-s interstimulus interval is illustrated for a pulse train with different pulse train durations. Note that a 300-ms duration pulse train caused an increase in I_{to} to a new steady-state value (reverse use dependence), while the 5-ms pulse train caused a use-dependent decrease in I_{to}. Reproduced with permission from Gilliam FR III, Starmer CF, Grant AO: Blockade of rabbit atrial sodium channels by lidocaine. Characterization of continuous and frequency-dependent blocking. Circ Res 1989; 65:723–739. Copyright 1989 American Heart Association. Reproduced with permission from Simurda J, Simurdova M, and Christé G: Use-dependent effects of 4-aminopyridine on transient outward current in dog ventricular muscle. Pflugers Arch 1989; 415:244–246.*

While a close correlation exists between the magnitude of Na^+ current blockade and the reduction of the upstroke of the action potential, the correlation between the magnitude of K^+ current blockade and the increase in action potential duration is poor (Colatsky et al, 1990; Hondeghem and Snyders, 1990; Jurkiewicz and Sanguinetti, 1993; Rasmusson et al, 1994). One reason for this lack of correspondence lies in the complex nature of repolarization, with multiple currents contributing to repolarization, as alluded to above. In addition, the difference in kinetics of drug-channel interaction, the dependence on the conformational state to which binding occurs, the lack of specificity of antiarrhythmic drug action, and the different rate dependence of different currents as discussed above also complicate this extrapolation. For example, analysis of the kinetics of K^+ channels shows that antiarrhythmic drugs can bind either to the closed state of the channel, the open or inactive state of the channel, or to more than one state of the channel depending on the compound and channel type (Kirsch and Drewe, 1993; Campbell et al, 1993b; Rasmusson et al, 1994). If a drug binds solely to the closed state of a K^+ channel, then the drug will likely display reverse use dependence. If a drug binds to the open or inactive state of the channel, the drug will likely display use dependence. If the drug binds to both the closed and open state, then there may be little "use dependence" detectable.

As experience with antiarrhythmic drugs has grown, it has become clear that these drugs are capable of not only suppressing cardiac arrhythmias, but also of causing them (Zipes, 1988a and 1988b; Akhtar et al, 1990; Akiyama et al, 1991). At least two different mechanisms underlying proarrhythmic events readily come to mind. As the active and passive properties of the reentrant loop and surrounding myocardium are nonuniform, then Na channel blocking compounds may lead to disparate effects on conduction in the reentrant circuit and surrounding tissue. Thus, a given concentration of antiarrhythmic drug may lead to conduction slowing in the reentrant circuit sufficient to cause termination of a reentrant arrhythmia and, yet, lesser degrees of conduction slowing in another area of the myocardium sufficient to cause reinitiation of another reentrant arrhythmia. In the case of K^+ channel blockade, the relatively small and directionally opposite currents are so closely balanced that blockade of a K^+ channel could upset the balance, resulting in net inward current and triggered activity. With the increased understanding of the currents that contribute to the plateau, one may be able to define which K^+ currents are best suited to blockade and what drug association/dissociation properties (kinetics) are ideally suited to maximizing drug effects on repolarization while minimizing the likelihood of generating triggered activity.

Targeting a Specific Channel May Alter the Integrated Electrophysiologic Properties of the Heart

It is well known that tetrodotoxin is a highly specific blocker of the Na^+ channel, and yet its administration is associated with a shortening of the action potential as well as a reduction in the amplitude and upstroke velocity of the action potential (Kiyosue and Arita, 1989). In this instance, the effect on repolarization reflects the blockade of the small population of noninactivating sodium channels that contribute to the plateau phase of the action potential (Fozzard and Hanck, 1992). Similarly, block of I_{to} allows the plateau phase to shift to more positive potentials (Campbell et al, 1993a and 1993b), thereby increasing the outwardly directed $I_{Na/Ca}$ and altering the sustained phase of I_{Ca} and the activation of I_{Ks} (Rasmusson et al, 1990; Qu et al, 1993), thereby affecting the entire phase of repolarization.

Sequence Homology Among Ion Channels

Advances in our understanding of the functional properties of ion channels has more recently been paralleled by advances in our understanding of the functional role of different amino acid residues within the different peptides. Information about structure and function of different cloned channels has led to the classification of different superfamilies of K^+ channels (Pongs, 1992). For example, many of the K^+ channels belong to a superfamily whose putative design consists of six membrane-spanning segments (S1 to S6) (Fig. 2). This family of voltage-gated channels is related to, but distinct from, the family of K^+ channels whose members include the inward rectifier and adenosine triphosphate-regulated K^+ channels, which contain only two membrane-spanning regions (Ho et al, 1993; Kubo et al, 1993a and 1993b) as well as another family which consists of a single membrane-spanning segment (Folander et al, 1990).

Structure-function studies of voltage-sensitive K^+ channels as

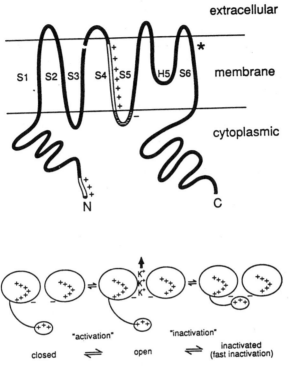

Figure 2. *Schematic representation of a K^+ channel polypeptide is depicted in the upper panel. The putative transmembrane-spanning segments (S1 to S6) are predicted from hydropathy analyses and the short hydrophobic segment between S5 and S6 is believed to form a portion of the channel pore. S4, with every third or fourth amino acid being positively charged, has been proposed to be the voltage sensor. The NH$_2$-terminal region contains a few basic residues that are involved in fast inactivation. The COOH-terminal region including part of S6 is believed to underlie slow inactivation. A model of K^+ channel function is depicted in the lower panel. Channel activation is voltage dependent and is responsible for the channel moving from the closed to open state, thereby allowing K^+ ions to diffuse down their electrochemical gradient through their pore region. Shortly after undergoing transition to the open state, fast inactivation develops for some K^+ channels (I_{to}). Inactivation involves the movement of a cytoplasmic ball depicted with negative charges (NH$_2$ terminus) toward the pore region or vestibule, binding to a site in the S4 to S5 linker near the mouth of the pore, thereby occluding the pore and preventing further ion permeation through the pore. Reproduced with permission from Jan LY, Jan YN: Structural elements involved in specific K^+ channel functions. Ann Rev Physiol 1992; 54:537–555.*

well as other ion channels have shown that this class of channels are tetramers (Pongs, 1992; Jan and Jan, 1992) (Fig. 2). Each subunit consists of six hydrophobic membrane-spanning segments, designated S1 to S6, with the NH_2 and COOH-termini located on the cytoplasmic side of the membrane. H5, a short hydrophobic segment composed of 20 amino acids between S5 and S6, is believed to form a portion of the channel pore and is highly conserved in K^+ channels. Numerous mutagenesis studies indicate that H5 forms the channel pore and contains multiple binding sites for ions and open channel blockers. S4, with every third or fourth amino acid being positively charged (lysine or arginine), has been proposed to be the voltage sensor in these voltage-gated K^+ channels (Pongs, 1992; Jan and Jan, 1992). In addition, the S4 to S5 linker region has been proposed to constitute the activation gate. Two different mechanisms appear to be responsible for inactivation. N-type inactivation is rapid and appears to be the result of a "ball-and-chain" mechanism, with the first 20 to 30 amino acids acting as the ball and the S4 to S5 linker near the mouth of the pore acting as the receptor for the ball (Jan and Jan, 1992; Pongs, 1992; Tseng-Crank et al, 1993; Comer et al, in press). C-type inactivation is slower and appears sensitive to mutations in the S6 region and the cytoplasmic carboxy-terminal domain (Pongs, 1992).

Using a combination of biophysical measurements and site-directed mutagenesis experiments, investigators have determined the molecular basis of toxin and drug binding to ion channels and identified novel molecular mechanisms for modulation of ion channel function. Specifically, they have demonstrated that specific amino acids within the tetramer serve as binding sites for different drugs such as tetraethylammonium (TEA) and toxins such as charybdotoxin and dendrodotoxin (Pongs, 1992). While detailed electrophysiologic studies have been done with different drugs on different K^+ channels with many different antiarrhythmic drugs, only certain binding characteristics lend themselves to a prediction of drug binding to a specific amino acid within the clone. For example, those drugs whose blocking mechanism is attributed to open channel block are likely to bind to sites within the pore region or H5. Apart from the quaternary TEA molecule, which binds to a threonine residue near the inner mouth of the pore as well as an external site, there are few reports of comparable data on binding sites for antiarrhythmic drugs using the site-directed mutagenesis approach. The assignment of a quinidine binding site to a residue at the inner mouth of the pore region was determined from the similarities in value of the effective electrical distance of TEA binding determined in experiments on other K^+ channel types (Shaker B) (Snyders et al, 1992b). Hydrophobic residues near the mouth of the pore may be involved in binding the hydrophobic domains of quinidine by a mechanism that is similar to that for binding of quaternary ammonium compounds with lipophilic side chains, such as with the external binding of TEA.

Sequence homologies among ion channel proteins may well explain the relative nonspecificity of currently available drugs; for example, it is now recognized that verapamil blocks I_K and I_{Na} (Davies et al, 1992; Lewis et al, 1992; Ragsdale et al, 1992) at concentrations not much higher than that required to block I_{Ca}, and that flecainide blocks I_K at concentrations roughly the same or slightly higher than those required to block I_{Na} (Follmer and Colatsky, 1990). Similarly, roughly the same concentrations of quinidine block I_{Na}, I_K and I_{Ca} (Salata and Wasserstrom, 1988).

The similarities among molecular structures characterized to date suggest that specificity of drug action will be difficult to achieve. However, the actual availability of target-specific drugs, such as digitalis, argues that specificity is an achievable goal. Recently, a series of drugs thought to be highly specific for the rapid component of the delayed rectifier current (I_{Kr}) have entered clinical trials (Roden, 1993). Both in vitro and in vivo studies strongly suggest that these compounds, which include dofetilide and E4031 (Carmeliet, 1993; Jurkiewicz and Sanguinetti, 1993), do not produce significant effects on other ion channels in the heart, or elsewhere, although exhaustive studies of this question have yet to be performed. A complementary DNA that encodes I_{Kr} behavior has not yet been cloned, and further studies of the tissue- and disease-dependent expression of this ion channel are only now underway. Further cloning of potential targets and understanding of which epitopes on the channel proteins are important to effect a desired pharmacologic response may lead to further identification of channel-specific drugs.

The Future of Drug Design (see also Ch. 16)

Rational drug design using computers is a promising new approach in new drug development (Martin, 1991; Livingstone, 1991;

Carrupt et al, 1991). In general, the following techniques are used. A three-dimensional structure of the macromolecule with an identification of the location and specification of the chemical nature of preferred interaction sites on the molecule is required. A known or hypothetical three-dimensional structure of the binding site is used in association with molecular graphics design and/or search of three-dimensional structures to identify templates to which to add the required groups. The final method searches data bases of substituent constants to design an analog with the physical properties that would maximize the likelihood for biologic activity. Other techniques such as the molecular electrostatic potential of drugs use stereoelectronic complementarity between the binding molecule and the receptor to explain molecular recognition and specificity. In this approach, the contributing intermolecular forces are hydrophobic and electrostatic. While productive in design of other agents, these techniques have yet to be applied successfully to the design of new antiarrhythmic agents. In part, lack of progress in this area reflects the unavailability of crystalline structure for membrane bound ion channels. Despite the absence of three-dimensional structure, the identification of a large number of toxins that bind selectively and with high affinity to different ion channel types (Table 2) strongly suggests that drug design that targets a drug to act on specific molecular targets represents a readily attainable goal.

As alluded to previously, antiarrhythmic drug design that targets drugs to specific membrane proteins faces a unique set of problems. Factors that need to be addressed include desired modification of channel function, appropriate association/dissociation kinetics, conformationally-specific drug binding, and specificity of drug binding to a particular K^+ channel family (Rasmusson et al, 1994). Specificity of drug binding requires identification of nonhomologous protein sequences as potential drug-binding sites. Analysis of the hydrophobic regions of different K^+ channels has demonstrated a striking degree of sequence homology between K^+ channels of a given superfamily (Pongs, 1992). For example, if the pore region represents an optimal drug-binding site, then, given the high degree of sequence homology between the H5 regions of different K^+ channels (Fig. 3), it is unlikely that blocking compounds will show much specificity based solely on drug interactions with the H5 segment. Such homologies may well explain the relative nonspecificity of some currently available drugs; for example, open channel blockers such as quinidine that probably

Table 2
Channel Inhibitors/Activators-Toxins

Channel Type	Inhibitor/Activator	Reference
Ca^{2+} Channel		
L-type	Calciseptine (blocker)	5
SR Ca^{2+} Release	Ryanodine (blocker)	13
	Imperatoxin-activator (activator)	15
	Imperatoxin-inhibitor (blocker)	15
Cl^- Channel		
Small Conductance	Chlorotoxin (blocker)	6
K^+ Channel		
Voltage Dependent	α-Dendrodotoxin (blocker)	1
	MCD Peptide (blocker)	14
Ca^{2+} Activated		
Apamin Sensitive	Apamin (blocker)	3,12
	Leiurotoxin I (blocker)	3
Apamin Insensitive	Charybdotoxin (blocker)	9
	Iberiotoxin (blocker)	7
	Kaliotoxin (blocker)	4
Na^+ Channel	Tetrodotoxin (blocker)	11
	Neurotoxin IV (inhibitor of inactivation)	8
	Brevetoxin (activator)	2
	Aconitine (activator)	10
	Batrachotoxin (activator)	11
	Pyrethroids (activators)	11

1. Benishin et al, 1988.
2. Catterall and Gainer, 1985.
3. Chicchi et al, 1988.
4. Crest et al, 1992.
5. de Weille et al, 1991.
6. DeBin et al, 1993.
7. Galvez et al, 1990.
8. Kopeyan et al, 1985.
9. Miller et al, 1985.
10. Muroi et al, 1990.
11. Narahashi, 1986.
12. Robertson and Steinberg, 1990.
13. Sutko et al, 1985.
14. Taylor et al, 1984.
15. Valdivia et al, 1992.

HOMOLOGY IN PORE REGION AMONG VARIOUS K⁺ CHANNEL CLONES

```
             S5                      H5                      S6
Sh    AVYFAEAGSENSFFKSIPDAFWWAVVTMTTVGYGDMTPVGFWGKIVGSLC
RCK1  -------EEAE-H-S----------S---------Y--TIG--------
RCK4  ------DEPTTH-Q-------------------K-IT-G--------
HK1   ------DEPTTH-Q-------------------K-IT-G--------
HK2   ------DNQGTH-S-------------------R-ITVG--------
DRK1  L-F---KDEDDTK-----AS----TI---------IY-KTLL-----G--
```

Figure 3. *Similarities of the pore lining region of the HK1, HK2, and various other K⁺ channels. Sequence of the putative pore region (proline to proline) of HK1 and HK2 (Snyders et al, 1992a and 1992b; Tamkun et al, 1991; Stuhmer et al, 1989; Tempel et al, 1987; MacKinnon and Yellen, 1990; Kamb et al, 1988; Frech et al, 1989; Hartmann et al, 1991; Stuhmer, 1991; Catterall, 1992).*

bind to the pore region block different K^+ currents (Snyders et al, 1992b; Balser et al, 1991; Rasmusson et al, 1994). If specificity of drug binding is deemed to be a desirable property of antiarrhythmic agents, then areas of sequence nonhomology of functional importance in the peptide will need to be identified as areas to explore as potential drug-binding sites.

The Moving Target Problem

Even as specific molecular targets are identified, whose block leads to circumscribed, desirable effects, a number of lines of evidence suggests that the pathophysiologic basis of cardiac arrhythmias may change over time, i.e., drugs may be aimed at a "moving target." Hence, a drug that appears effective at one point in time may become ineffective or may actually provoke arrhythmias at another. The clinical evidence that best supports this contention is derived from the Cardiac Arrhythmia Suppression Trial (CAST), in which the death rate among patients on encainide or flecainide therapy remained elevated for the duration of the study (Echt et al, 1991a). This occurred despite the fact that these two agents demonstrated marked suppression of ventricular premature beats. As discussed in detail elsewhere (Strauss, 1994), one would have anticipated that most of the proarrhythmic effects of drugs would have occurred early during treatment. However, the deaths in the active treatment groups were equally distributed throughout the period of drug treatment, perhaps reflecting a change in the clinical setting, such as progression of myocardial ischemia. It is well recognized that perturbations such as ischemia, congestive heart failure, stretch, neurohumoral activation, or electrolyte abnormalities can acutely alter the electrophysiologic properties of the heart and its response to drugs (Grant et al, 1984; Snyders et al, 1992a; Lue and Boyden, 1992; Beuckelmann et al, 1993; Strauss, 1994). The development of a new arrhythmogenic mechanism could lead to a potentiation of the depressant effects in this new setting as well as proarrhythmia or failure of arrhythmia control.

In summary, while the prospect for new antiarrhythmic drug development appears promising, the path appears more convoluted than is the case of drug design for action against other membrane proteins such as receptors. This derives from the complex nature of the pathophysiologic mechanisms underlying cardiac arrhythmias, the problems associated with identification of appropriate areas of the membrane proteins necessary for achieving specificity of drug binding, and the need to address optimal drug association/dissociation properties to maximize therapeutic potential. Although the pessimist may despair, the continued advances in this field offer hope of favorable outcomes.

Chapter 4

Electrophysiologic Mechanisms for Cardiac Arrhythmias

The Sicilian Gambit describes a logical framework for understanding the means for the termination or prevention of cardiac arrhythmias. Its premise is that from a knowledge of the cellular electrophysiologic mechanism causing an arrhythmia, a vulnerable parameter can be ascertained, the alteration of which would have an antiarrhythmic effect. The purpose of this chapter is to review the electrophysiologic mechanisms that have been shown to cause arrhythmias and to indicate possible vulnerable parameters. This will serve as a background for the discussion of drug actions on targets and on specific arrhythmias in subsequent chapters.

The Normal Transmembrane Action Potential

The transmembrane potentials of normal sinoatrial and atrioventricular node, ventricular specialized conducting, and atrial and ventricular myocardial fibers were determined some years ago (e.g., Hoffman and Cranefield, 1960). As an example, the canine Purkinje fiber (Fig. 1) has a high resting membrane potential, rapid phase 0 depolarization, three phases of repolarization, and the ability to depolarize during phase 4 such that spontaneous activity can be initiated. The

From *Antiarrhythmic Therapy: A Pathophysiologic Approach* edited by Members of the Sicilian Gambit © 1994, Futura Publishing Co., Inc., Armonk, NY.

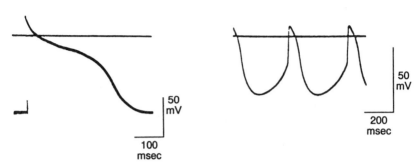

Figure 1. *Left panel: Purkinje fiber action potential, having a rapid upstroke and three prominent phases of repolarization. Right panel: Sinus node action potential having a lower membrane potential, a slower phase 0 upstroke, and marked depolarization during phase 4, generating a spontaneous rhythm. Reproduced with permission from Rosen MR: Mechanisms of arrhythmias: Contributions of cellular electrophysiology. In Josephson ME, Wellens HJJ (eds): Tachycardias: Mechanisms and Management. Mt. Kisco, NY: Futura Publishing Co., 1992.*

action potential provides a basis for comprehending the determinants of the electrocardiogram that reflect extracellular current generated by local adjacent differences in intracellular potential. Specifically, the electrocardiographic QRS complex reflects rapid phase 0 depolarization and conduction in myocardium; the ST segment and T wave reflect phases 1 to 3 of myocardial repolarization. Some instances of automaticity are explained by phase 4 depolarization in specialized conducting fibers. Moreover, it is understood that, in nodal tissues, the resting membrane potential is less negative and the action potential upstroke lower in its velocity than in Purkinje fiber, and in the sinus node, phase 4 depolarization occurs consistently, thereby determining the onset of the cardiac impulse.

Studies using the voltage-clamp technique (in which the transmembrane voltage is controlled and the currents flowing inward or outward across the membrane are measured) permitted investigators to determine the ionic origins of the transmembrane potential (e.g., Hille, 1992). The resting potential is attributed to a transmembrane potassium K^+ ion gradient (as in Purkinje fibers where $[K^+]_o$ is approximately 4 mmol/L and $[K^+]_i$ is about 30 times greater). The rapid phase 0 upstroke of the action potential is the result of Na^+ entering the cell, and the three phases of repolarization are associated with Ca^{2+} and, to a lesser extent, Na^+ entering and with K^+ leaving the cell by as many as eight different channels. The various channels and their contribution to the action potential are reviewed in Ch. 2, Figure 1.

In sinus and atrioventricular nodes, the membrane potential is low and the upstroke of the action potential is the result of Ca^{2+} entry (Fig. 1). Phase 4 depolarization in the sinus node is attributed to the pacemaker current I_f (DiFrancesco et al, 1986) and to the decay of I_K (Brown, 1982).

Classification of Cellular Mechanisms of Cardiac Arrhythmias

A general schema for the classification of the electrophysiologic mechanisms causing cardiac arrhythmias is shown in Table 1 (Hoffman and Rosen, 1981). This schema subdivides the general causes of arrhythmias into two: abnormalities in impulse initiation and abnormalities in impulse conduction. Each of these divisions has subclassifications. Both abnormalities may also occur simultaneously.

Table 1
Classification of Electrophysiologic Mechanisms Causing Cardiac Arrhythmias

Abnormal Impulse Initiation
  Automaticity
    Normal automaticity
    Abnormal automaticity
  Triggered Activity
    Early afterdepolarizations
    Delayed afterdepolarizations
Abnormal Impulse Conduction
  Conduction block leading to ectopic pacemaker "escape"
  Unidirectional block and reentry
    Ordered reentry
    Random reentry
  Reflection
Simultaneous Abnormalities of Impulse Generation and Conduction
  Impaired conduction caused by phase 4 depolarization
  Parasystole

Modified from Hoffman BF, Rosen MR: Cellular mechanisms for cardiac arrhythmias. Circ Res 1981; 49:1–15.

Arrhythmias Caused by Abnormal Impulse Initiation

The term "impulse initiation" is used to indicate that an electrical impulse can arise in a single cell or group of closely coupled cells through depolarization of the cell membrane and, once initiated, spread through the rest of the heart. There are two major causes for the impulse initiation that may result in arrhythmias: automaticity and triggered activity. Each has its own unique cellular mechanism resulting in membrane depolarization.

Automaticity

There are two kinds of automaticity. Normal automaticity is found in the primary pacemaker of the heart—the sinus node—as well as in certain subsidiary or latent pacemakers that can become the pacemaker under conditions that are described later. Impulse initiation is a normal property of these latent pacemakers. On the other hand, abnormal automaticity only occurs in cardiac cells when there have been major (abnormal) changes in their transmembrane potentials; in particular, partial loss of resting potential. This property of abnormal automaticity is not confined to any specific latent pacemaker cell type but may occur almost anywhere in the heart.

Normal automaticity

The normal site of impulse initiation is the sinus node. The cause of normal automaticity in the sinus node is a spontaneous decline in the transmembrane potential during diastole, referred to as the pacemaker potential, phase 4, or diastolic depolarization (we use the terms interchangeably). This is depicted in Ch. 2, Figure 1. There is evidence that diastolic depolarization results from the turning on of an inward current called "i_f" that is activated after repolarization of the sinus node action potential (Brown and DiFrancesco, 1980; Di-Francesco and Ojeda, 1980; DiFrancesco, 1990). The i_f current is carried by Na^+ and K^+ as shown by ion substitution experiments; the reversal potential of the current is intermediate between the Na^+ and K^+ equilibrium potentials (DiFrancesco, 1990). From the voltage-clamp studies, it is known that the i_f channels are inactivated at positive membrane potentials, begin to activate after hyperpolarization to around -40 mV, and are fully activated after hyperpolarization to around -100 mV (Yanigihara and Irisawa, 1980; DiFrancesco, 1986; DiFrancesco et al, 1986). Since the maximum diastolic potential of the sinus node pacemaker cells is between -60 and -70 mV, the i_f current is turned on during repolarization to this level, although it is not fully activated at the maximum diastolic potential. Activation of i_f also has a time dependency and, therefore, this inward current continues to increase after complete repolarization, causing the progressive fall in the membrane potential during phase 4. However, an important role for a time-dependent decrease in a potassium conductance, I_K, in causing spontaneous diastolic depolarization also has been proposed (Brown, 1982; Brown et al, 1982). In addition, activation of both T- and L-type inward calcium currents (Reuter, 1984; Bean, 1985) during diastolic depolarization contributes to phase 4 depolarization (Hagiwara et al, 1988; Doerr et al, 1989). Therefore, there may be no single pacemaker current in the sinus node but, rather, a number of currents may contribute to the expression of automaticity (Irisawa and Giles, 1990).

In the normal heart, cells with pacemaking capability are located not only in the sinus node, but in some parts of the atria and ventricles. However, they are not pacemakers while the sinus node is functioning normally. These are referred to as latent or subsidiary pacemakers (Fig. 2). Since spontaneous diastolic depolarization is a normal property of these cells, the automaticity generated by them is classified as normal. In the atria, subsidiary pacemakers are located along the crista terminalis (Hogan and Davis, 1968), at the junction of the inferior right atrium and inferior vena cava (Jones et al, 1978; Rozanski and Lipsius, 1985; Rozanski et al, 1983), at the orifice of the coronary sinus (Wit and Cranefield, 1977), and in the atrial muscle that extends into the tricuspid and mitral valves (Wit et al, 1973; Bassett et al, 1976; Rozanski, 1987). In the atrioventricular junction, atrioventricular nodal cells possess the intrinsic property of automaticity (Kokubun et al, 1980), although there is still some uncertainty as to the exact location of these pacemakers in the node (James et al, 1979). In the ventricles, latent or subsidiary pacemakers are found in the His-Purkinje system where Purkinje fibers have the property of spontaneous diastolic depolarization (Weidmann, 1956; Hoffman and Cranefield, 1960). The intrinsic Purkinje fiber pacemaker rate is less than the rate

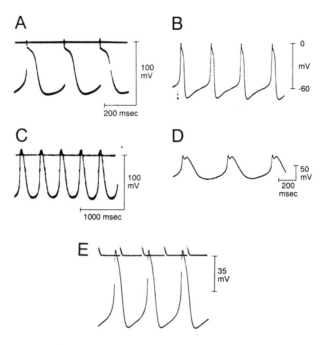

Figure 2. *Transmembrane potentials recorded in isolated superfused preparations from some subsidiary pacemaker cells with the property of normal automaticity. Spontaneous diastolic depolarization that developed in the absence of overdrive suppression is shown in each panel. A: Atrial fiber in crista terminalis in the presence of isoproterenol. Reproduced with permission from Hogan PM, Davis LD: Evidence for specialized fibers in the canine right atrium. Circ Res 1968;23: 387–396. Copyright 1968 American Heart Association. B: Atrial fiber in the inferior right atrium. Reproduced with permission from Rozanski GJ, Lipsius SL: Electrophysiology of functional subsidiary pacemakers in canine right atrium. Am J Physiol 1985; 249:H594–H603. C: Atrial fiber in ostium of coronary sinus in the presence of norepinephrine. Reproduced with permission from Wit AL, Cranefield PF: Triggered and automatic activity in the canine coronary sinus. Circ Res 1977; 41:435–445. Copyright 1977 American Heart Association. D: Atrial fiber in stretched mitral valve leaflet. Reproduced with permission from Wit AL, Fenoglio JJ Jr, Wagner BM, Basset AL: Electrophysiological properties of cardiac muscle in the anterior mitral valve leaflet and the adjacent atrium in the dog. Possible implications for the genesis of atrial dysrhythmias. Circ Res 1973; 32:731–745. Copyright 1973 American Heart Association. E: Atrioventricular nodal fiber of the rabbit heart after the atrioventricular node was separated from the atrium. Reproduced with permission from Wit AL, Rosen MR: Cellular electrophysiology of cardiac arrhythmias. In Josephson ME, Wellens HJJ (eds): Tachycardias: Mechanisms, Diagnosis, Treatment. Philadelphia, PA: Lea & Febiger, 1984, pp. 1–27.*

of atrial and junctional pacemakers, and decreases from the His bundle to the distal Purkinje branches (Hope et al, 1976).

The membrane currents responsible for normal spontaneous diastolic depolarization at ectopic sites have also been studied. The most thorough analyses have been done on the pacemaker current in Purkinje cells using voltage-clamp techniques. These studies have shown the presence of an i_f pacemaker current, as in the sinus node (DiFrancesco, 1981a and 1981b, 1985). Other currents are also likely to contribute to the pacemaker potential in Purkinje cells (Noble, 1984; DiFrancesco and Noble, 1985; DiFrancesco, 1985; Gintant and Cohen, 1988). A membrane current similar to the i_f pacemaker current in Purkinje fibers may also be involved in the pacemaker activity in atrial and atrioventricular junctional pacemakers (Earm et al, 1983; Carmeliet, 1984; Kokubun et al, 1980 and 1982).

In the normal heart in sinus rhythm, subsidiary pacemaker activity is suppressed by the more rapid rate of sinus node impulse initiation and overdrive suppression (Vassalle, 1977). The mechanism of overdrive suppression has been characterized in microelectrode studies on isolated Purkinje fiber bundles exhibiting pacemaker function. It is mostly mediated by enhanced activity of the Na^+/K^+ exchange pump that results from driving a pacemaker cell faster than its intrinsic spontaneous rate. During normal cardiac rhythm, the sinus node drives the latent pacemakers at a faster rate than their normal (intrinsic) automatic rate. As a result, the intracellular Na^+ of the latent pacemakers is increased to a higher level than would be the case were the pacemakers firing at their own intrinsic rate. This is the result of Na ions entering the cells during each action potential upstroke. The rate of activity of the sodium pump is largely determined by the level of intracellular Na^+ concentration (Glitsch, 1979), so that pump activity is enhanced during high rates of stimulation (Vassalle, 1970). Since the sodium pump moves more Na^+ outward than K^+ inward, it generates a net outward (hyperpolarizing) current across the cell membrane (Gadsby and Cranefield, 1979). When subsidiary pacemaker cells are driven faster than their intrinsic rate (such as by the sinus node), the enhanced outward pump current hyperpolarizes the membrane potential and suppresses spontaneous impulse initiation in these cells that, as described before, is dependent on the net inward current. Another mechanism that may suppress subsidiary pacemakers, in addition to overdrive suppression, is the electrotonic interaction between the pacemaker cells and nonpacemaker cells in the surrounding myocardium (van Capelle and Durrer, 1980). A shift in the site of impulse initiation to one of the regions where subsidiary pacemakers are located that results in arrhythmias would be expected to happen when any of the following occurs.

1. The rate at which the sinus node activates subsidiary pacemakers falls considerably below the intrinsic rate of the subsidiary pacemakers. Once overdrive suppression is removed by sinus node inhibition, the subsidiary pacemaker with the fastest rate becomes the site of impulse origin (Vassalle, 1977).
2. Inhibitory electrotonic influences between nonpacemaker and pacemaker cells are interrupted. Any event that decreases intercellular coupling between latent, subsidiary, pacemaker cells, and surrounding nonpacemaker cells may remove the inhibitory influence of electrotonic current flow on the latent pacemakers and allow them to fire at their intrinsic rate (van Capelle and Durrer, 1980). Coupling might be reduced by fibrosis that can separate myocardial fibers.
3. Impulse initiation in subsidiary pacemakers is enhanced. This may result from the effects of sympathetic stimulation. The flow of current between partially depolarized myocardium and normally polarized latent pacemaker cells also might enhance automaticity (Katzung et al, 1975) as can inhibition of the electrogenic Na/K pump (Rosen et al, 1973a and 1973b). A decrease in the extracellular potassium level also enhances normal automaticity (Vassalle, 1965), as does acute stretch (Deck, 1964).

Abnormal automaticity

Atrial and ventricular myocardial cells do not normally show spontaneous diastolic depolarization and do not initiate spontaneous impulses even when they are not excited for long periods of time by propagating impulses. However, when the resting potentials of working atrial or ventricular myocardial cells are reduced sufficiently, spontaneous diastolic depolarization may occur and cause repetitive impulse initiation, a phenomenon called depolarization-induced automaticity or abnormal automaticity (Fig. 3). The reduction of the membrane potential may be a result of cardiac disease. The level of membrane potential at which abnormal automaticity occurs is in a range between -70 and -30 mV (Hauswirth et al, 1969; Katzung and Mor-

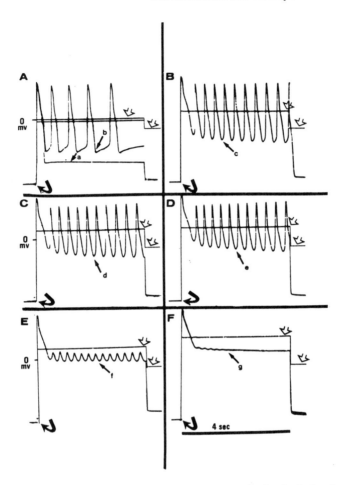

Figure 3. *Effects of depolarizing membrane currents applied only during the action potential on the membrane potential and automatic firing of a guinea pig papillary muscle. Panel A: Two superimposed traces are shown. Trace a (black arrow) shows a single action potential at the left induced by a stimulus in a normally polarized cell. Trace b (black arrow) shows abnormal automaticity in the same cell after membrane potential was depolarized by 20 mV with a current pulse (open arrow). Panels B through F: The effects of further depolarization on the abnormal automaticity. In each panel, the black arrows point to the membrane potential and the open arrows point to the current pulse. Reproduced with permission from Imanishi S, Surawicz B: Automatic activity in depolarized guinea pig ventricular myocardium. Circ Res 1976; 39:751–759. Copyright 1976 American Heart Association.*

genstern, 1977; Imanishi and Surawicz, 1976; Brown and Noble, 1969). The upstrokes of the spontaneously occurring action potentials generated by abnormal automaticity can be caused by either Na^+ or Ca^{2+} inward currents or, possibly, a mixture of the two depending on the level of the depolarized membrane potential and whether or not the fast inward sodium current is completely inactivated or not. In Purkinje fibers, enhanced automaticity may also occur over the range of membrane potentials between the normal high level (around -90 mV) and the low level at which abnormal automaticity occurs (around -60 mV). At these intermediate levels of membrane potential, there is no sharp distinction between normal and abnormal automaticity. Such a distinction is not a problem in atrial or ventricular cells in which normal automaticity does not occur. A low level of membrane potential is not the only criterion for defining abnormal automaticity. If this were so, the automaticity of the sinus node would have to be considered abnormal. Therefore, an important distinction between abnormal and normal automaticity is that the resting membrane potential of fibers showing the abnormal type of activity is reduced from the normal level. For this reason, we do not classify automaticity in the atrioventricular node or valves, where membrane potential is normally low, to be abnormal automaticity.

A likely cause of automaticity at depolarized membrane potentials in muscle is deactivation of the delayed rectifier K current (Katzung and Morgenstern, 1977; Noble and Tsien, 1968). Under normal circumstances, an action potential activates this current, which deactivates slowly on repolarization. The outward current generated repolarizes membranes. As the current deactivates, spontaneous diastolic depolarization occurs. If either Na or Ca channels are reactivated after the preceding action potential, the spontaneous depolarization caused by K channel deactivation may lead to an upstroke caused by current flowing through one of these channels (depending on the level of the membrane potential) (Katzung and Morgenstern, 1977). Experiments on depolarized human atrial myocardium from dilated atria also indicate that calcium-dependent processes may contribute to abnormal pacemaker activity at low membrane potentials (Escande et al, 1987a and 1987b; Kimura et al, 1988). The mechanism may be similar to the one causing the transient inward current responsible for delayed afterdepolarizations (see the section entitled "Arrhythmias Caused by Triggered Activity").

In the heart, myocardial fibers with low resting potentials and a propensity for abnormal automaticity will not express that rhythm if the sinus node drives them faster than their intrinsic abnormal automatic rate. An abnormal automatic focus should manifest itself and cause an arrhythmia when the sinus rate decreases below the intrinsic rate of the focus or when the rate of the focus increases above that of the sinus node, as was discussed for latent pacemakers with normal automaticity. At normal sinus rates, there may be little overdrive suppression of pacemakers with abnormal automaticity (Dangman and Hoffman, 1983). As a result, even transient sinus pauses or occasional long sinus cycle lengths may permit an ectopic focus with a slower rate than the sinus node to capture the heart for one or more beats. It is also possible that the depolarized level of membrane potential at which abnormal automaticity occurs might cause entrance block into the focus and prevent it from being overdriven by the sinus node, even when impulses initiated in the focus can leave it (unidirectional block) (Ferrier and Rosenthal, 1980). This would lead to parasystole, an arrhythmia caused by a combination of abnormal impulse conduction and initiation. The firing rate of an abnormally automatic focus might also be increased above that of the sinus node, for example, by sympathetic stimulation, leading to arrhythmias in the absence of sinus node suppression or conduction block between the focus and surrounding myocardium. The automatic rate of an abnormal pacemaker is also a direct function of the level of membrane potential (see Fig. 3) so that more severely depolarized regions are likely to have rates faster than that of the sinus node.

Effects of electrical stimulation on arrhythmias caused by automaticity

In the heart, in situ, it is not routinely possible to obtain direct electrical recordings from an arrhythmogenic source that enables one to determine the electrophysiologic mechanism causing an arrhythmia, although some success has been attained with highly specialized techniques (Cramer et al, 1977). Therefore, indirect approaches have evolved to determine the mechanism. Among these approaches is the use of electrical stimulation of the heart to study arrhythmias.

Overdrive by either the sinus node or electrical stimuli exerts an inhibitory effect on the normal automatic mechanism of subsidiary pacemakers (overdrive suppression) that is primarily the result of enhanced Na/K pump activity (Vassalle, 1970 and 1977). When overdrive is applied during an ongoing arrhythmia caused by normal automaticity, the rate of the arrhythmia is expected to be transiently suppressed immediately after overdrive is stopped. The transient pause after overdrive should be followed by a gradual speeding up of the rhythm until the original rate is resumed. The duration of the transient pause and the time required for resumption of the original rate is expected to be directly related, within limits, to the rate and duration of the overdrive (Vassalle, 1970). It is important to stress that the arrhythmia caused by normal automaticity cannot be terminated, but only suppressed transiently. In addition, automaticity cannot be initiated by overdrive stimulation. On the other hand, arrhythmias caused by abnormal automaticity should not be suppressed by overdrive unless the overdrive period is long and the rate of overdrive is fast (Hoffman and Dangman, 1982). Short periods of overdrive can even result in a transient speeding of the rate of impulse generation (overdrive acceleration) (Hoffman and Dangman, 1982). Like normal automaticity, arrhythmias caused by abnormal automaticity typically are not started or stopped by overdrive stimulation.

The characteristics of the response of arrhythmias caused by automaticity to premature stimulation are also sometimes useful in distinguishing automaticity from other arrhythmogenic mechanisms. Of major importance is the fact that automatic rhythms caused by either normal or abnormal automaticity cannot be started or terminated by stimulated, premature impulses. This is in contrast to reentry and some forms of triggered activity. Other than that, premature impulses induced at different times during diastole may transiently perturb an automatic rhythm for a few cycles (Bonke et al, 1969; Dangman and Hoffman, 1985; Klein et al, 1972 and 1973).

Vulnerable parameters of automaticity

Tachycardias resulting from enhanced automaticity at ectopic sites may require pharmacologic treatment. The goal is to suppress the rate of firing of the ectopic pacemaker without doing the same to the sinus node pacemaker, thereby restoring the site of impulse initiation to the sinus node (Table 2). Modification of the rate of an enhanced normally automatic focus can result from interventions that change, singly or in concert, the maximum diastolic potential, the rate of phase 4 depolarization, the voltage of the threshold potential, or

Table 2

Classification of Arrhythmogenic Mechanisms at the Cellular Level in Terms of Vulnerable Parameters

Mechanisms of Arrhythmia	Vulnerable Parameter (Antiarrhythmic Effect)	Ionic Currents Most Likely to Modulate Vulnerable Parameter
Automaticity		
Enhanced normal automaticity	Phase 4 depolarization (decreased)	I_f; I_{Ca-T} (block) $I_{K(ACh)}$ (activate)
Abnormal automaticity	Maximum diastolic potential (hyperpolarize) or	I_K; $I_{K(ACh)}$ (activate)
	Phase 4 depolarization (decrease)	I_{Ca-L}; I_{Na} (block)
Triggered activity based on:		
Early afterdepolarizations	Action potential duration (shorten) or early afterdepolarizations (suppress)	I_K (activate) I_{Ca-L}; I_{Na} (block)
Delayed afterdepolarizations	Calcium overload (unload) or delayed afterdepolarizations (suppress)	I_{Ca-L} (block) I_{Ca-L}; I_{Na} (block)
Reentry		
Primary impaired conduction (long excitable gap) due to depressed Na$^+$ channels	Decrease excitability and conduction	I_{Na} (block)
Primary impaired conduction (long excitable gap) due to slow calcium current	Decrease excitability and conduction	I_{Ca-L} (block)
Primary impaired conduction (long excitable gap) due to anisotropy	Decrease excitability and conduction	Gap junction (block)
Conduction encroaching on refractoriness (short excitable gap)	Effective refractory period (prolong)	I_K (block) I_{Na}; I_{Ca-L} (increase)

(continued)

Table 2 *(continued)*

Mechanisms of Arrhythmia	Vulnerable Parameter (Antiarrhythmic Effect)	Ionic Currents Most Likely to Modulate Vulnerable Parameter
Other mechanisms		
Reflection	Excitability (decrease)	I_{Na}; I_{Ca-L} (block)
Parasystole	Phase 4 depolarization (decrease)	I_f (block) (if maximum diastolic potential high)

Modified from The Sicilian Gambit: A new approach to the classification of antiarrhythmic drugs based on their actions on arrhythmogenic mechanisms. Circulation 1991; 84: 1831–1851.

the action potential duration. A change in one is likely to affect some of the others. The most likely vulnerable parameter, however, appears to be the phase 4 depolarization, with the target being the membrane channels responsible for the pacemaker current. Block of those channels and the resulting decrease in inward current and spontaneous diastolic depolarization would seem to be an effective antiarrhythmic intervention. One difficulty might be to decrease pacemaker current in the ectopic pacemakers without doing the same thing to the sinus node. Thus, the development of a drug specific for ectopic pacemakers is dependent on identifying differences in channel properties between sinus node and ectopic pacemakers and then taking advantage of these differences to target a drug only to the ectopic mechanism.

For abnormal automaticity, an obvious vulnerable parameter is the reduced diastolic membrane potential that is the cause of the abnormal firing (Table 2). In pathologic situations, the exact alterations in membrane channels causing depolarization are not yet known. For example, in Purkinje fibers surviving on the subendocardial surface of experimental infarcts one day after coronary occlusion, the depolarization of maximum diastolic potential is associated with a significant reduction of intracellular potassium, but it is not known how this potassium is lost (Dresdner et al, 1987). Therefore, a successful drug intervention to prevent the loss has not yet been devised. The depolarization, in addition, cannot be completely accounted for by the reduction in intracellular potassium. There is also a change in membrane conductance indicating alteration of properties of membrane channels (presumably I_{K1}) that have not yet been firmly identified (Dresdner et al, 1987; Kline et al, 1992). When they are, a pharmacologic agent might be devised to restore channel function to normal and, as a result, hyperpolarize the membrane potential. An additional vulnerable parameter, in the absence of hyperpolarizing the membrane, is obviously the spontaneous diastolic depolarization of the depolarized cells. Suppressing it might be done by targeting a drug to any of the membrane channels that are involved in causing it.

Arrhythmias Caused by Triggered Activity

Triggered activity is a term used to describe impulse initiation in cardiac fibers that is dependent on afterdepolarizations (Cranefield and Aronson, 1974; Cranefield, 1977; Cranefield and Aronson, 1988). Afterdepolarizations are oscillations in membrane potential that follow the upstroke of an action potential.

Delayed afterdepolarizations and triggered activity

Delayed afterdepolarizations are oscillations in membrane potential that occur after repolarization (Fig. 4). A triggered impulse is initiated when a delayed afterdepolarization depolarizes the membrane potential to the threshold potential for activation of the inward current responsible for the upstroke of the action potential. Afterdepolarizations do not always reach threshold, so that triggerable fibers may sometimes be stimulated at a regular rate without becoming rhythmically active. Probably the most important influence that causes subthreshold delayed afterdepolarizations to reach threshold is a decrease in the cycle length (an increase in the rate) at which action potentials occur. Therefore, arrhythmias triggered by delayed afterdepolarizations can be expected to be initiated by either a spontaneous or pacing-induced increase in the heart rate. A triggered action potential is also followed by an afterdepolarization that may or may not reach threshold. When it does not reach threshold, only one triggered impulse occurs. Quite often, the first triggered action potential is followed by a short or long "train" of additional triggered action potentials, each arising from the afterdepolarization caused by the previous action potential.

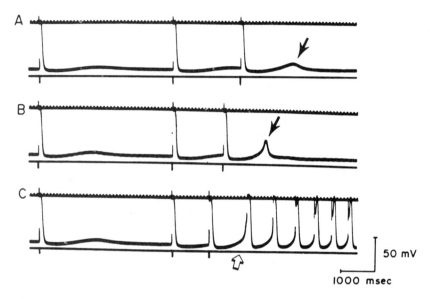

Figure 4. *Effects of premature stimulation on afterdepolarization amplitude and triggering. Each panel shows transmembrane potentials recorded from a Tyrode's superfused preparation of atrial muscle from the canine coronary sinus. The first two action potentials, from left to right, are the last action potentials in a train of 10 stimulated at a basic cycle length of 4000 ms. The third action potential results from a premature stimulus. The afterdepolarizations following the prematurely stimulated action potentials are pointed out by the arrows. In panel C, the afterdepolarizations attain threshold and a triggered rhythm occurs. Reproduced with permission from Wit AL, Cranefield PF: Triggered and automatic activity in the canine coronary sinus. Circ Res 1977; 41:435–445. Copyright 1977 American Heart Association.*

Delayed afterdepolarizations usually occur under a variety of conditions in which there is an increase in Ca^{2+} in the myoplasm and the sarcoplasmic reticulum above normal levels (sometimes referred to as Ca overload). The most widely recognized cause of delayed afterdepolarization-dependent triggered activity is digitalis toxicity (Davis, 1973; Ferrier et al, 1973; Ferrier and Moe, 1973; Rosen et al, 1973a and 1973b; Hashimoto and Moe, 1973; Hogan et al, 1973; Aronson and Cranefield, 1974). Cardiac glycosides cause delayed afterdepolarizations by inhibiting the Na/K pump. In the presence of toxic amounts of digitalis, this effect results in an increase in intracellular Na^+ (Deitmer and Ellis, 1978; Lee and Dagostino, 1982). An increase in intracellular Na^+, in turn, causes an increase in intracellular Ca^{2+} through the Na^+/Ca^{2+} exchange mechanism (Reuter and Seitz, 1968; Mullins, 1979 and 1981). Other interventions that increase intracellular Na^+ by either inhibiting Na^+ extrusion or by increasing Na^+ entry into cells may also lead to an increase in cellular Ca^{2+} and delayed afterdepolarizations for a similar reason. In addition to digitalis, catecholamines are widely recognized as a cause of delayed afterdepolarizations in atrial, ventricular, and Purkinje fibers (Wit and Cranefield, 1976; Wit and Cranefield, 1977; Rozanski and Lipsius, 1985; Boyden et al, 1984; Belardinelli and Isenberg, 1983; Lazzara and Marchi, 1989). Catecholamines may cause delayed afterdepolarizations by increasing the slow inward, L-type calcium current (Reuter, 1984). In addition, catecholamines enhance uptake of Ca^{2+} by the sarcoplasmic reticulum that may lead to the occurrence of delayed afterdepolarizations (Morad and Rolett, 1972; Fabiato and Fabiato, 1975; Fabiato, 1983).

Delayed afterdepolarizations and triggered activity are usually caused by an oscillatory membrane current called the transient inward current that is distinct from the pacemaker currents (Aronson et al, 1973; Lederer and Tsien, 1976; Hiraoka, 1977; Aronson and Gelles, 1977; Kass et al, 1978a and 1978b; Karagueuzian and Katzung, 1982; Vassalle and Mugelli, 1981; Lipsius and Gibbon, 1982; Eisner and Lederer, 1979; Tseng and Wit, 1987; Lipp and Pott, 1988). The secondary rise in myoplasmic Ca^{2+} after repolarization causes the transient inward current. Two possible mechanisms are being actively considered. The first is that the calcium released from the sarcoplasmic reticulum after repolarization acts on the sarcolemma to increase its conductance to ions that flow into the cell down a concentration gradient through membrane channels (Kass et al, 1978a). It has been suggested that this transient inward channel is a nonselective cation channel (Kass et al, 1978a; Cannell and Lederer, 1986; Colquhoun et al, 1981; Ehara et al, 1988). The second mechanism proposed for the origin of the transient inward current is that the rise in calcium causes the inward transient inward current through an electrogenic (rheogenic) exchange of Ca^{2+} for Na^+ (Mullins, 1979; Eisner and Lederer, 1985; Lipp and Pott, 1987). In either case, the charge carrier for the transient inward current that causes delayed afterdepolarizations in a normal extracellular environment appears to be mainly Na^+.

Under any of the conditions that cause delayed afterdepolarizations, the transient inward current is elicited by the action potential that precedes the delayed afterdepolarization. Transient inward current is maximal at around −60 mV and diminishes at more positive and more negative membrane potentials (Kass et al, 1978a; Karagueuzian and Katzung, 1981; Arlock and Katzung, 1985; Vassalle and Mugelli, 1981). As a result of the dependence of the transient inward current on the level of membrane potential, the amplitude of delayed afterdepolarizations and, therefore, the possibility of triggered activity are influenced by the level of membrane potential at which the action potentials occur. In the digitalis toxic Purkinje system, there is a "window" of membrane voltage for maximum diastolic potential, which is between approximately −75 to −80 mV, at which the amplitude of delayed afterdepolarizations tends to be greatest (Ferrier, 1980; Wasserstrom and Ferrier, 1981).

The voltage-time course of action potentials also controls the characteristics of delayed afterdepolarizations, with longer action potential durations favoring their occurrence (Fig. 5) (Henning and Wit, 1984). The prolongation of the duration of membrane depolarization increases intracellular Ca by increasing the flow of inward calcium current leading to an increase in the transient inward current (Coraboeuf, 1980; Kass and Scheuer, 1982). Other mechanisms may also be involved. Drugs like quinidine, which prolong action potential duration, may increase delayed afterdepolarization amplitude (Wit et al, 1990b), while drugs like lidocaine, which shorten action potential duration, may decrease delayed afterdepolarization amplitude (Sheu and Lederer, 1985).

Increasing the amount of time the membrane is maintained in the depolarized state enhances the amplitude of the transient inward current and causes it to occur more quickly. This explains the important effect of the rate of stimulation on delayed afterdepolarizations (Rosen et al, 1973b; Ferrier et al, 1973; Wit and Cranefield, 1976 and 1977; Saito et al, 1978; Aronson, 1981; El-Sherif et al, 1983; Nordin et al, 1985). Decreasing the drive cycle length increases the amplitude of delayed afterdepolarizations and tends to decrease their coupling interval to the action potential (Rosen et al, 1973b; Ferrier et al, 1973; Wit and Cranefield, 1977; Saito et al, 1978). As a result, there is a direct relationship between the drive cycle length at which triggered impulses are initiated, and the coupling interval between the first triggered impulse and the last stimulated impulse that induces them, i.e., as the drive cycle length is reduced, the first triggered impulse occurs earlier with respect to the last driven action potential. A decrease in the length of even a single drive cycle (i.e., a premature

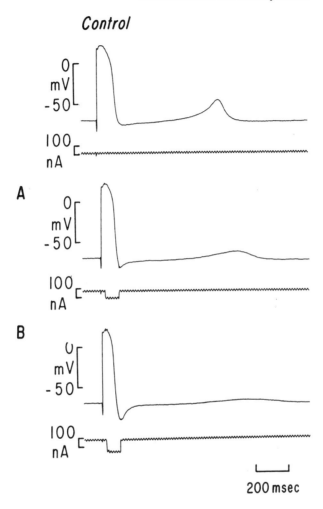

Figure 5. *The effects of action potential duration on the amplitude of the delayed afterdepolarization in an atrial fiber from the canine coronary sinus. In each panel, the top trace is the transmembrane potential recording and the bottom trace shows the current injected through a second microelectrode that was used to alter the action potential duration. The top panel (control) shows the unaltered action potential and delayed afterdepolarization that followed it. Panels A and B show that when action potential duration was decreased by passing a repolarizing current pulse through the microelectrode, the amplitude of the delayed afterdepolarization was reduced.*

impulse) also results in an increase in the amplitude of the delayed afterdepolarization that follows the premature cycle, and can cause triggered activity (Fig. 4). The increased time during which the membrane is in the depolarized state at shorter stimulation cycle lengths or after premature impulses increases Ca^{2+} in the myoplasm and the sarcoplasmic reticulum, thereby increasing the transient inward current that is responsible for the increased afterdepolarization amplitude.

Early afterdepolarizations and triggered activity

Early afterdepolarizations occur when membrane potential does not follow the trajectory characteristic of normal repolarization but suddenly shifts in a depolarizing direction (Fig. 6). Early afterdepolarizations may appear at the plateau level of membrane potential, which is usually more positive than -60 mV, or they may appear later during phase 3 of repolarization. Under certain conditions, early afterdepolarizations can lead to "second upstrokes" (Cranefield, 1975; Cranefield, 1977) or action potentials. When an early afterdepolarization is large enough, the decrease in membrane potential leads to an increase in net inward (depolarizing) current, and a second action potential occurs prior to complete repolarization of the first (Fig. 6). The second action potential occurring during repolarization is triggered in the sense that it is evoked by an early afterdepolarization that, in turn, is induced by the preceding action potential. The second action potential may also be followed by other action potentials, all occurring at the low level of membrane potential characteristic of the plateau or at the higher level of membrane potential of late phase 3. The sustained rhythmic activity may continue for a variable number of impulses and terminates when repolarization of the initiating action potential returns membrane potential to a high level.

The major differentiation between triggered activity caused by early afterdepolarizations and abnormally automatic rhythms may be that the former results from interruption of repolarization and the latter from steady depolarization of the membrane to a similar range of potentials. Otherwise, some of the mechanisms and characteristics of triggered rhythms caused by early afterdepolarizations may be identical to those of abnormal automaticity (see below). The rhythmic activity that is triggered by an early afterdepolarization may well be

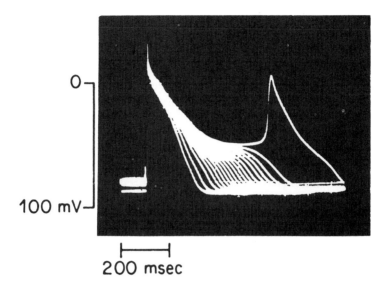

0 ⌐

100 mV ⌐

⊢————⊣
200 msec

Figure 6. *Quinidine-induced early afterdepolarizations recorded from an isolated, superfused bundle of canine Purkinje fibers. Superimposed action potentials during exposure to quinidine are shown. The control recording in the absence of quinidine is the shortest duration action potential of the series of superimposed action potentials. During exposure to quinidine, the early afterdepolarization delayed repolarization, manifesting itself mainly during phase 3 until, finally, a second action potential was triggered. Reproduced with permission from Roden DM, Hoffman BF: Action potential prolongation and induction of abnormal automaticity by low quinidine concentrations in canine Purkinje fibers. Relationship to potassium and cycle length. Circ Res 1985; 56:857–867. Copyright 1985 American Heart Association.*

triggered in its mechanism of onset, but automatic during the subsequent impulses (Damiano and Rosen, 1984).

Early afterdepolarizations and triggered activity occur under a variety of conditions that delay repolarization of the action potential. Most often, early afterdepolarizations occur more readily in Purkinje fibers than in ventricular or atrial muscle. Agents that increase inward current, such as aconitine, prolong the action potential duration and cause early afterdepolarizations (Cranefield and Aronson, 1988). In contrast, other agents cause early afterdepolarizations and triggered activity by blocking outward K^+ current, which also delays repolarization (Damiano and Rosen, 1984). Because the experimental arrhythmias caused by agents known to induce early afterdepolarizations, such as cesium, resemble torsades de pointes, it has been proposed that clinically occurring torsades is caused by early afterdepolarizations (Brachman et al, 1983). Antiarrhythmic drugs that prolong the duration of the action potential of Purkinje fibers (e.g., sotalol [Strauss et al, 1970; Carmeliet, 1985; Hiromasa et al, 1988], N-acetyl procainamide [Dangman and Hoffman, 1981], clofilium [Gough et al, 1988], and quinidine [Roden and Hoffman, 1985; Davidenko et al, 1989]) can cause early afterdepolarizations and triggered activity when administered to isolated preparations of Purkinje fibers, particularly when the rate of stimulation is low and the K^+ concentration in the superfusate is less than normal. Both the d (no β-receptor blockade) and the l (β-blocking) forms of sotalol prolong the action potential duration by inhibiting the repolarizing K current, I_K (Carmeliet, 1985). The prolongation of the action potential by quinidine leading to early afterdepolarizations is also related to quinidine's blocking effect on the outward membrane repolarizing K^+ current (Colatsky, 1982).

Normally, the net outward membrane current during repolarization shifts membrane potential progressively in a negative direction, and the final rapid phase of action potential repolarization takes place. An early afterdepolarization occurs when, for some reason, the current-voltage relationship is altered to cause outward current during repolarization to approach or attain 0, at least transiently. Such a shift can be caused by any of the factors discussed previously, which either decrease outward current or increase inward current. If the change in the current-voltage relationship results in a region of net inward current during the plateau range of membrane potentials (Trautwein, 1970), it could lead to a secondary depolarization (a triggered action potential) during the plateau or phase 3 by activating a regenerative inward current.

The early afterdepolarizations that occur during late repolarization, at membrane potentials negative to about -60 mV (phase 3), probably have different ionic mechanisms than those that occur earlier during the plateau phase. These early afterdepolarizations appear to result at least partly from a Na^+ current flowing through tetrodotoxin-(TTX-) sensitive channels (Coulombe et al, 1980). Early afterdepolarizations occurring in the plateau range of membrane potentials (-50 mV to 0 mV) can result from increased activation of the L-type calcium current (January and Riddle, 1989). Other outward and inward currents may also be involved in the control of early afterdepolarizations occurring during the plateau.

Triggered activity initiated by an early afterdepolarization may consist of only a second upstroke or it may be more sustained. When it persists for a number of action potentials, the mechanism for the perpetuation of the rhythmic activity is uncertain. It may involve the same membrane currents that cause abnormal automaticity or the membrane currents that cause delayed afterdepolarizations (Cranefield and Aronson, 1988).

The ionic current responsible for the upstrokes of the action potentials during triggered activity caused by early afterdepolarizations is determined by the level of membrane potential at which the action potentials occur. Triggered action potentials occurring during the plateau phase and early in phase 3, at a time when most fast Na^+ channels are still inactivated, most likely have upstrokes caused by the inward L-type calcium current. At higher membrane potentials during late phase 3 of repolarization, where there is partial reactivation of the fast Na^+ channels, fast responses predominate. Current flowing through both L-type calcium channels and partially reactivated fast Na^+ channels may be involved over intermediate ranges of membrane potential.

Effects of electrical stimulation on arrhythmias caused by triggered activity

Triggered arrhythmias caused by delayed afterdepolarizations in the heart can be initiated by either overdrive stimulation or programmed premature stimulation (Rosen et al, 1980; Rosen and Reder, 1981). Extrasystoles or the first beats of tachycardias caused by delayed afterdepolarization-dependent triggered activity initiated by stimulation are predicted to occur late in the cardiac cycle (Rosen et al, 1980). There is a direct relationship between the cycle length of a period of stimulation that induces triggered activity dependent on delayed afterdepolarizations and the coupling interval of the first beat of tachycardia to the last stimulated impulse. As the pacing cycle length decreases, the coupling interval from the last stimulated impulse to the first impulse of tachycardia decreases. Failure to show the direct relationship, however, cannot be taken as proof that the arrhythmia is not caused by triggered activity since slow conduction into or out of the triggerable focus can distort it. During initiation of triggered activity with premature stimuli, there is often no significant effect of the premature stimulus coupling interval on the coupling interval of the first triggered impulse to the premature impulse (Johnson and Rosen, 1987).

Triggered arrhythmias caused by delayed afterdepolarizations, unlike automatic arrhythmias and like reentrant arrhythmias, can be terminated by electrical stimulation. Single premature impulses may terminate triggered arrhythmias, but termination is infrequent and not usually reproducible at the same critical premature cycle length. On the other hand, overdrive stimulation terminates triggered arrhythmias more easily. Termination requires a critical rate and duration of overdrive as it does with reentry (Rosen and Reder, 1981; Wit et al, 1981; Moak and Rosen, 1984; Johnson et al, 1986). Overdrive stimulation may cause acceleration of triggered arrhythmias followed by gradual slowing and termination, or rapid overdrive may cause abrupt termination. Overdrive stimulation that does not terminate triggered activity does not entrain the arrhythmia (Vos et al, 1989; Furukawa et al, 1990).

Arrhythmias caused by early afterdepolarizations cannot be induced by overdrive pacing or by one or several prematurely stimulated impulses. Early afterdepolarization-induced triggered activity is facilitated by long cycle lengths and, therefore, this kind of triggered activity should be initiated by slowing the basic heart rate or by the occurrence of a long pause. Pacing the heart at faster rates causes disappearance of the short-lasting salvos of tachycardia caused by early afterdepolarizations. When the pacing is stopped the salvos reappear. Triggered arrhythmias caused by early afterdepolarizations might not only occur in salvos but might also be sustained. Some sustained arrhythmias might be terminated by premature stimuli, but this is a relatively rare occurrence. The effects of premature stimulated impulses that do not terminate the arrhythmia are expected to be the same as their effects on automatic impulse initiation (Damiano and Rosen, 1984). Some arrhythmias also might be terminated by overdrive pacing, but termination is not the usual effect. When termination does not occur, overdrive is not expected to cause any significant effect on the rhythm; the response should be more similar to an arrhythmia caused by abnormal automaticity (Dangman and Hoffman, 1983) than normal automaticity, which is readily overdrive suppressed (Vassalle, 1970).

Vulnerable parameters of triggered
activity

Delayed afterdepolarizations.   The vulnerable parameter of triggered activity caused by delayed afterdepolarizations is calcium overload and, therefore, triggered activity can be prevented by reducing
the intracellular calcium (Table 2). This can be done in a number of
ways. Drugs that block the L-type calcium current are highly effective
in preventing triggered impulses (Ferrier et al, 1973; Wit and
Cranefield, 1977; Gough et al, 1984; Mary-Rabine et al, 1980). Calcium
can also be decreased by altering some of the characteristics of the
action potential. Decreasing action potential duration, for example,
decreases inward calcium current and abolishes delayed afterdepolarizations (Henning and Wit, 1984; Sheu and Lederer, 1985). Decreasing
inward sodium current during the upstroke of the action potential also
reduces intracellular calcium and delayed afterdepolarizations (Rosen
and Danilo, 1980; Karagueuzian and Katzung, 1981; Elharrar et al,
1978; Hewett et al, 1983; Wasserstrom and Ferrier, 1981; Sheu and
Lederer, 1985). Drugs that block Na-Ca exchange, such as doxorubicin
(Binah et al, 1983), and drugs that alter the release of calcium from the
sarcoplasmic reticulum, such as caffeine and ryanodine, can inhibit
triggered activity (Paspa and Vassalle, 1984; Aronson et al, 1985).

Early afterdepolarizations.   The vulnerable parameter for triggered activity caused by early afterdepolarizations is the prolonged
action potential duration and a rational approach to the termination
or prevention of the triggered arrhythmias is to shorten the duration
(Table 2). This might be done by targeting pharmacologic agents to
enhance outward currents or reduce inward currents. In the case of
antiarrhythmic drugs that prolong action potential duration as part
of their therapeutic effect, there are special considerations. Prolongation of duration is probably most needed at the rapid heart rates
caused by a tachyarrhythmia and not during the slower rate of sinus
rhythm. It is the slower rate that favors the occurrence of the triggered
arrhythmias. The problem, therefore, is to promote drug-channel interactions that prolong action potential duration only at rapid rates.
In addition to shortening action potential duration, it might be possible to prevent triggered activity by preventing the triggered action
potentials themselves. This might be done with drugs that block the

inward current causing the triggered action potential, drugs that block the L-type calcium channels, or drugs that block fast sodium channels.

Abnormal Impulse Conduction

The second major heading of arrhythmia mechanisms in Table 1 is abnormal impulse conduction. Abnormal impulse conduction causes reentrant excitation, a mechanism for arrhythmias that does not depend on the generation of impulses by cells.

Arrhythmias Caused by Reentry

During reentrant excitation, an excitation wave is able to reexcite a region of the heart a number of times rather than only once as in sinus rhythm. In reentry, the circulating (reentrant) impulse travels over a route that leads it back to its point of origin. This route is called the reentrant circuit. The reentrant circuit may be an anatomic structure such as a loop of fiber bundles in the peripheral Purkinje system. The anatomic circuit has a central obstacle that prevents the impulse from taking a "shortcut" that would stop reentry. The circuit may also be functional and its existence, size, and shape may be determined by electrophysiologic properties of cardiac cells rather than an anatomically defined pathway. The central inexcitable region of a functional circuit is often the result of refractoriness of cells in the center of the circuit rather than a real obstacle. The size and location of an anatomically defined reentrant circuit obviously remains fixed and results in what may be called ordered reentry. The size and location of reentrant circuits dependent on functional properties rather than anatomy may also be fixed (ordered), but they also may change with time, leading to random reentry. Random reentry is probably most often associated with atrial or ventricular fibrillation, whereas ordered reentry can cause most other types of arrhythmias (Hoffman and Rosen, 1981).

Role of slow conduction

A condition necessary for reentry is that the impulse be delayed sufficiently in the reentrant pathway to allow the regions of the circuit in front of it to recover from refractoriness. In the case of rapidly conducting impulses, sufficient delay might occur if the pathway is long enough so that, while the impulse is travelling at a normal velocity, enough time passes to allow recovery of excitability. Reentry is facilitated when conduction is slow since such long pathways are then not necessary. A low conduction velocity can be a consequence of alterations of active membrane properties determining the characteristics of inward currents depolarizing the membrane during the action potential or it can be a consequence of passive properties governing the flow of current between cardiac cells.

The depolarization phase or upstroke of the action potential of atrial, ventricular, and Purkinje fibers results from the opening of specific membrane channels (fast sodium channels) through which sodium ions rapidly pass from the extracellular fluid into the cell (Fozzard, 1979). A reduction in this inward current, leading to a reduction in the rate or amplitude of depolarization during phase 0, may decrease axial current flow, slow conduction, and lead to reentrant excitation (Cranefield, 1975). Such a reduction in Na^+ current may result from the inactivation of sodium channels. The inward Na^+ current, amplitude, and rate of rise of premature action potentials initiated during repolarization (relative refractory period) are reduced because the Na^+ channels are only partly reactivated (Weidmann, 1955). Premature activation of the heart can, therefore, induce reentry because premature impulses conduct slowly in regions of the heart where the cardiac fibers are not completely repolarized (where Na^+ channels are to some extent inactivated) or where reactivation of Na^+ channels is delayed.

Conduction slow enough to facilitate reentry might also occur in cardiac cells with persistently low levels of resting potential (which may be between -60 and -70 mV) caused by disease. At these resting potentials, some Na^+ channels are inactivated (Weidmann, 1955), and, therefore, unavailable for activation by a depolarizing stimulus. Also, at these resting membrane potentials, recovery from inactivation is markedly prolonged and extends beyond complete repolarization (Gettes and Reuter, 1974). The magnitude of the inward current during phase 0 of the action potential is reduced and, consequently, both the speed and amplitude of the upstroke are diminished, decreasing axial current flow and slowing conduction significantly. Such action potentials with upstrokes dependent on inward current flowing via partially inactivated Na^+ channels are sometimes referred to as "depressed fast responses." Further depolarization and inactivation of the Na^+ channel shift threshold potential to more positive voltages, thereby decreasing the excitability of cardiac fibers to such an extent that conduction velocity decreases further and a site of unidirectional conduction block may evolve (Dodge and Cranefield, 1982). Thus, in a diseased region with partially depolarized fibers, there may be some areas of slow conduction and some areas of conduction block, depending on the level of resting potential. This combination may cause reentry.

Although the fast sodium channel may be largely inactivated at membrane potentials near -50 mV, the L-type calcium channel is not inactivated and is still available for activation (Cranefield, 1975). Under certain conditions, in cells with resting potentials less than -60 mV (such as when membrane conductance is very low or when catecholamines are present), this normally weak inward calcium current may give rise to regenerative action potentials that propagate very slowly and are prone to block. The propagated action potential, dependent on inward calcium current, is referred to as the "slow response" (Cranefield, 1975). Slow response action potentials can occur in diseased cardiac fibers with low resting potentials, but they also occur in some normal tissue of the heart, such as cells of the sinus and atrioventricular nodes where the maximum diastolic potential is normally less than about -70 mV (Cranefield, 1975; Zipes and Mendez, 1973).

The slow conduction that facilitates the occurrence of reentry can also be caused by factors other than a decrease in inward current during the transmembrane action potential. An increased resistance to axial current flow (resistance to current flow in the direction of propagation) decreases the magnitude and spread of axial current along the myocardial fiber and may decrease conduction velocity (Spach et al, 1981 and 1982). The extent and distribution of the gap junctions in normal myocardium have a profound influence on axial resistance and conduction. The myocardium is better coupled in the direction of the long axis of its cells and bundles (because of the high frequency of the gap junctions) than the direction transverse to the long axis (because of the low frequency of gap junctions). This is reflected in a lower axial resistivity in the longitudinal direction than in the transverse direction (Roberts et al, 1979; Clerc, 1976). Therefore, conduction through atrial and ventricular myocardium is much more rapid in the longitudinal direction, owing to the lower resistivity, than in the transverse direction. Thus, cardiac muscle is anisotropic; its conduction properties vary depending on the direction in which they are measured. Spach et al (1981, 1982, 1986) have classified anisotropy into two major subdivisions: uniform and nonuniform. Uniform anisotropy is characterized by an advancing wavefront that is smooth in all directions (longitudinal and transverse to fiber orientation), indicating relatively tight coupling between groups of fibers in all directions, although coupling is "tighter" in the longitudinal than in the transverse direction (Spach et al, 1988). Nonuniform anisotropy has been defined by Spach et al (1982) as tight electrical coupling between cells in the longitudinal direction, but recurrent areas in the transverse direction in which side-to-side electrical coupling of adjacent groups (unit bundles) of parallel fibers is absent. Therefore, propagation of normal action potentials transverse to the long axis is interrupted such that adjacent bundles are excited in a markedly irregular sequence or "zigzag conduction" (Spach et al, 1982; Spach and Dolber, 1986). The slow conduction associated with nonuniform anisotropy may lead to reentry, as is discussed later. The morphologic basis for nonuniform anisotropic properties is often the separation of fascicles of muscle bundles in the transverse direction by fibrous tissue that forms longitudinally oriented insulating boundaries (Spach et al, 1982; Spach and Dolber, 1986). Similar connective tissue septa cause nonuniform anisotropy in some normal cardiac tissues such as crista terminalis and the interatrial band in adult atria or ventricular papillary muscle, as well as pathologic situations in which fibrosis in the myocardium occurs (chronic ischemia).

In addition to the structural features of the cellular interconnections influencing axial current flow and conduction as expressed in the anisotropic properties of cardiac muscle, the intercellular resistance may also increase because of an increase in gap junctional resistance that results from a decrease in the conductance of the junctions (Rudy and Quan, 1987; Quan and Rudy, 1990). Perhaps the most important influence on gap junctional resistance in pathologic situations is the level of intracellular calcium; a significant rise increases resistance to current flow through the junctions and eventually leads to physiologic uncoupling of the cells (DeMello, 1975; Hess and Weingart, 1980). Intracellular calcium increases during ischemia and may be a factor causing slow conduction and reentry.

Unidirectional block of impulse conduction

Unidirectional block, block of conduction in one direction along a bundle of cardiac fibers, but maintained conduction in the other direction, is necessary for the occurrence of most forms of reentry (Wit and Cranefield, 1978). Unidirectional block in part of the circuit leaves a return pathway through which the impulse conducts to reenter previously excited areas. There are a number of mechanisms that might cause unidirectional block. Like the causes of slow conduction, they involve both active and passive electrical properties of cardiac cells.

One cause of the unidirectional block that enables the initiation of reentry is regional differences in recovery of excitability. When differences in effective refractory period duration exist in adjacent areas, conduction of an appropriately timed premature impulse may be blocked in the region with the longest refractory period, which becomes a site of unidirectional block, while continuing through regions with shorter refractory periods (Fig. 7) (Janse et al, 1969; Mendez et al, 1969; Sasyniuk and Mendez, 1971). Therefore, the unidirectional block caused by regional differences in excitability is actually a result of transient block; block occurs in the antegrade direction in one pathway while conduction is successful in the retrograde direction. This kind of unidirectional block can cause initiation of reentry in both anatomic functional circuits. For reentrant arrhythmias to arise because of regional differences in refractory periods, a premature depolarization that initiates reentry is as necessary a requirement as the conditions allowing perpetuation of reentrant activation; both a "trigger" (the premature impulse) and a "substrate" (the reentrant circuit) are needed. The mechanism causing the premature depolarization may be quite different from the arrhythmia it initiates; it might arise spontaneously by automaticity or it might be a result of triggered activity. The premature impulse might also be induced by an electrical stimulus during programmed stimulation protocols.

Unidirectional conduction block in a reentrant circuit can also be persistent and independent of premature activation. Persistent unidirectional block is often associated with depression of the transmembrane potentials and excitability of cardiac fibers. There are several possible mechanisms for the persistent unidirectional block in a region

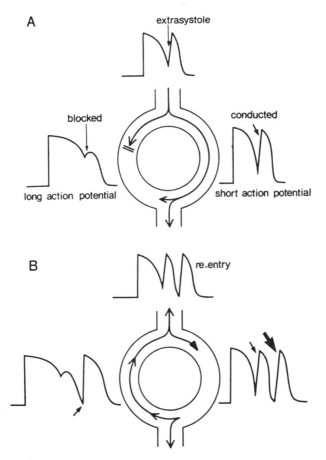

Figure 7. *Diagram of reentry caused by dispersion in refractory periods. A ring of cardiac tissue is shown and the pattern of conduction is indicated by the arrows. Action potentials with different durations, located in different regions of the ring, are diagrammed. Panel A shows the conduction pattern of a premature impulse (extrasystole) initiated at the top. The impulse is blocked in the region of the ring with the long action potential (at the left), while conduction succeeds through the region of the ring with the short action potentials (at the right). Panel B shows a continuation of the propagation pattern begun in Panel A. The impulse that succeeded in conducting through the ring from the right reached the area of block after it recovered excitability, excited it, and then returned to its site of origin as a reentrant impulse. Reproduced with permission from Wit AL, Janse MJJ: The Ventricular Arrhythmias of Ischemia and Infarction. Electrophysiological Mechanisms. Mt. Kisco, NY: Futura Publishing Co, 1993.*

where action potentials are depressed. These mechanisms are discussed in detail in other publications (Cranefield, 1975; Fozzard, 1979; Dodge and Cranefield, 1982; Wit and Janse, 1992).

Characteristics of reentrant circuits

Ordered reentry implies a circuit that has a fixed size and location (Hoffman and Rosen, 1981). The circuit can be comprised of a well-defined anatomic pathway, an anatomic circuit. Functional circuits (dependent on cellular electrophysiologic properties rather than anatomy) might also cause ordered reentry if the electrophysiologic properties crucial for reentry are confined to a specific location, and reentry only occurs in that location.

There are a number of examples of anatomic circuits that cause ordered reentry. Reentrant circuits in the Wolff-Parkinson-White syndrome are comprised of the atria, atrioventricular conducting system (atrioventricular node and His bundle), ventricles, and an accessory pathway connecting atria and ventricles (Gallagher et al, 1978; Durrer et al, 1967). The reentrant circuit causing bundle branch reentry, comprised of the bundle branches that communicate proximally through the His bundle and distally through ventricular myocardium, is another example of an anatomic circuit causing ordered reentry (Janse, 1971; Akhtar et al, 1974; Lyons and Burgess, 1979). A third example of an anatomic circuit is the band of circumferential muscle bundles around the natural obstacle provided by the orifice of the tricuspid valve (Frame et al, 1986 and 1987; Boyden et al, 1989a). Reentry causing atrial flutter can be initiated in this region in a canine model. If conduction is markedly slowed, and/or refractory period duration considerably shortened as discussed previously, the length of reentrant circuits needed to permit anatomic reentry may be very much shorter than the previous examples. In experiments in vitro, reentry has been demonstrated to occur in small anatomic circuits (circumference of 10 to 20 mm) composed of Purkinje bundles from the ventricular conduction system, when conduction was depressed by exposure of the bundles to an environment containing elevated K^+ concentration (Wit et al, 1972b). Other mechanisms for slow conduction that we discussed (anisotropy and cellular uncoupling) may also operate in anatomic circuits, thereby allowing reentry to occur in a small circuit. In fact, in almost all anatomically defined reentrant circuits, the path is anisotropic and must be because of the anatomic structure of the myocardium. There thus will be one or more components of the path in which conduction slows.

An important feature of an anatomically defined, ordered reentrant circuit is that there exists a gap of either partially or completely excitable tissue between the crest of the circulating reentrant impulse and the relative refractory "tail." This means that there is a segment of the reentrant circuit that is excitable while the reentrant impulse is travelling around the circuit. As a result, impulses originating outside the reentrant circuit can invade the circuit through this gap and influence the reentrant rhythm, sometimes terminating the reentrant arrhythmia. Such invading impulses may arise spontaneously outside the circuit or may be initiated by electrical stimulation.

In addition to ordered reentry in circuits with anatomically defined conducting pathways, ordered reentry may also occur in functional circuits, e.g., circuits that are formed because of electrophysiologic properties of the cardiac cells and not by a predetermined anatomic pathway. In the leading circle model of functional reentry described by Allessie and coworkers (1973, 1976, 1977), the reentrant impulse circulates around a central area that is kept refractory because it is constantly bombarded by impulses propagating toward it from all sides of the circuit (Fig. 8). The circumference of the smallest (leading) circle around the functional obstacle may be as little as 6 to 8 mm and represents a pathway in which the efficacy of stimulation of the circulating wavefront is just sufficient to excite the tissue ahead that is still in its relative refractory phase. Conduction through the functional reentrant circuit is slowed, because impulses are propagating in partially refractory tissue. In the leading circle model, no gap of fully excitable tissue exists between crest and tail of the circulating wave, and resetting or termination by prematurely stimulated impulses might be difficult. Functional reentrant circuits of the leading circle type may also change their size and location and, if they do, would fall under the general category of random reentry (discussed below).

Reentry caused by anisotropy can also occur without well-defined anatomic pathways and might be classified as functional. However, unlike the functional characteristic that leads to the leading circle type of reentry, that is, a difference in membrane properties such as refractory periods in adjacent areas, in functional reentry caused by anisotropy, the functional characteristic is the difference in effective axial resistance to impulse propagation dependent on fiber direction. Reen-

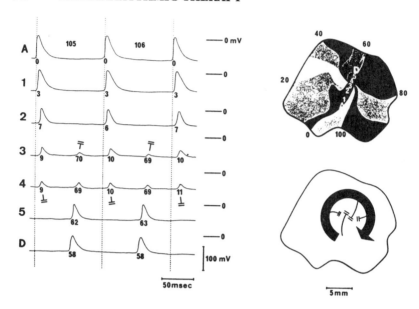

Figure 8. *Leading circle reentry in atrial myocardium. At the top right is a diagram of activation of a piece of left atrial muscle during tachycardia that was induced by premature stimulation. The activation pattern is indicated by the isochrones (0 to 100 ms) for one complete revolution of the wavefront. The diagram at the bottom right is the same piece of atrial myocardium with the reentrant pattern of activation indicated by the thick black arrow. The small curved lines toward the center indicate wavefronts colliding in the center. At the left are displayed transmembrane potentials recorded at the seven sites indicated on the upper right diagram (A, 1 to 5, D). Reproduced with permission from Allessie MA, Bonke FIM, Schopman FJG: Circus movement in rabbit atrial muscle as a mechanism of tachycardia. III. The "leading circle" concept: A new model of circus movement in cardiac tissue without the involvement of an anatomical obstacle. Circ Res 1977; 41:9–18. Copyright 1977 American Heart Association.*

try caused by anisotropy is classified as anisotropic reentry (Spach et al, 1988; Dillon et al, 1988).

Experiments have shown that anisotropy is a cause of reentrant excitation in the healing and healed phases of myocardial infarction that results in ventricular tachyarrhythmias (Dillon et al, 1988). The origin of these tachycardias in a canine model of infarction is often from reentrant circuits in the epicardial muscle that survives on the surface of a transmural infarct and which forms the epicardial border zone (Wit et al, 1982; Ursell et al, 1985; El-Sherif et al, 1977a and 1977b;

El-Sherif et al, 1981; Cardinal et al, 1988). These surviving myocardial fibers are arranged parallel to one another in fascicles (Ursell et al, 1985). Because of the parallel orientation of the myocardial bundles, the epicardial border zone in canine infarcts is anisotropic (Dillon et al, 1988; Cardinal et al, 1988; Ursell et al, 1985). The anisotropy is mostly nonuniform because of the separation of the muscle fiber bundles. The slow activation in the reentrant circuit, enabling reentry to occur, is a consequence of the nonuniform anisotropic properties of the cardiac muscle in which the circuit forms. The high axial resistance between myocardial fiber bundles in the transverse direction is the major cause of slow conduction (Gardner et al, 1985; Dillon et al, 1988; Kramer et al, 1985). Impulse propagation during reentry in this anisotropic matrix occurs both parallel and transverse to the long axis. In regions of the circuit in which activation is occurring parallel to the fibers, conduction is fast (approximately 0.5 M/sec) and isochrones are widely separated and oriented perpendicular to the long axis of the fibers (Fig. 9). In the regions of the circuit where activation occurs transverse to the long axis, the isochrones are bunched closely together and are oriented parallel to the long axis of the fibers indicating very slow activation (as slow as .05 M/sec). These closely bunched isochrones sometimes form part of the lines of apparent block in the activation maps, and when they do, they can be called pseudoblock (Dillon et al, 1988). These lines of block are located in regions with a high degree of nonuniform anisotropy where the slowing of transverse conduction is most severe. The regions of fast and slow conduction in anisotropic reentrant circuits cause them to be elliptical. In contrast, in the leading circle mechanism, conduction around the entire circuit may be slower than normal because the wavefront is conducting in relatively refractory myocardium and the circuit may be circular. There is a dispersion of anisotropy in the epicardial border zone, that is, some regions have a greater degree of nonuniform anisotropy than others. The stable lines of block and ordered reentry associated with monomorphic sustained ventricular tachycardia form in regions with a high degree of nonuniform anisotropy because, in these regions, transverse conduction is slow enough to allow stable reentry. In infarcts that have no region with sufficient nonuniform anisotropy, sustained tachycardia cannot occur, although there may be nonsustained tachycardia or fibrillation caused by random reentry (see below). Stability of anisotropic reentrant circuits is also assisted by the presence of a completely excitable gap that does not occur in

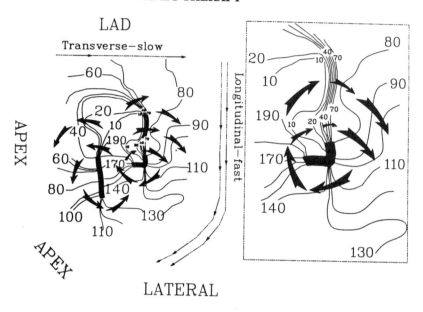

Figure 9. *Anisotropic reentry in the epicardial border zone of a healing canine myocardial infarct. The orientation of the muscle fiber bundles is indicated. At the left is a diagram of a figure of eight reentrant circuit with isochrones drawn at 10 ms intervals. The arrows show that the wavefront, beginning at the 10 ms isochrone, splits into two wavefronts, one of which moves to the right and then down toward the lateral apex, and the other, which moves to the left and then down toward the apex. The two wavefronts coalesce and they return to their point of origin. At the right is an enlargement of the right-hand loop of the circuit. In the reentrant circuit, propagation in the longitudinal direction is rapid, as indicated by the widely spaced isochrones, while it is very slow in the transverse direction as indicated by the very closely spaced isochrones. This is characteristic of anisotropic reentry. Reproduced with permission from Wit AL, Janse MJJ: The Ventricular Arrhythmias of Ischemia and Infarction. Electrophysiological Mechanisms. Mt. Kisco, NY: Futura Publishing Co, 1993.*

the leading circle functional circuit. The excitable gap is caused by the sudden slowing of conduction velocity and decrease in the wavelength of excitation as the reentrant impulse turns the corner from the fast longitudinal direction to the slow transverse direction or vice versa (Schalij, 1988; Lammers et al, 1987).

In random reentry, the circuit changes its size, shape, and location for each reentrant revolution. Therefore, the reentrant circuit must be a functional one. Both the leading circle mechanism and anisotropic reentry may sometimes be random. Another model of functional reentrant excitation that can cause random reentry is called spiral wave reentry (Jalife et al, 1991). This is a form of reentry in which the excitation wave is in the form of a rotor. The inner tip of the rotor circulates around a disk of quiescent myocardium. The marked curvature of the rotor slows down its propagation because of increased electrical load. Random reentry is associated mostly with atrial or ventricular fibrillation. Experimental studies in which excitation patterns have been mapped during these arrhythmias have shown that it is exceptional if an impulse follows the same route more than once. Rather, areas are continuously reexcited by different wavefronts (Allessie et al, 1985; Janse et al, 1980).

Reflection

The term "reflection" has been used to describe a form of reentry in a linear bundle in which two excitable regions are separated by an area of depressed conduction (Cranefield, 1975). During reflection, excitation occurs slowly in one direction along the bundle and is followed by continued propagation and excitation occurring in the opposite direction. One form of reflection may, in fact, be microreentry based on a functional longitudinal dissociation within the depressed segment (Cranefield, et al, 1973; Schmitt and Erlanger, 1928; Wit et al, 1972a). A fundamentally different mechanism for reflection has been proposed, where antegrade and retrograde transmission along the bundle occurs through the same fibers, as compared to functional longitudinal dissociation where antegrade and retrograde transmission are in different fibers (Cranefield, 1975; Cranefield et al, 1971; Antzelevitch et al, 1980; Jalife and Moe, 1981; Rozanski et al, 1984).

Effects of electrical stimulation on reentrant excitation

The initiation of arrhythmias by overdrive or programmed stimulation can be used as an indicator of a reentrant mechanism if other characteristics are also present that eliminate the probability of triggered activity dependent on delayed afterdepolarizations. The arrhythmia results because, at a critical premature coupling interval or stimulation rate, unidirectional block occurs in a potential reentrant circuit and slow conduction is induced to occur around that circuit. Additional evidence that the arrhythmia is caused by reentry is the ability to directly demonstrate that induction of the arrhythmia is related to a critical amount of slow conduction in the region where the arrhythmia originates, such as the critical prolongation in atrioventricular nodal conduction time associated with the initiation of atrioventricular nodal reentrant tachycardia (Goldreyer and Damato, 1971; Bigger and Goldreyer, 1970) or fractionation of electrograms during initiation of ventricular tachycardia. Slowing of conduction is sometimes manifested as an inverse relationship between the premature impulse coupling interval and the interval from the premature impulse to the first impulse of tachycardia (Goldreyer and Bigger, 1971; Bigger and Goldreyer, 1970; Josephson, 1992). At shorter premature coupling intervals, slower conduction around the circuit results in the inverse relationship.

Another feature of reentrant arrhythmias is that they can be terminated by overdrive or premature stimulation. This is not specific for reentry, since triggered activity caused by delayed afterdepolarizations can also be terminated. The termination of reentry by stimulation can only be demonstrated in stable, sustained tachyarrhythmias, the initiation of which is dependent on the transient block and slow conduction caused by an initiating event such as a premature impulse. As with initiation, termination by overdrive requires a critical rate and duration of the stimulation train, while termination with stimulated premature impulses requires a critical coupling interval between the premature impulse and the previous impulse of the tachyarrhythmia. Failure to terminate an arrhythmia by stimulated impulses does not alone eliminate reentry as a mechanism for the arrhythmia. Termination of reentry requires that the stimulated impulse can enter the reentrant circuit to cause block of the reentrant wavefront, and this requires that the circuit has an excitable gap. Functional circuits caused by the leading circle mechanism and some anatomic circuits may not have a gap of excitability that allows a premature impulse to penetrate into the circuit. If a tachycardia is very rapid, the excitable gap also may be very small, preventing easy penetration by stimulated impulses.

The response of an arrhythmia to a prematurely stimulated impulse or to a period of overdrive that does not terminate it may still provide information useful for determining the mechanism of the arrhythmia. The concept of entrainment describes the effects of overdrive stimulation on tachycardias caused by reentrant excitation (Waldo et al, 1983 and 1987), while other arrhythmogenic mechanisms cannot be entrained.

Vulnerable parameters of reentrant excitation

There are a number of different ways that pharmacologic agents might act effectively to abolish reentrant excitation (Table 2). In general, drugs might prevent the initiation of reentry if such initiation is triggered by a transient event such as a premature impulse, or a drug might prevent the perpetuation of reentry. Both effects might be dependent on similar drug actions on electrophysiologic properties of cardiac fibers. The main goal is to cause block of the circulating impulse in the reentrant circuit. The way this might be accomplished is dependent to a large extent on the properties of the circuit itself; is it anatomic or functional, how large is the excitable gap, and what is the cause of the slow conduction in the circuit. If the excitable gap is long, there is little likelihood that prolonging refractoriness will stop reentry. Block might be caused by targeting the ion channel responsible for the upstroke of the action potentials causing slow activation. If they have depressed fast responses, a drug that decreases inward sodium current might be effective. If they have slow responses, a drug that decreases L-type calcium current might be effective. However, if the action potential upstroke is not responsible for the slow conduction, such as in anisotropic reentry, targeting inward current channels is not predicted to be effective. In this case, perhaps drugs that decrease cellular coupling would be appropriate. At the present time, no antiarrhythmic drugs with this specific property are available. If the excitable gap is short, block might also be brought about by prolonging the time course of recovery of excitability of cells in the circuit so that the circulating wavefront encounters refractory tissue in the reentrant pathway and dies out. This might be done by targeting channels that control the time course of repolarization. However, the effectiveness of this approach is predicted to depend on the size of the excitable gap in the circuit. It seems unreasonable to expect a drug that prolongs refractoriness to be effective in causing conduction block in a circuit with a large, completely excitable gap, although it may be effective in a circuit with a small excitable gap. The effectiveness is further determined by the nature of the circuit; i.e., whether it is anatomic or functional. In a functional circuit, the size of the circuit can change after alterations in refractoriness by a drug to permit reentry to continue, while in an anatomic circuit, this may not be the case. The conclusion, therefore, is that although the vulnerable parameter in reentry is certainly conduction in the reentrant circuit, the precise target of drugs depends specifically on the mechanism causing reentry, as will be discussed in subsequent chapters.

Ischemia and Infarction

Because of the preponderant role of ischemic heart disease in the occurrence of cardiac arrhythmias, this final section of this chapter considers mechanisms of arrhythmogenesis in the setting of ischemia and infarction. A variety of mechanisms have been associated with the arrhythmias induced by acute ischemia and infarction. These include enhanced normal automaticity, abnormal automaticity, interactions across segments of depressed excitability, afterdepolarizations, and reentry secondary to circus movement. Each of these mechanisms can arise from a variety of underlying causes such as structural changes and changes in the functional anatomy (changes in cable properties), changes in excitatory currents, and changes extrinsic to the heart, such as in autonomic nervous innervation.

Acute ischemia is an unstable situation with rapid changes in electrophysiologic parameters that, therefore, are difficult to study. The mechanism of single premature beats occurring in this setting may be reentry, which may require that a normally occurring supraventricular excitation be blocked in some directions and that activity along alternate pathways reexcites the tissue (Pogwizd and Corr, 1987). Another possibility would be a nonreentrant mechanism the nature of which has not yet been clearly elucidated (Janse et al, 1980). Characteristically, the ventricular tachycardias are irregular and polymorphic and most often nonsustained, which suggests that a potential site of block changes its location from beat to beat; this is consistent with the rate-dependency of excitability in depolarized tissue. There is also a strong tendency to degenerate into ventricular fibrillation.

The electrophysiologic alterations induced by myocardial ischemia include a marked decrease in resting membrane potential, amplitude of the action potential, upstroke velocity of phase 0 ($\dot{V}_{max}$), and action potential duration as studied in isolated hearts of pigs and dogs perfused according to the Langendorff technique (Janse, 1986; Janse et al, 1980; Janse and van Capelle, 1982; Janse et al, 1986; Kleber et al, 1978). In these experiments, the spread of activation during spontaneous ventricular premature depolarizations that occur in the first 10 minutes following coronary occlusion was mapped. The earliest epicardial activity was recorded from normal tissue close to the ischemic border and the earliest ectopic activity was recorded from the subendocardium. Whenever activity from the subendocardial Purkinje system was recorded, it preceded myocardial activity during a premature beat; in no instance was activity recorded that bridged the gap between late activity during a sinus beat and early ectopic activity. In most experiments, the extracellular space of the ischemic zone had a markedly negative potential. As a result of the ischemia, K^+ accumulated in the interfiber space in the epicardium. This partially depolarized the cells, and this depolarization caused current flow between the depolarized and normal cells such that the latter were depolarized to threshold.

After about 15 to 30 minutes, central ischemic areas become inexcitable (Downar et al, 1977). On a regional basis, transient recovery of electrical activity may occur (Janse et al, 1986). Concurrent with these changes of the action potential, changes in cellular refractoriness occur. After an initial decrease, the refractory period increases beyond the control state (Penkoske et al, 1978; Russell and Oliver, 1978). Conduction velocity shows a transient increase during the early phase of ischemia. With ongoing ischemia, there is a marked decrease in conduction velocity (Janse et al, 1986), and occurrence of local conduction block (Williams et al, 1974) accompanied by a marked regional dispersion of slowing of conduction (Janse et al, 1986). These inhomogeneities in conduction velocity and refractoriness are the pathophysiologic basis for the arrhythmias in the early phase of ischemia, which most probably depend on reentry as demonstrated by mapping experiments (Janse, 1987; Janse et al, 1980; Pogwizd and Corr, 1987).

It has also been suggested that some ectopic activity in the early phase of ischemia might originate from Purkinje fibers since Purkinje fiber activity precedes ventricular muscle activity during spontaneous ventricular extrasystoles (Janse et al, 1986; Bagdonas et al, 1961). These extrasystoles might originate from Purkinje fibers overlying the region of infarction either by microreentry or reflection or by triggered activity emerging from either early or delayed afterdepolarizations. It is likely that Purkinje fibers that are not hypoxic because of their proximity to well-oxygenated cavitary blood but that are exposed to substances that leak away from ischemic myocardium can develop triggered activity. However, all these possibilities remain speculative and await demonstration in the intact heart (Wit and Janse, 1993).

During the later phase of ischemia, delayed afterdepolarizations and triggered activity seem to dominate. They rarely cause sustained ventricular tachyarrhythmias (Cranefield and Aronson, 1988; Dangman et al, 1988; Friedman et al, 1973; Horowitz et al, 1976; January and Fozzard, 1988; Sakai et al, 1989; Scherlag et al, 1974). Delayed afterdepolarizations are related to ischemia-induced intracellular calcium overload (Cranefield and Aronson, 1988; January and Fozzard, 1988; Kass et al, 1978a and 1978b; Noble, 1984; Thandroyen et al, 1988) and other consequences of ischemia, such as damage of membrane function by lysophosphatidylcholine (Pogwizd et al, 1986; Zeiler et al, 1987). These alterations lower the diastolic membrane potential that may cause spontaneous, calcium-triggered, repetitive depolarizations in a range of membrane potentials of -60 to -65 mV (Dresdner et al, 1987; El-Sherif et al, 1983). Such electrical activity may reach the normal myocardium or it may be blocked in the surrounding tissue. Multiform ectopic rhythms based on triggered activity during myocardial ischemia are frequent and may secondarily initiate reentrant arrhythmias (Janse et al, 1980; Kaplinsky et al, 1979a and 1979b; Pogwizd and Corr, 1986).

A hypothetical scenario for the mechanism of ventricular premature beats has been presented by Janse et al (1986). A supraventricular impulse may propagate through a Purkinje strand towards the ischemic zone and be blocked close to the border. The more centrally located ischemic myocardium may be activated in a 2:1 fashion with great delay over another pathway. Excitability in the ischemic area is depressed to a variable degree. Delayed activity in the central ischemic zone cannot propagate back to the normal Purkinje fibers close to the border, but electrotonic currents can be transmitted via the unresponsive cells and reexcite the Purkinje fibers. Another explanation is that the electrotonic current may trigger repetitive activity based on delayed afterdepolarizations (Janse and van Capelle, 1982). This electrotonic current is provided by the "injury current" flowing from ischemic cells showing delayed repolarization via a segment of inexcitable ischemic cells in the border zone to normally perfused cells with suppressed automaticity. This proposed mechanism resembles the mechanism of reflection that has been studied in in vitro preparations (Antzelevitch et al, 1980).

The arrhythmias occurring during phase 1a (within 10 minutes of coronary occlusion) are related to a marked increase in refractory period, conduction delay, and threshold for excitation. During phase 1b (12 to 30 minutes after occlusion), there is a partial recovery of these parameters (Horacek et al, 1984). It is likely that 1b arrhythmias may be related to release of endogenous catecholamines. These catecholamine effects occur between 15 and 20 minutes of ischemia and may be the cause for improvement in action potential amplitude and upstroke potential and a shortening of the refractory period (Penny, 1984; Schömig et al, 1984). Therefore, mechanisms other than reentry (such as abnormal automaticity) might be the cause of 1b arrhythmias, as discussed by Wit and Janse (1993).

Subacute and Chronic Phase of Myocardial Infarction

Despite the vast literature on the incidence of these arrhythmias after infarction, less is known about their mechanisms. The genesis of sustained ventricular tachycardia or fibrillation is complex. Two different mechanisms may play a role. The arrhythmias may either be based on chronic electrophysiologic abnormalities or on a new episode of ischemia either in the area of previous myocardial infarction or remote from it (Breithardt et al, 1989). These events are modulated to a great extent by the autonomic nervous system (Locati and Schwartz, 1987; LaRovere et al, 1988). It is generally thought that spontaneous ventricular premature depolarizations initiate sustained ventricular tachyarrhythmias by creating unidirectional block and slow conduction. Although our understanding of the events that occur after premature ventricular depolarizations or artificially introduced premature activations has been greatly advanced during the last decade, less is known about the mechanisms that underlie the initiating ventricular premature depolarizations. Observations of the spontaneous onset of sustained ventricular tachycardia in experimental models (El-Sherif et al, 1985) and in man (Berger et al, 1988) may help to better understand the underlying mechanisms.

El-Sherif et al (1985) induced experimental myocardial infarction by a one-stage ligation of the left anterior descending coronary artery in dogs. They observed that reentrant excitation occurred "spontaneously" one to five days later during a regular sinus or atrial rhythm in four dogs. A tachycardia-dependent Wenkebach conduction sequence in a potential reentrant pathway was the initiating mechanism and was the basis for both manifest and concealed reentrant extrasystolic rhythms. This process could be repetitive, giving rise to a reentrant tachycardia, or it resulted in a single reentrant cycle in a repetitive pattern, giving rise to a reentrant extrasystolic rhythm. The in vitro correlates of these extracellular electrograms has been previously demonstrated in transmembrane recordings from cells in the ischemic epicardial layer (El-Sherif and Lazzara, 1979). These cells showed variable degrees of partial depolarization, reduced action potential amplitude, and decreased upstroke velocity. They also showed the phenomenon of postrepolarization refractoriness where full recovery of responsiveness outlasted the action potential duration.

A major issue is whether the isolated (or sometimes repetitive) ventricular extrasystoles after myocardial infarction are in some way related to the site involved in the generation of sustained ventricular tachycardia, e.g., by representing a "one-beat" type of reentry, or whether these extrasystoles are independent and originate at a site remote from the potential reentry circuit. In the latter case, they might still originate from an area belonging to the infarct but might have mechanisms different from reentry or may even arise from the normal myocardium. The mechanisms might increase normal or abnormal automaticity or triggered activity.

Chapter 5

The Sicilian Gambit Approach to Antiarrhythmic Drug Actions

Pharmacokinetic Information Important for the Use of Antiarrhythmic Drugs

The Role of Pharmacokinetics in the Evaluation of Antiarrhythmic Therapy

It is well recognized that there is tremendous heterogeneity among patients in response to drug therapy of any kind. Antiarrhythmic drugs have especially narrow margins between the doses required for efficacy and those that produce cardiovascular or noncardiovascular toxicity. Hence, monitoring plasma concentrations to ensure that they remain within a prescribed therapeutic range has become an important part of the management of patients receiving antiarrhythmic drugs. However, this approach does have certain limitations. First, for some drugs, a suitable "therapeutic range" of effective and well-tolerated plasma concentrations may not be identified; drugs with extensive tissue distribution (e.g., amiodarone; Mason, 1987) and those with variably produced active metabolites (e.g., propafenone;

From *Antiarrhythmic Therapy: A Pathophysiologic Approach* edited by Members of the Sicilian Gambit © 1994, Futura Publishing Co., Inc., Armonk, NY.

Siddoway et al, 1987; Funck-Brentano et al, 1990) are examples. Second, an occasional patient will tolerate (and actually require) "supra-therapeutic" concentrations for arrhythmia suppression. Finally, and most importantly, much of the serious toxicity associated with antiarrhythmic drug use (e.g., proarrhythmic effects) can occur at usual doses and plasma concentrations in those individuals who are especially susceptible. Sometimes, such individual susceptibility may occur for readily identifiable reasons. For example, hypokalemia increases the risk for torsades de pointes (McKibbon et al, 1984; Roden et al, 1986). Similarly, the use of potent depressors of sodium channel-dependent conduction (e.g., flecainide) may be entirely safe in the subject with a normal heart or conceivably even in a patient convalescing from a myocardial infarction, until some intercurrent factor, such as ischemia, stretch, or neurohumoral activation, alters the electrophysiology of normal and abnormal tissue in such a way as to enable drug-facilitated reentry (Ruskin, 1989; Echt et al, 1991a; Akiyama et al, 1991).

Interpretation of Plasma Drug Concentrations

While monitoring plasma concentrations should be a routine part of management of patients receiving some antiarrhythmic drugs, clinical decisions should be made not merely on the basis of a low or high plasma level, but on the clinical response of the patient. Side effects developing at low drug doses raise three possibilities:

1. the symptoms may be due to some intercurrent factor and not the drug;
2. plasma drug concentrations may be low, but the patient may be particularly susceptible to certain side effects; or
3. plasma concentrations of drug or active metabolite(s) may be elevated despite low drug doses; impaired drug disposition or drug interactions, discussed further below, are then the likely explanation.

When plasma concentration monitoring is readily available, distinguishing among these possibilities is usually straightforward. When plasma concentration monitoring is not available, other findings (e.g., electrocardiographic changes) may give some indication of elevated drug concentrations or excess drug effect.

Conversely, the failure of a patient to respond to therapy with high doses of a drug should raise a similar set of possibilities, which may be distinguished by measurement by plasma drug concentrations, as follows:

1. the patient may not be taking or absorbing the drug;
2. the patient may be clearing the drug (by metabolism or by elimination of unchanged drug) especially rapidly;
3. the drug may not be delivered to its important site of action; or
4. the arrhythmia may be absolutely or relatively resistant to the drug.

An example of failure of drug delivery is the improper administration of adenosine, which can lead to apparent adenosine resistance; because adenosine is so rapidly eliminated from the circulation, it must be administered as a rapid bolus through a large bore catheter (Camm and Garratt, 1991). If a drug appears to be ineffective, side effects are absent, and anticipated side effects are readily manageable, cautious increases in dose may be entertained, even in the face of usual plasma concentrations; for example, a subset of patients in whom usual concentrations of lidocaine are ineffective but in whom supratherapeutic concentrations are effective and tolerated has been described (Alderman et al, 1974). It is possible that this phenomenon reflects the increased protein binding of lidocaine in some patients with acute myocardial infarctions (Kessler et al, 1984). The problem with this approach is that some serious side effects, such as pulmonary toxicity with amiodarone or proarrhythmia with flecainide (Morganroth and Horowitz, 1984), occur at higher doses even in the absence of premonitory symptoms.

Alterations in drug absorption, distribution, and elimination have been well described and have clear implications for the management of patients receiving drug therapy of any type. Patients with advanced heart failure may fail to absorb drugs or may fail to distribute doses normally. Thus, for example, toxicity during lidocaine loading can be avoided in this group by reducing the size of the loading doses (Thompson et al, 1973). The concept that the effect of some drugs may be mediated in whole or in part by active metabolites is now well established in clinical practice (Woosley and Roden, 1983; Turgeon et al, 1990), as is the idea that drug doses should be reduced with impairment of the function of drug-clearing organs. Thus, for example, either procainamide or its active metabolite N-acetylprocainamide, or both, may accumulate to toxic concentrations in patients with renal disease (Drayer et al, 1977); in this situation, the appropriate approach is to monitor plasma concentrations and to adjust procainamide dose to avoid toxic concentrations of either the parent drug or the active metabolite. Interestingly, it was the observation of arrhythmia suppression at very low procainamide concentrations in this setting that raised the possibility that N-acetylprocainamide might exert antiarrhythmic effects on its own. Other studies also showed that procainamide and N-acetylprocainamide exert different pharmacologic effects (Dangman and Hoffman, 1981); the metabolite is devoid of sodium channel blocking properties but, like the parent drug, prolongs action potential duration. These clinical and basic studies then provided the rationale for the synthesis and development of a series of potent methanesulfonanilide action potential prolonging analogs of N-acetylprocainamide that prolong potential duration (Lumma et al, 1987).

It is increasingly recognized that one especially undesirable aspect of the use of multiple medications in a single patient ("polypharmacy") is the exponentially-increasing risk of drug interactions. Some drug interactions are in fact readily predictable and drug doses can be adjusted prospectively (or the offending combinations avoided). The acceleration of quinidine or mexiletine elimination by drugs such as phenytoin, rifampicin, or phenobarbital is an example (Data et al, 1976). Monitoring drug concentrations and anticipating the use of high doses to maintain drug efficacy is one appropriate clinical approach here. Similarly, a pharmacokinetic interaction between digoxin and quinidine is by now so well established that digoxin doses should be routinely halved, and plasma concentrations monitored, if quinidine is added.

Many drugs are prescribed as racemates, 50:50 mixtures of mirror image forms (enantiomers) which may produce different pharmacologic effects (Turgeon et al, 1990). For example, β-blockade during propafenone therapy is determined by one enantiomer, S-(+)-propafenone. Although one could argue that the use of specific enantiomers would be more desirable than the use of racemates, specific enantiomers are more difficult to manufacture, and racemization may occur in vivo for some drugs. Thus, the use of enantiomer-specific therapy should be reserved for those situations in which one enantiomer is responsible for some form of adverse drug effects, while the other retains desirable effects. This rationale underlies the development of d-sotalol as an antiarrhythmic agent. Both enantiomers block K^+ channels and prolong action potentials, but the l-enantiomer is a much more potent β-blocker (Carmeliet, 1985).

Isoenzyme-Specific Drug Metabolism

The concept of the liver as a nonspecific drug-metabolizing sponge is being replaced by an understanding of the individual isozymes that are responsible for the metabolism of specific drugs. Advances in knowledge in this area have led to the identification of relatively common heritable patterns of aberrant drug metabolism and the identification of drug interactions that may occur only in some patients on a genetic basis. It has been recognized for over 30 years that drug conjugation by N-acetylation of a number of drugs, including procainamide, hydralazine, and isoniazid, varies among individuals (Price-Evans et al, 1960; Drayer and Reidenberg, 1977). In slow acetylators, drug-induced lupus during procainamide therapy is more common than in rapid acetylators (Woosley et al, 1978). The defects in the specific enzyme system, N-acetyltransferase, are now being elucidated at the molecular level (Blum et al, 1990). The most common hepatic isozyme responsible for oxidative metabolism is P4503A4. Importantly, P4503A4 is inhibited by a number of drugs, including erythromycin, ketoconazole, and many calcium channel blockers (Peck et al, 1993). The effects of inhibition of the function of any isozyme in a given patient are determined by at least two factors: one, the activity of other pathways for clearance of a given drug and, two, the relative activities and potencies of the parent drug and any metabolites whose formation may be inhibited. Thus, for example, inhibition of P4503A4 by erythromycin or ketoconazole can lead to marked accumulation of the antihistamine terfenadine, because alternate pathways for drug elimination are not generally present (Peck et al, 1993; Honig et al, 1992 and 1993). The resultant very high plasma concentrations of terfenadine have been associated with torsades de pointes (which has also been observed in patients with advanced liver disease—in whom P4503A4 function may be perturbed—as well as in patients taking terfenadine overdoses). Inhibition of P4503A4 by calcium channel blockers may be used to advantage in patients receiving cyclosporine in that, because cyclosporine elimination is impaired, doses (and, thus, drug cost) can be reduced.

Polymorphic Drug Metabolism

While functional P4503A4 and N-acetyltransferase can be identified in all patients (albeit to variable extents), some patients completely lack certain functional enzymes. The best-studied example, and one which has had considerable impact in antiarrhythmic therapy, is the P4502D6 polymorphism (Eichelbaum and Gross, 1990). In the late 1970s, it was recognized that 5% to 10% of British subjects lacked the ability to biotransform debrisoquine, an antihypertensive, to its inactive 4-hydroxy metabolite. In these "poor metabolizers," usual doses of debrisoquine caused markedly elevated plasma debrisoquine concentrations and hypotension (Mahgoub et al, 1977; Idle et al, 1978). Debrisoquine 4-hydroxylase, now termed P4502D6, is absent in 5% to 10% of Caucasians, but the defect is seen in only 1% to 2% of Orientals. P4502D6 can be completely inhibited by very low doses of quinidine (which is not thought to be a substrate), as well as by a number of other commonly prescribed drugs that are P4502D6 substrates, including metoprolol, propafenone, and fluoxetine. It is important to note that pharmacokinetic interactions based on these drugs will only occur in extensive metabolizer subjects, that is, in those in whom active enzyme (which can be inhibited) is present. Moreover, although poor metabolizer subjects might display aberrant responses during initiation of drug therapy, it is the much larger extensive metabolizer group that is at risk for side effects when inhibitors are added during long-term therapy. The clinical consequences of the poor metabolizer trait, and of the use of P4502D6 inhibitors in extensive metabolizers, are determined by the guidelines listed below.

Alternate Elimination Pathways Present

The elimination of flecainide is partly renal and partly by P4502D6 to inactive metabolites. Therefore, the presence of the poor metabolizer trait, or the concomitant use of a P4502D6 inhibitor, ordinarily causes no major increase in plasma concentrations (Mikus et al, 1989; Birgersdotter et al, 1992). However, at least in theory, flecainide would accumulate (with potential toxicity) in a poor metabolizer subject with renal failure (Beckmann et al, 1988).

P4502D6-Dependent Biotransformation to Active Metabolites

Codeine is ordinarily biotransformed by P4502D6 to the potent active metabolite morphine; therefore, poor metabolizer subjects or those receiving inhibitors may experience less analgesia than extensive metabolizer subjects (Caraco et al, 1993). Encainide is another example of a drug whose effects are mediated at least in part by the P4502D6-dependent formation of active metabolites (Woosley et al, 1988).

P4502D6-Dependent Biotransformation to Less Active Metabolites

Propafenone exerts two major effects in vitro: sodium channel blockade and β-blockade (Funck-Brentano et al, 1990). P4502D6-dependent metabolism results in the formation of the major metabolite 5-hydroxypropafenone, which is equipotent to the parent drug in blocking sodium channels but less potent as a β-blocker. In poor metabolizers, or in extensive metabolizers receiving inhibitors, propafenone produces significantly greater β-blockade (Lee et al, 1990; Mörike and Roden, 1994). This may be desirable in some patients, but in others, it may increase side effects; in poor metabolizers, plasma propafenone concentrations are elevated and side effects are significantly more common, perhaps reflecting at least, in part, intolerance to β-blockade (Siddoway et al, 1987).

Pharmacokinetic Considerations for New Drugs

Contemporary drug development often includes in vitro assessment of the potential role of specific isozymes, of individual enantiomers, and of active metabolites in mediating drug effect; parallel information should be sought in clinical studies, as directed by this preclinical work. This might include studies in subjects with specific enzyme deficiencies, and the evaluation of isozyme-specific drug interactions. The clinical evaluation of new compounds should also obviously include studies of drug disposition, particularly in patients with common diseases that may affect drug disposition (such as heart failure, renal disease, hepatic disease). It is also important, based on the above considerations, that appropriate methods to measure plasma concentrations of drug and relevant metabolites should be developed very early, and used routinely in a drug development program.

The critical information that is required before widespread trials can be undertaken with a new drug entity is the range of doses required to produce efficacy and the range of doses that may be associated with toxicity. Obviously, should these overlap substantially, further development of a specific compound might be undesirable. Thus, dose-ranging studies, which determine both minimally effective and maximally tolerated doses and plasma concentrations in that patient population for which a given drug is intended, are crucial in early drug development (Echt et al, 1991b).

The field of pharmacokinetics evolved in the 1950s, when methods were developed to measure concentrations of drugs in plasma and urine, and to correlate these concentrations with desirable and undesirable drug effects. As these first principles have been applied by clinical investigators, important new standards in the care of patients have emerged. More fundamentally, the intensive study of plasma drug concentrations over time, and the relationship between drug concentrations and drug effects, has resulted in important new knowledge about the factors that determine the widely-recognized diversity in response to drug therapy.

The Sicilian Gambit Approach to Antiarrhythmic Drugs

The purpose of the Gambit is to develop a framework for applying the knowledge from basic and clinical research to the most sound and effective treatment of patients with arrhythmias. This demands that the framework organize the tremendous amount of information that is known about the pharmacology and the clinical pharmacology of the drugs that may be used to treat arrhythmias. To be useful, the framework must be more than a simple listing or structureless catalog of the information. It should have a scientifically and/or clinically based structure that first guides the physician to the most relevant information that is not restricted in application to small subsets of the population. For example, a framework that catalogs drugs according to their effects on the shape of an action potential or the surface electrocardiogram provides limited information about the useful actions of drugs and pertains more to toxic effects of the drugs. Furthermore, the framework should be expandable and allow for the revision and update of information about old drugs and the orderly addition of new drugs and new drug actions.

The initial Sicilian Gambit (1991) proposed a two-dimensional tabular framework for drug actions (Fig. 1). The pharmacologic actions that could be expected with antiarrhythmic drugs form columns and the drugs are listed in rows in order of their predominant antiarrhythmic action. This yields a figure with the predominant drug action appearing along a diagonal. Additional relevant actions are included in the figure and appear as deviations from the diagonal. Subsequently, the figure was expanded to include additional useful information for each drug's effects on heart rate, electrocardiographic intervals, ventricular performance, and side effect potential (Fig. 1) (Schwartz and Zaza, 1992).

At the second Gambit meeting, the statement was made that individuals with extreme points of view could suggest that, in light of the fact that only three drugs to date have been suggested to reduce the incidence of sudden death in the postinfarction period (β-blockers, sotalol, and amiodarone), all other drugs should be deleted from the figure. However, this would ignore the role of drugs in patients with symptomatic arrhythmias: e.g., adenosine for selected supraventricular tachycardias. Another suggestion was that the list should be expanded to include all antiarrhythmics currently in use or being tested. The latter, encyclopedic information *is* available to interested parties through the *Current Drugs* series published by Current Drugs, Ltd., in London. In any event, the consensus of the group was that Figure 1 in its present form provides a framework for the approach individuals can use, and should be presented as such, as an admittedly incomplete example.

The drug actions (Fig. 1) are in two major groups: in vitro actions and clinical actions. The in vitro actions are subdivided into the effects on channels, receptors, and pumps, i.e., the major determinants of cardiac electrophysiology. Each drug's relative potency to alter the channel, receptor, or pump (at clinically relevant doses) is indicated

DRUG	CHANNELS Na Fast	CHANNELS Na Med	CHANNELS Na Slow	Ca	K	I_f	RECEPTORS α	β	M2	A1	PUMPS Na-K ATPase	CLINICAL EFFECTS Left ventricular function	Sinus Rate	Extra-cardiac	CLINICAL EFFECTS PR interval	QRS width	JT interval
Lidocaine	○											→	→	⊘			↓
Mexiletine	○											→	→	⊘			↓
Tocainide	○											→	→	●			↓
Moricizine	●(I)											↓	→	○		↑	
Procainamide		●(A)			⊘							↓	→	●	↑	↑	↑
Disopyramide		●(A)			⊘				○			↓	→	⊘	↑↓	↑	↑
Quinidine		●(A)			⊘		○		○			→	↑	⊘	↑↓	↑	↑
Propafenone		●(A)						⊘				↓	↓	○	↑	↑	
Flecainide			●(A)	○								↓	→	○	↑	↑	
Encainide			●(A)									↓	→	○	↑	↑	
Bepridil	○			●	⊘							?	↓	○			↑
Verapamil	○			●		⊘						↓	↓	○	↑		
Diltiazem				⊘								↓	↓	○	↑		
Bretylium					●		▧	▧				→	↓	○			↑
Sotalol					●			●				↓	↓	○	↑		↑
Amiodarone	○			○	●		⊘	⊘				→	↓	●	↑		↑
Alinidine					⊘	●						?	↓	●			
Nadolol								●				↓	↓	○	↑		
Propranolol	○							●				↓	↓	○	↑		
Atropine									●			→	↑	⊘	↓		
Adenosine										□		?	↓	○	↑		
Digoxin										□	●	↑	↓	●	↑		↓

Relative potency of block: ○ Low ⊘ Moderate ● High   A = Activated state blocker
□ = Agonist ▧ = Agonist/Antagonist   I = Inactivated state blocker

Figure 1. *This figure summarizes the important actions of drugs on membrane channels, receptors, and ion pumps in the heart as well as on the electrocardiogram, sinus rate, and left ventricular function. Most of these drugs are already marketed as antiarrhythmic agents, but some are not yet approved for this purpose and others are no longer being used. There is no listing for proarrhythmia because, under appropriate circumstances, all antiarrhythmic drugs may be proarrhythmic. With this in mind, be aware that this figure, like all drugs, should be used with*

by the shading of the symbol. Antagonistic effects are shown with circles, agonists with open triangles, and drugs with both agonist and antagonist potential are designated with solid triangles. The likelihood of clinically effective doses of the drugs to alter left ventricular function, sinus heart rate, electrocardiographic intervals (PR, QRS, or JT) is shown with arrows. If clinical experience is limited or contradictory, a question mark is indicated. Shaded circles are used to indicate the relative potency for extracardiac side effects such as hepatitis or other organ toxicity. Note that proarrhythmic potential is not listed. The major reasons for not including this information are that there is very limited comparative data available and all antiarrhythmic drugs have this potential in some patients. In many cases, it is related more to the individual patient than it is to the specific drug.

←_____

caution; it is certain to raise some controversy. For areas such as the clinical and electrocardiogram effects, the information available is so voluminous and diverse that the figure unavoidably includes some degree of subjectivity. Accordingly, the shading of the symbols and the direction of the arrows should not be taken as absolute. Moreover, the clinical information presented refers to the patient who does not have importantly compromised left ventricular function prior to drug administration. For the section on channels, receptors, and pumps, the actions of drugs on sodium (Na), calcium (Ca), potassium (I_K), and I_f channels are indicated. No attempt is made here to indicate effects on different channels within the Na, Ca, or K groups. Sodium channel blockade is subdivided into three groups of actions characterized by fast ($\tau < 300$ ms), medium ($\tau = 300$ to 1500 ms), and slow ($\tau > 1500$ ms) time constants for recovery from block. This parameter is a measure of use-dependence and predicts the likelihood that a drug will decrease conduction velocity of normal sodium-dependent tissues in the heart and perhaps the propensity of a drug for causing bundle branch block or proarrhythmia. The rate constant for onset of block might be even more clinically relevant. Blockade in the inactivated (I) or activated (A) state is indicated. Drug interaction with receptors (α, β, muscarinic subtype 2 [M_2] and adenosine [A1]) and drug effects on the sodium-potassium pump (Na/K ATPase) are indicated. Circles indicate blocking actions; unfilled squares indicate agonist actions; and filled/unfilled squares indicate combined agonist/antagonist actions. The intensity of the action is indicated by shading. The absence of a symbol indicates lack of effect. The use of a question mark (?) indicates uncertainty concerning effect. The arrows in the clinical effect and electrocardiogram section indicate direction; no quantitative differentiation has been made between weak and strong effects. The effects listed for electrocardiogram, left ventricular function, sinus rate, and "extracardiac" are those that may be seen at therapeutic plasma levels. Deleterious effects that may appear with concentrations above the therapeutic range are not listed. Modified with permission from Schwartz PJ, Zaza A: The Sicilian Gambit revisited. Theory and practice. Eur Heart J 1992; 13(suppl F):23–29.

Sodium Channel Blockers

Drugs that predominantly act to block sodium channels can be used for their ability to slow conduction and are, therefore, selected to treat reentrant arrhythmias. The drugs are listed in Figure 1 in order of their time constants for recovery from block. The drugs are grouped according to time constants as either fast (<300 milliseconds), medium (300 to 1500 milliseconds), and slow (>1500 milliseconds). This is an index of their potential for causing prolongation of normal intracardiac conduction, i.e., QRS widening. Their selectivity for actions on ischemic (depolarized) or injured tissue is at least partially determined by their relative block of inactivated compared to activated channels. Lidocaine and its congeners tocainide and mexiletine have similar electrophysiologic actions and the differences in their clinical applications are determined by their clinical pharmacology and adverse effect profiles. Figure 1 also indicates the selectivity for the specific channel state during which the sodium channel is blocked. In interpreting this aspect of the figure, the reader should be aware that some controversy exists concerning lidocaine block of channels. The initial argument that lidocaine bound to the inactivated state of the Na^+ channel (e.g., Cahalan, 1978; Yeh, 1978) was questioned based on experiments suggesting block of the open channel state (Wang et al, 1987; McDonald et al, 1989). Similar arguments have been presented for drugs such as propafenone (Kohlhardt et al, 1989). In sum, it is safe to say that lidocaine block appears to persist through activated and inactivated channel states and that further information is needed to sort out whether "pure" block during one or another channel state occurs. It is important to sort out these issues as they have a direct impact on whether a drug will or will not show a propensity to block the Na channel in diseased, partially-depolarized tissues.

The increased time constants for onset of and recovery from block for drugs such as flecainide and propafenone explain the prolongation of the QRS interval that occurs at physiologic heart rates (Woosley et al, 1984; Morganroth and Horowitz, 1984). It also is consistent with the episodes of sustained monomorphic ventricular tachycardia induced by these drugs, presumably because of their increased propensity to slow conduction and to activate new reentrant circuits (Anastasiou-Nana et al, 1987). Note the additional but different ancillary actions of these two drugs. The additional action of some drugs to block the delayed rectifier potassium channel is thought to contribute to the efficacy of flecainide (Follmer and Colatsky, 1990), procainamide, quinidine (Balser et al, 1987b), and disopyramide in the treatment of patients with supraventricular arrhythmias (Sonnhag et al, 1988; Colatsky et al, 1990). Likewise, the additional effect of propafenone to block β-adrenergic receptors may contribute to its efficacy in treating patients with these arrhythmias (Lee et al, 1990). The polymorphic metabolism of propafenone, flecainide, encainide (Buchert and Woosley, 1992), and mexiletine (Broly et al, 1991) is due to inherited deficiency of the hepatic cytochrome P4502D6 and leads to highly variable dose-response relationships, especially for the β-blocking actions of propafenone (Lee et al, 1990).

Quinidine is listed in the group of sodium channel blockers because it is traditionally prescribed for this action. However, it is likely that much of its clinical efficacy is due to its effects on potassium channels (Roden et al, 1988) and the resulting increase in refractoriness of atrial and ventricular muscle.

Calcium Channel Blockers

The calcium channel blockers that are used for the treatment of arrhythmias are listed in Figure 1 with symbols indicating their relative potency for cardiac calcium channels. The darker symbol for verapamil indicates its greater potency for slowing atrioventricular node conduction (Mitchell et al, 1982). Although bepridil is often used for the treatment of angina, it is well known to have efficacy as an antiarrhythmic agent due to its effects on calcium and/or potassium channels (Dietrich et al, 1985).

Potassium Channel Blockers

Bretylium, sotalol, and amiodarone are listed as potassium channel blockers in Figure 1 because it is generally assumed that their primary antiarrhythmic activity results from their block of the delayed rectifier potassium channel (Colatsky et al, 1990). This action results in prolongation of the QT interval and myocardial refractoriness. They also have other actions that contribute to their clinical effects and perhaps their antiarrhythmic efficacy. This is especially true for amiodarone that has at least five different actions (Follmer et al, 1990).

It is important to recognize that the potassium channels are members of a superfamily of channel proteins and that drugs acting here may block multiple potassium channels (Wible et al, 1993). The clinical relevance of actions on these other potassium channels is not well understood, although, in general, there is an association between block of the delayed rectifier, I_K, and the ability to induce torsades de pointes (Colatsky et al, 1990).

I_f Blockers

There are no drugs used clinically to specifically block the I_f current that is responsible for maintaining sinus rate. Alinidine is the prototypic experimental agent in this class at this time. There are drugs being developed that should be useful in slowing heart rate without producing β-receptor blockade (Goethals et al, 1993). It is hoped that these drugs will have a role in the treatment of angina or in reducing myocardial damage during infarction without negative inotropic effects.

β-Receptor Antagonists

Although there are many β-receptor antagonists available, only two are listed in Figure 1 because these have been studied more completely for their antiarrhythmic efficacy than the others. There is considerable evidence that propranolol has actions other than β-receptor blockade that can be antiarrhythmic (Thompson et al, 1990). Because of its ability to shorten action potential duration in vitro and in man, we have indicated that this is likely to be due to an effect on sodium channels (although other currents may be involved).

Muscarinic Antagonists

Drugs such as atropine that block the muscarinic M_2-receptor subtype speed the heart rate and can be useful in the treatment of bradyarrhythmias. Drugs that lack the centrally mediated vagomimetic effect of atropine have been tested (Boudet et al, 1991) in the past, but none is currently in development.

Digoxin is listed with the drugs affecting muscarinic receptors because its antiarrhythmic actions are considered to be predominantly due to its vagomimetic effects in the atrioventricular node. Its other direct effects on the sodium-potassium (Na/K) pump are thought to be responsible for its inotropic effects.

Adenosine Receptors

Adenosine is a highly specific and rapidly acting agonist for purinergic receptors in the atrioventricular node and can be used to treat reentrant arrhythmias such as paroxysmal supraventricular tachycardia (DiMarco et al, 1985). Figure 1 indicates its lack of other effects. As newer A1 specific drugs become available, the figure can be easily modified.

Advantages of the Gambit Approach

The major advantage to the Gambit framework for considering the actions of antiarrhythmic drugs is that it does not discard useful information. For example, if one considers quinidine as a Vaughan Williams Class "Ia" drug, then one only knows that it blocks sodium channels and lengthens action potential duration. Yet, the Gambit framework teaches that quinidine blocks the activated state of the sodium channel preferentially. Also, because the time constant for recovery from block is in the middle range, it is not likely to widen the normal QRS at clinically useful doses and usual heart rates (Campbell, 1983). In addition, Figure 1 shows that it also blocks the delayed rectifier potassium channel and will therefore increase cardiac refractoriness and is capable of causing torsades de pointes. Figure 1 also indicates that quinidine blocks M_2 receptors and can therefore accelerate ventricular rate in atrial fibrillation (Mirro et al, 1980). An additional subtle, but clinically relevant, point is also included in Figure 1. Many fail to remember that quinidine blocks α-receptors (Schmid et al, 1974). This is the potentially desirable action responsible for the reduction in afterload (Mahmarian et al, 1987) that distinguishes it from the other sodium channel blockers. However, this action can also lead to serious orthostatic hypotension when quinidine is combined with vasodilators such as nifedipine (Bowles et al, 1993). Clearly, the Gambit conveys far more of the relevant pharmacology of the drugs than other approaches.

Another advantage of Figure 1 is that it includes information about the potency of drugs with regard to the different states of the sodium channel and their rates of recovery from block. This allows one to compare the potential of a series of drugs to have depressant effects on the normal or diseased conduction system.

The tabular approach is also useful if one wishes to quickly review a list of drugs with a common action. For example, one may want to consider which drugs are likely to cause torsades de pointes. In this case, one can scan the list of drugs that block potassium channels and find that the following drugs may be capable of causing torsades de pointes: procainamide, disopyramide, quinidine, flecainide, bepridil, bretylium, sotalol, and amiodarone. One would have to read further to learn why some are more or less likely to do so.

Disadvantages or Limitations of the Gambit Approach

No approach can be all inclusive, and much information must, of necessity, be omitted. The Sicilian Gambit listing in Figure 1 includes more clinically relevant information than any other system that is available, but it still has limitations. For example, it fails to consider differences in the action of drugs on ventricular muscle versus atrial tissue versus Purkinje fibers. It also does not include information on the possible actions of these drugs in the central nervous system that could be antiarrhythmic (Verrier, 1986). It fails to consider the other eight (or more) potassium channels that could be affected by these drugs (Tamkun et al, 1991). It does not adequately explain all of the exceptions that are apparent when one delves into the clinical experience with these drugs. For example, one could expect that amiodarone would cause torsades de pointes as frequently as any other drug that prolongs repolarization by blocking potassium channels. In fact, it only rarely, if ever, causes torsades de pointes (Mattioni et al, 1989). Yet, to its credit, the Gambit approach tells one that amiodarone also blocks calcium and sodium channels, and either of these actions could block the early afterdepolarizations that are likely to be responsible for torsades de pointes (January and Riddle, 1989).

Some may consider Figure 1 too complete and too complex. However, it contains much of the valuable information that is necessary for a more complete understanding of the pharmacology of these highly complex drugs. It more accurately reflects the "real world" complexity of the treatment of arrhythmias and should convey a level of humility to physicians who may wish to master the treatment of patients with these drugs. Physicians should not be lured into the false sense of security that a simple shorthand such as the Vaughan Williams classification might engender.

In summary, Figure 1 is an expandable framework for the basic and clinical information that is essential for the logical approach to the selection of drugs for the treatment of patients with arrhythmias. Physicians and students should refer to it when making therapeutic decisions and when anticipating or interpreting the response of patients to these drugs. Modification and expansion of the figure are readily accomplished per the dictates of increasing knowledge and desirability of change.

SECTION II

Clinical Arrhythmias:
Identification of Critical Components and Vulnerable Parameters

Chapter 6

Clinical Electrophysiologic Evaluation of Arrhythmias and of Antiarrhythmic Drug Actions

The clinical electrophysiologic profile of an antiarrhythmic drug suggests the spectrum of its antiarrhythmic effect and its proarrhythmic potential. However, a comprehensive assessment of electropharmacology is essential in order to characterize the full range of drug actions (Zipes, 1985). Individual studies performed on patients are necessarily brief and selective. Sufficient information can only be gathered by conducting a large series of clinical studies. Apart from the general reasons, common to all drug development programs, clinical studies of antiarrhythmic drugs are needed because electrophysiologic effects differ among species (Colatsky, 1990) and because there is no animal model that completely simulates the clinical arrhythmia. Clinical studies are also key to the development of an antiarrhythmic drug because the proarrhythmic potential of the drug and the best method for its administration and guide to its monitoring may emerge only from such studies (Zipes, 1988b).

Drug effects on electrophysiologic parameters can be derived

From *Antiarrhythmic Therapy: A Pathophysiologic Approach* edited by Members of the Sicilian Gambit © 1994, Futura Publishing Co., Inc., Armonk, NY.

Table 1
Problems and Limitations of Clinical Electrophysiologic Studies

Clinical Study	Limited dose range (one dose) Limited measurements (one) Coarse tool

Heterogeneous Patients	"Normals"
	No tachycardia, but:
	   Sinus node disease
	   His-Purkinje disease
	Congenital abnormality:
	   Wolff-Parkinson-White syndrome
	Conduction
	Tachycardia substrates

Study Design	No control No placebo No randomization Not blind Numbers small

from the scalar electrocardiogram (including the signal averaged electrocardiogram) and from intracardiac recordings coupled with programmed stimulation (an electrophysiology study). Although clinical electrophysiologic assessment is an important step in the characterization of an antiarrhythmic drug, there are often difficulties with the interpretation of such studies that relate to the clinical constraints of the study, patient selection, and study design (Table 1).

The Electrocardiogram

It is well known that drugs with electrophysiologic activity may affect the electrocardiogram. Such effects were the original basis for the division of the Vaughan Williams Class I into three subgroups. It was realized that the local anesthetic/membrane stabilizing drugs demonstrated considerable differences in respect of their effect on the scalar electrocardiogram (Table 2) and, in 1979, Harrison proposed the division of Class I into subgroups A, B, and C, based mainly on clinical observation (Harrison, 1985). Most of these differences may be due to the kinetics of Class I drugs, i.e., the rate of binding and dissociation from sodium channels (onset and offset of channel block)

Table 2
Subclassification of Vaughan Williams Class I Drugs According to Their
Effects on the Electrocardiogram

	Class IA Quinidine Disopyramide	Class IB Lidocaine Mexiletine	Class IC Flecainide Encainide
PR	±	0	+
QRS	+	−	+ +
JT	+	0	0
QT	+ +	−	+

(Vaughan Williams, 1984). Class IB agents have short time constants of binding and short recovery times with rapid dissociation from sodium channels (less than one second) (Campbell, 1983). Class IC agents exhibit slow kinetics, whereas Class IA drugs have intermediate kinetics (Vaughan Williams, 1984). The fast onset-offset kinetics of Class IB drugs mean that a normal diastole is long enough to permit detachment of the drug from most sodium channels in a way that the QRS complex duration remains unaltered in sinus rhythm (Vaughan Williams, 1991). The QRS complex duration prolongs after administration of Class IC drugs, whereas Class IA drugs have an intermediate effect. Thus, differences in the kinetics of Class I drugs were thought to confirm the subgrouping based on clinical observations. A major problem with this synthesis of drug actions is that Vaughan Williams Class IA and IC drugs overlap to a large extent in t 'r effects on the sodium channel (Honerjager, 1990). Other classifica ns dividing drugs according to their effect on surface electrocardiogram have also appeared (e.g., Milne et al, 1984).

The general effect of an antiarrhythmic drug on three broad categories of electrophysiologic phenomena can be recognized from the electrocardiogram: sinus (and sometimes idiojunctional and idioventricular) automaticity; conduction within the atrium (P wave duration), atrioventricular conduction system (PR interval duration), intraventricular conduction system and ventricles (QRS complex duration); and recovery of the ventricles (QT/JT intervals), atrioventricular conduction system (ventricular rate in response to atrial fibrillation), and sometimes atrium (TPa duration) (Debbas et al, 1984). However, surface electrocardiogram measurements do not accurately reflect many of these parameters, particularly those that are rate dependent. The accuracy of measurements made from clinical electrocardiographic recordings is also compromised by the slow recording speed used for clinical records (25 or 50 mm/s). Despite these drawbacks, the depressant effect on automaticity, the slowing of His-Purkinje conduction, and the prolongation of ventricular recovery of various antiarrhythmic drugs have been well documented using the surface electrocardiogram. A particular advantage of using the electrocardiogram is that it can be recorded using portable tape recorders, patient-triggered event monitors, or on electrocardiographic machines in any hospital or office to which a patient presents. Thus, transient arrhythmias or evanescent electrophysiologic and electropharmacologic effects can be easily recorded.

The Signal Averaged Electrocardiogram

Noise-free amplification of the electrocardiogram can be achieved by averaging techniques (Breithardt et al, 1991). Late potentials on the signal averaged electrocardiogram can often be demonstrated in patients with ventricular arrhythmias. Drug effects on the signal averaged electrocardiogram have been described (Kulakowski et al, 1993; Lombardi et al, 1992). Both powerful sodium channel blockers and potassium channel blockers tend to emphasize late potentials by prolonging the duration of the signal averaged electrocardiogram. It has sometimes been possible to correlate this effect with clinical efficacy, but this may be due to the fact that the effect on the signal averaged electrocardiogram depends on the presence of a drug, which is usually given to responders. In such circumstances, drug efficacy depends heavily on compliance and the effect on the signal averaged electrocardiogram may reflect this. As yet, drug effects on the signal averaged electrocardiogram do not help the clinician to choose between antiarrhythmic drugs and have not formed the basis of any classification of antiarrhythmic drugs.

Clinical Electrophysiologic Study

An electrophysiologic study is usually performed in order to provoke, diagnose, and document a clinical arrhythmia (Wellens et al, 1985). The technique involves the insertion of multiple electrodes, on one or more electrode leads, into the cavities of the heart. The electrodes are carefully positioned to record activity from relevant cardiac structures, such as the His bundle, and to stimulate appropriate areas of the heart. Programmed stimulation is used to control heart rate and measure the duration of cardiac refractoriness, to induce and terminate arrhythmias, and to explore their mechanism. Intracardiac recordings are used to define cardiac activation (electrogram recording) and recovery (monophasic action potential recording). Tools available to the clinical electrophysiologist, such as multipole and steerable catheters, have been substantially improved in recent years because of the need to accurately localize tissue that can be ablated to achieve relief from arrhythmia (Jenkins et al, 1993). A major component of clinical electrophysiologic testing is programmed stimulation to induce clinical tachycardia (Wellens et al, 1985). After the administration of a potentially effective antiarrhythmic drug, repeat programmed stimulation may be unable to induce the tachycardia. This technique has been used to confirm the likely efficacy of antiarrhythmic regimens prior to the discharge of a patient from the hospital (Camm and Katritsis, 1992; Mason, 1993).

Clinical electrophysiologic testing allows the determination of the effect of drugs on the following parameters: conduction time (between any two fixed points); refractoriness (relative, functional, and effective) of atrial, atrioventricular nodal, His-Purkinje, accessory pathway, or ventricular tissue (Table 3); pacemaker periodicity and recov-

Table 3

Clinical Electrophysiologic Effects of Antiarrhythmic Drugs

Drug	Sinus Period	Node Rec	Atrium		Atrio-ventricular Node		Ventricle		Acc Path	
			Cond	Refr	Cond	Refr	Cond	Refr	Cond	Refr
Adenosine	−	?	?	−	+	+	0	0	±	−
Quinidine	−	+	+	+	±	±	+	+	+	+
Flecainide	−	+	+	±	+	+	+ t	±	+	+
Sotalol	−	+	0	+	+	+	0	+ b	−	+

Period: periodicity; Rec: recovery; Cond: conduction; Refr: refractoriness; +: increase; −: reduction; ±: variable effect; 0: no effect; ?: unknown effect; t: tachycardia dependent; b: bradycardia dependent.

Table 4

Electrophysiologic Parameters Derived from Clinical Electrophysiologic Study

Automaticity	Sinus node (atrioventricular junctional) recovery time
Conduction (Rate-dependency)	PA, AH, HV intervals
	Atrial, ventricular, His bundle, and accessory potential electrogram duration
	Interval between any two points, e.g., His bundle to right bundle
Recovery (Rate-dependency)	Effective and functional refractory periods of atrium, atrioventricular node, His-Purkinje tissue, accessory connection and ventricle
	Monophasic action potential duration in atrium or ventricle
	Postrepolarization refractoriness (effective refractory period—monophasic action potential)
Tachycardia Characteristics	Rate, conduction time(s), and refractoriness of component parts
	Mechanism and site of origin
	Inducibility (by stimulation, exercise, or drug/catecholamine infusion)
	Drug sensitivities including suppression of inducibility
Tissue Characteristics	Decremental versus "all or none"
	Electropharmacologic type (e.g., verapamil sensitive)

ery after overdrive suppression; and the duration (and shape) of the monophasic action potential recorded from atrial and ventricular tissue. In addition, in diseased hearts, the clinical electrophysiologic effects (conduction and refractoriness) of antiarrhythmic drugs on different tachycardia circuits can be established (Table 4). Critical components of tachycardia mechanisms can also be documented and abnormal tissue characteristics and responses can be defined.

Similarities and Differences between Antiarrhythmic Drugs

The Touboul Classification

A major property of many antiarrhythmic drugs is depression of conduction in all or part of the atrioventricular conduction system.

Most drugs suppress either atrioventricular nodal conduction (increase the AH interval) or His-Purkinje conduction (the HV interval). This differential effect formed the basis of an antiarrhythmic drug classification (Fig. 1) proposed by Touboul et al (1979). Class I drugs, which include adenosine, β-blockers, calcium antagonists, and digitalis glycosides prolong atrioventricular nodal conduction. Class 2 drugs, such as procainamide and flecainide, depress conduction in the His-Purkinje system. This class is subdivided on the basis of the drug effect on His-Purkinje refractoriness. Class 3 drugs, which include propafenone and amiodarone, prolong both components of the atrioventricular conduction system to a similar degree. Physicians have found this classification useful in part (Milne et al, 1984; Camm and Ward, 1981). For example, Class I drugs are useful for the control of the ventricular rate in atrial fibrillation and some Class 2 drugs may produce complete heart block in susceptible patients.

Electrophysiologic testing indicates that some drugs are, from a clinical perspective, target specific (such as adenosine for the atrioventricular node and other adenosine-sensitive areas), whereas others,

TOUBOUL CLASSIFICATION OF ANTIARRHYTHMIC DRUGS

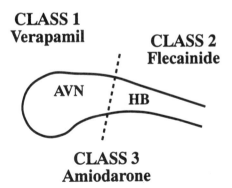

CLASS 1
Verapamil

CLASS 2
Flecainide

AVN   HB

CLASS 3
Amiodarone

Figure 1. *The Touboul classification of antiarrhythmic drugs is based on their effect on atrioventricular conduction. Drugs such as verapamil, which impair atrioventricular nodal conduction, belong to Class 1, whereas drugs, such as flecainide, which predominantly affect His-Purkinje conduction, belong to Class 2. Drugs, such as amiodarone, which modify both atrioventricular nodal and His-Purkinje conduction, are placed in Class 3.*

such as amiodarone, have effects almost everywhere in the heart (equivalent to a broad spectrum effect). For empiric management strategies, broad spectrum antiarrhythmic drugs have considerable appeal.

Differential Effects

The majority of antiarrhythmic drugs slow conduction (for example, flecainide), increase refractoriness (for example, amiodarone), or do both (for example, quinidine). Some drugs, such as mexiletine or pentosamide, shorten refractoriness and do little to conduction velocity (Fig. 2). Clinical electrophysiologic testing has confirmed observations from the basic laboratory that some drugs have more marked effects in the atrium than in the ventricle (Colatsky, 1990) (for example, ibutilide or dofetilide), but other drugs act only in the ventricle (lidocaine, tocainide, and mexiletine). Whereas some drugs (encai-

Electrophysiological Characterization of Antiarrhythmic Drugs

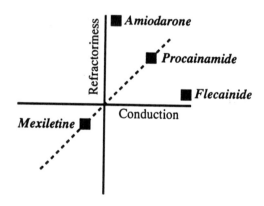

Figure 2. *In broad clinical electrophysiologic terms, antiarrhythmic drugs are perceived as capable of modifying either refractoriness or conduction or both. For example, amiodarone predominantly prolongs refractoriness and has little effect on conduction velocity. Conversely, flecainide slows conduction (increases conduction time), but does not greatly affect refractoriness. These interrelationships are conveniently displayed on a two-dimensional plot of refractoriness versus conduction (time), an example of which is illustrated in this figure.*

nide) affect predominantly antegrade accessory pathway conduction, it may be that others (flecainide) predominantly suppress retrograde conduction.

Rate-Dependency

As in the basic laboratory, it has been possible in clinical studies to demonstrate that the electrophysiologic effect of some antiarrhythmic drugs is rate dependent. Recent work has shown that the interaction of sodium and calcium channel blockers with their receptors is time- and voltage-dependent and can be explained by molecular models of antiarrhythmic drug action. One such model is based on drug binding to a constant affinity channel receptor, with receptor access determined by channel gating (guarded receptor hypothesis) (Grant et al, 1984). According to this model, it is assumed that the frequency-dependent blockade of the sodium channel induced by Class I antiarrhythmic drugs results from a periodic ligand-receptor reaction between drug molecules (ligands) and channel binding sites.

Hondeghem and Katzung (1977) have proposed another model based on the so-called modulated receptor hypothesis. This is based on observations that drugs enter the sarcolemmal channels and bind in or near the sodium channels only during certain phases of the action potential (Weidmann, 1955), such as when the channel gates are used (use-dependence) or when they are inactivated (voltage-dependence). A typical example can be provided by the sodium channels of the Purkinje fibers. Purkinje cells have sodium channels in at least three states: open or activated during depolarization (phase 0), inactivated during repolarization (plateau of the action potential, phase 2 and 3), and resting, i.e., closed but able to be opened in late diastole. Drugs such as quinidine and procainamide have the highest affinities for the activated state, blocking the sodium channels when they are open. Lidocaine and mexiletine, on the other hand, have the highest affinities during the inactivated state, although block of the activated state also occurs (Hondeghem, 1987). These drugs also shorten the action potential duration by decreasing the sodium residual or window current or by increasing potassium conductance (Zipes, 1989). This effect results in shortening of the duration of the inactivated state and the opportunity of the drug to produce inactivation state-dependent block of the sodium current. Sodium channel blockade by most sodium blockers is therefore use dependent and is more prominent at more rapid heart rates or rates of stimulation and after long periods of stimulation. At slower rates, increased time is spent in diastole and a greater proportion of receptors become drug free. The preference of the fast sodium blockers for the inactivated state of sodium channels has been used to explain, in part at least, the negligible effect of these agents on atrial arrhythmias, since the short action potential duration of atrial muscle cells has a relatively short inactivated state.

Quinidine primarily reduces the potassium current at negative membrane potentials, and block becomes less pronounced during depolarization. Thus, this kind of block of outward channels actually exhibits reverse use-dependence (Hondeghem and Snyders, 1990) in a way that blocks increases during diastole (phase 4) and declines during the plateau of the action potential, resulting in less block with increasing use. Sodium channel blockade is more prominent at fast heart rates, whereas potassium channel blockade and prolongation of action potential duration is most marked at slow heart rates (Roden and Hoffman, 1985). Indeed, recent work in humans (Nademanee et al, 1990) confirmed that quinidine increases the action potential duration and ventricular refractoriness, but these effects are diminished with increased heart rate. The drug prolonged the QRS duration in a use-dependent manner. Consequently, quinidine is mainly a sodium blocking agent during tachycardias, but a potassium blocker at slow heart rates, becoming less effective during tachycardias and proarrhythmic during bradycardias or after long diastolic intervals such as compensatory postextrasystolic pauses. Amiodarone, a drug with prominent potassium channel blocking properties, exhibits a different behavior with increased potassium current block during depolarization (Balser et al, 1987a) and lengthening of the action potential duration almost to a similar extent during sinus rhythm and tachycardia (Anderson et al, 1989). The fact that prolongation of the action potential duration is not much increased by bradycardia might partly explain the low incidence of torsade de pointes with this agent (Hondeghem and Snyders, 1990).

Thus, the positive rate-dependency of electrophysiologic effects may well render drugs specifically active during tachycardia but not during normal sinus rhythm, whereas negative rate-dependency may promote arrhythmogenic effects at slow heart rates.

Improved Clinical Electrophysiologic Assessment

The clinical development of antiarrhythmic drugs generally has not included a comprehensive electrophysiologic assessment. Failure to incorporate such studies has been due to the lack of expectation from physicians and regulatory authorities, coupled with the diversion of increasingly limited funds towards the funding of large scale clinical trials. Increasingly, clinical electrophysiologic studies included in a drug development program have been restricted to the documentation of the ability of the drug to suppress the inducibility of an arrhythmia.

Patient Populations

The majority of patients who undergo invasive electrophysiologic tests have presented to the clinic with palpitations, syncope, or manifest tachyarrhythmias. Very few "normal" subjects are studied because of the invasive nature of the test and the risks entailed in instrumenting the heart. However, some patients with syncope or palpitations prove to have no discernible electrophysiologic abnormality and such patients may constitute a near normal group for the study of an antiarrhythmic drug. However, it is also important to study patients with diseased hearts. In this respect, the electrophysiologic effects of antiarrhythmic drugs given to patients with bundle branch block (or other manifestations of His-Purkinje disease), sinus node disease, and accessory pathway conduction should be documented. Exaggerated effects, such as sinus node arrest in patients with sinus node disease or complete heart block in patients with His-Purkinje disease, are frequently revealed (Ward and Camm, 1987; Bergfeldt et al, 1985; Twidale et al, 1988).

The large number of studies in patients with tachycardia offers an important opportunity to investigate the effects of drugs on specific aspects of tachycardia substrates. For example, the electrophysiologic effect on large sections of a reentrant circuit can be investigated. Specifically, the drug action on slowly conducting or abnormal tissue can be measured. In particular, tissue that generates abnormal electrograms (fractionated or delayed) or has an abnormal pattern or duration of repolarization could be carefully sought out and studied. The possibility of achieving this has been recently improved by the development of highly maneuverable mapping catheters and multipole (sometimes orthogonal) electrode arrays (Jenkins et al, 1993).

There are some well-characterized components of potential reentrant substrates on which antiarrhythmic agents should be tested. These include accessory atrioventricular connections, including concealed decremental varieties, "Mahaim" fibers, and fast and slow atrioventricular nodal pathways.

Autonomic Challenge

There is abundant evidence that the autonomic nervous system plays a fundamental role in the genesis of cardiac arrhythmias (Schwartz and Priori, 1990), that some antiarrhythmic drugs have marked autonomic effects, and that autonomic factors modulate the efficacy and proarrhythmic potential of many antiarrhythmic drugs (Jazayeri et al, 1989).

Several antiarrhythmic drugs have been assessed in patients who have undergone cardiac transplant and others have been administered after autonomic blockade with muscarinic antagonists (atropine) and β-blockers (propranolol) (Bexton et al, 1983b; Alboni et al, 1985 and 1988; Paparella et al, 1986; Cappato et al, 1993). In this way, the direct and associated autonomic effects of drugs such as quinidine, disopyramide, propafenone, and digoxin have been evaluated in the clinical setting (Bexton et al, 1983a).

Physical Maneuvers

Simple physical maneuvers, such as exercise or head-up tilt, result in changes in the balance of autonomic effects on the heart (relative excess of sympathetic over parasympathetic activity). When antiarrhythmic drugs are evaluated in such circumstances, their electrophysiologic effects may be different to those observed in supine, resting conditions. For example, in the presence of atrial fibrillation, the frequency of antegrade conduction over an accessory atrioventricular connection is slowed with sodium channel blocking drugs, but if sympathetic stimulation occurs, this effect is greatly reduced (Klein et al, 1979).

Pharmacologic Challenge

Catecholamines reduce the efficacy of sodium channel blocking drugs, such as flecainide (Manolis and Estes, 1989) and I_{Kr} blocking drugs such as d-sotalol and dofetilide (Katritsis and Camm, 1993). Epinephrine (both α- and β-stimulation) has additional effects compared with isoproterenol alone (β-stimulation). Pretreatment with muscarinic agonists, such as oxotremorine, counteract the effect of I_{Kr} blockers at the level of the atrium. The electrophysiologic effects of antiarrhythmic drugs should be reassessed after catecholamine and, where appropriate, muscarinic agonist administration.

Monophasic Action Potential

Monophasic action potentials can be recorded from single or multiple points on the endocardial surface of the heart using contact or suction techniques (Franz, 1991). Recording from multiple sites allows aspects of the dispersion of recovery to be measured. Single site recording, coupled to programmed stimulation at the same site, allows postrepolarization refractoriness to be measured. Increased postrepolarization refractoriness, a phenomenon seen with some antiarrhythmic drugs such as quinidine, has been correlated with clinical efficacy in some situations. Some investigators have successfully used monophasic action potential recording techniques in patients with prolonged repolarization syndromes to demonstrate oscillations towards the end of the action potential that are reminiscent of the early afterdepolarizations seen in transmembrane action potential recordings. The effect of antiarrhythmic agents on these clinical potentials has not yet been fully elucidated, but the oscillations may represent an important vulnerable parameter.

Implications of Electrophysiologic Testing to the Sicilian Gambit

Electrophysiologic tests are key to the use of the Sicilian Gambit strategy in three ways:

1. the elucidation of tachycardia mechanisms, critical components, and vulnerable parameters;

2. the characterization of electrophysiologic effects of antiar-rhythmic drugs on normal and diseased tissues and on those tachycardia mechanisms that can be studied in the clinical laboratory; and
3. the specific diagnosis and description of tachycardia and the evaluation of antiarrhythmic therapies in individual patients.

In some cases, it is feasible to make an accurate diagnosis of tachycardia mechanism and to define the critical components and vulnera-

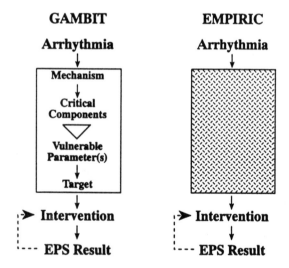

Figure 3. *The empiric approach to the evaluation of antiarrhythmic drug action by electrophysiologic study (EPS) involves the identification of the arrhythmia and a trial and error approach to the selection and assessment of antiarrhythmic therapy. The approach advocated in the Sicilian Gambit is a structured, iterative method by which an antiarrhythmic drug and a specific property is selected in order to target a particular vulnerable parameter. The EPS is used to assess the effect of the antiarrhythmic drug on the target tissues. If the effect is not as anticipated, the "diagnosis, mechanism, critical components, vulnerable parameter" cascade is reevaluated, a different dose or drug is selected, and the process is repeated until a satisfactory result is achieved.*

ble parameters of that mechanism in the clinical electrophysiology laboratory. An example is the Wolff-Parkinson-White syndrome where it is feasible to measure the accessory connection refractoriness relative to the tachycardia cycle length and deduce the length of the excitable gap at the accessory pathway. When the gap is short, a drug that prolongs accessory pathway refractoriness should be a successful therapy. This can be evaluated in the first instance by repeating the electrophysiologic test after acute administration of the drug as shown in Figure 3. In fact, this figure, which is specific to electrophysiologic testing, is a modification of the more "generic" Figure 2 described in Ch. 1, p. 7. "Electrophysiologic testing" is substituted for "clinical outcome." A detailed electrophysiologic profile is available for most antiarrhythmic drugs and those that might target a specific vulnerable parameter are known in many instances. Therefore, the clinical electrophysiologic study will fulfill a fundamental role in the Sicilian Gambit strategy. Such studies allow an immediate confirmation or denial of the success or otherwise of an individual prescription of an antiarrhythmic treatment. This clinical endpoint information should be very useful to confirm or reject the process by which therapy was selected. Repeated attempts to select therapy will, by an iterative process, eventually lead to the best fit of a particular therapy for a specific arrhythmia. By such means, the approach recommended by the Sicilian Gambit will eventually be indicated as a successful clinical approach. As knowledge accumulates about drug effects, tachycardia mechanisms, and their interaction, the treatment of arrhythmias in general will improve and the application of the principles of the Sicilian Gambit will become increasingly feasible.

Conclusions

Fundamental to the improvement of antiarrhythmic drug treatment is the ability to choose the correct drug for specific arrhythmias. Although progress in basic science will uncover more about the mechanisms of arrhythmias and the mechanisms of action of antiarrhythmic therapy, it is essential to relate this increasingly large knowledge base to the clinical management of arrhythmias. The Sicilian Gambit provides an intellectual structure to encourage the transfer of information from the cell to the bedside. Clinical electrophysiologic techniques are important practical methods that will facilitate the necessary clinical progress.

Chapter 7

The Concept of the Vulnerable Parameter and its Application to Specific Arrhythmias

In Chs. 1 and 6, we discussed the concept of the vulnerable parameter and how it relates to critical components of an arrhythmia. In this chapter, we refine the concept of the vulnerable parameter and give an example of how it can be used to aid in the selection of antiarrhythmic therapy.

The Vulnerable Parameter

Those critical components of an arrhythmogenic mechanism that are most readily and safely manipulated by pharmacologic agents to abolish the arrhythmia are defined as vulnerable parameters. Thus, there are two aspects of a component of an arrhythmia that identify it as a vulnerable parameter: one, a critical role in the arrhythmogenic mechanism and, two, susceptibility to modulation, pharmacologically or by other means.

For each arrhythmia category and its known or suspected mechanism, vulnerable parameters can be identified generally and initial therapeutic selections made accordingly. Table 2 on p. 53, modified from the Sicilian Gambit (1991), lists vulnerable parameters and target

From *Antiarrhythmic Therapy: A Pathophysiologic Approach* edited by Members of the Sicilian Gambit © 1994, Futura Publishing Co., Inc., Armonk, NY.

currents identified for the major categories of arrhythmia mechanisms. Among the critical components generally associated with an arrhythmia, the specific vulnerable parameter that can be successfully modulated in any individual patient will differ from that in another patient and even in the same patient at different times.

While critical components of arrhythmia mechanisms and the subset of critical components that comprise the vulnerable parameters targeted for pharmacologic modulation are composite properties of cells and cell aggregates, the actual targets of drug action generally are the subcellular units such as ion channels or receptors that regulate the traffic of ions. The terminology describing drug actions commonly identifies the actions on these fundamental units; e.g., sodium channel blockers, β-blockers, and calcium channel blockers. The concept of the vulnerable parameter serves as an intellectual link between the arrhythmia mechanism and the basic action of the pharmacologic agent. The recognition that conduction through the atrioventricular node, mediated by calcium current, is a critical component and a vulnerable parameter of the reentry mechanism of atrioventricular reentrant tachycardia explains the use of calcium blockers to block conduction in the reentry circuit and to terminate the arrhythmia. With the added information that β-blockers, muscarinic agonists, and adenosine all reduce excitatory calcium current, alternative pharmacologic approaches are rationalized within the same conceptual framework.

The rational process that guides enlightened pharmacotherapy for arrhythmias and the interaction of that process with empiricism is shown in Ch. 1, Figure 2, p. 7. This schema traces the process by which rational drug selection can be made when there is sufficient knowledge to identify a mechanism and the corresponding vulnerable parameters. When the state of knowledge precludes precise identification of the mechanism, often the case in clinical practice, there is generally recourse to empiricism both to guide therapy and to aid in the identification of mechanisms and vulnerable parameters.

Since the vulnerable parameters for any category of arrhythmia depend on the state of elucidation of the arrhythmia mechanism and on the available pharmacologic tools for modulation of the mechanism, vulnerable parameters represent ideas in evolution, changing with the acquisition of new knowledge and new means to affect the targets that regulate the various ion movements that determine the critical components of the arrhythmia mechanisms.

In summary, the vulnerable parameters are the conceptual

bridges between the known actions of agents on subcellular units and their therapeutic actions in abolishing arrhythmia mechanisms. The identification of vulnerable parameters and elucidation of their governance by specific ion movements provide a rational basis for drug selection and for drug development.

Application of the Vulnerable Parameter to a Specific Arrhythmia

The Wolff-Parkinson-White syndrome is the prototypical reentrant rhythm. Its pathway(s) has/have been clearly delineated during years of intensive study and, as a result, it offers a "textbook example" of how the pathophysiologic approach recommended by the Gambit can be applied to therapy. Moreover, not only is the pharmacologic treatment of the Wolff-Parkinson-White arrhythmias clearly understood in light of the Gambit, but so is the current therapy of choice, radiofrequency catheter ablation. A discussion of this arrhythmia is presented here as an example of how one can apply the Gambit philosophy to a clinical arrhythmia.

The Wolf-Parkinson-White syndrome is characterized by the presence of one or multiple accessory atrioventricular connections. If anterograde conduction over the accessory pathway occurs, the PR interval during sinus rhythm is short and the QRS complex is abnormal and begins with a delta wave. If the accessory pathway only conducts in the retrograde direction (so-called concealed accessory pathway), the electrocardiogram during sinus rhythm is normal, but the pathway forms a link in the reentrant circuit, which consists of the atrium, atrioventricular node, His-Purkinje system, ventricular myocardium, and accessory pathway.

Four different forms of tachycardias in the Wolff-Parkinson-White syndrome can be distinguished, as follows:

1. Reentry with anterograde conduction over the atrioventricular node and retrograde conduction over the accessory pathway (orthodromic atrioventricular reentrant tachycardia);
2. Reentry with anterograde conduction over the accessory pathway and retrograde conduction over the atrioventricular node (antidromic atrioventricular reentrant tachycardia);
3. Reentry with anterograde conduction over one accessory path-

way and retrograde conduction over another accessory pathway; and

4. Reentrant rhythms in the atria, notably atrial flutter and fibrillation, with anterograde conduction over the atrioventricular node and/or the accessory pathway.

In the Sicilian Gambit, atrioventricular reentrant tachycardia has been characterized in three ways:

1. Sodium channel-dependent reentry with a long excitable gap. In the presence of a long excitable gap, it is unlikely that K^+ channel blockers will prolong the refractory period to such an extent that the excitable gap will be closed and the tachycardia terminates because the circulating wavefront encroaches on its refractory tail. The critical component of a reentrant circuit with a long excitable gap is thought to be a segment with impaired conduction, which depends on partially inactivated Na^+ channels. The vulnerable parameter is conduction and excitability in that segment, which should be further depressed by Na^+ channel blocking agents so that block will occur and tachycardia be abolished. Such a segment could be the insertion of the accessory pathway into the ventricular muscle mass. The excitatory current provided by the thin accessory pathway must be distributed over a large number of ventricular muscle fibers and, therefore, the safety margin for conduction would be low at the junction. In an experimental model of the Wolff-Parkinson-White syndrome, where a large mass of atrial tissue was excited via a narrow strand of atrial tissue, unidirectional block was shown to occur at the junction of the narrow band with the large area, while conduction from the large atrial mass to the isthmus was still possible (De la Fuente et al, 1971). Any agent that would depress action potential amplitude and upstroke velocity, thus diminishing the stimulating efficacy of the wavefront in the isthmus, would enhance the degree of block. Thus, antidromic atrioventricular reentrant tachycardia should be terminated by Na^+ channel blockers. If we assume that the junction between accessory pathway and atrial tissue would also constitute a weak link for propagation in the retrograde conduction, Na^+ blockers would also be effective in orthodromic atrioventricular reentrant tachycardia.

2. Sodium channel-dependent reentry with a short excitable gap. Here, the vulnerable parameter is the refractory period, which should be prolonged. Obviously, the segment of the reentrant circuit that has the longest refractory period would be the most vulnerable. K^+ channel blockers are the drugs of choice, but Na^+ channel blockers with slow kinetics, which preferentially prolong the refractory period at rapid heart rates (Wang et al, 1993a), may be used as well. Ajmaline and procainamide have been shown to cause anterograde block in the accessory pathway in patients in whom the refractory period of that pathway is relatively long (Wellens et al, 1980a and 1982b). It is difficult to decide whether this effect is produced by diminishing the stimulating efficacy of the action potential at the junction of the accessory pathway and ventricle or by a true prolongation of the refractory period of the accessory pathway.

The distinction between long and short excitable gap reentry is difficult to make. If a tachycardia is easily entrained and terminated by electrical stimulation, there must be a sizable excitable gap. If electrical stimuli have no effect, the excitable gap is most likely short. Another way to distinguish between a short and a long excitable gap may be the response to ajmaline. When ajmaline, given intravenously in a dose of 50 mg, does not produce anterograde block in the accessory pathway, it is very likely that the refractory period of the accessory pathway is short, i.e., shorter than 270 milliseconds. Furthermore, patients with such short refractory periods have only a modest increase in refractory period duration following administration of Na^+ channel blockers (procainamide, ajmaline, quinidine) or of amiodarone (Wellens et al, 1980a). The ajmaline test is not only useful for identifying patients at high risk for sudden death when atrial fibrillation develops (because of the short refractory period of the accessory pathway, the ventricular rhythm during atrial fibrillation may resemble ventricular fibrillation), but may also identify patients in whom prolongation of the refractory period in the accessory pathway will not be very useful.

As already stated, in short excitable gap reentry, one should prolong the refractory period of that segment of the reentrant circuit that has the longest refractory period. It is by no means certain that that segment is the accessory pathway. In other words, the critical component of the circuit in short excitable gap reentry may well be another part of the reentrant circuit; for instance, the specialized conduction system.

3. Calcium channel-dependent reentry. The vulnerable parameter is conduction through the atrioventricular node, which should be depressed by calcium channel blockers. The atrioventricular node is clearly a critical component of the reentrant circuit that is highly vulnerable to pharmacologic attack.

Therapeutic Goals

There are three therapeutic goals in the Wolff-Parkinson-White syndrome: to abolish an existing tachycardia, to prevent recurrence of tachycardia, and to protect the ventricles against excessively rapid rates during atrial flutter and fibrillation.

Elimination of the accessory pathway by radiofrequency ablation accomplishes these goals and is the treatment of choice. It is unlikely that every patient with the Wolff-Parkinson-White syndrome in the world will undergo catheter ablation, and, therefore, drug treatment will not altogether disappear.

Drug Treatment to Abolish an Existing Tachycardia

While recognizing that the use of antiarrhythmic drugs varies from country to country, from hospital to hospital, and from physician to physician, there is some consensus regarding the most effective drug treatment in the Wolff-Parkinson-White syndrome (for references, see Wellens et al, 1980b; Camm 1989; Camm et al, 1992).

The first line of attack is to depress conduction through the atrioventricular node by calcium channel blockers (verapamil, diltiazem), by β-adrenoreceptor blockers (including sotalol), by vagal maneuvers, by digitalis, or by adenosine.

If drugs acting on the atrioventricular node do not work, drugs acting on the accessory pathway are given (Na^+ channel blockers, with the exception of mexiletine, lidocaine, and tocainide). If all drugs fail, and the tachycardia is symptomatic, cardioversion may be considered. It thus appears that clinical practice is in agreement with the

Sicilian Gambit approach insofar as the tachycardia is seen both as a calcium dependent- and a sodium-dependent reentrant arrhythmia.

Drug Treatment to Prevent Attacks of Tachycardia

Amiodarone seems to be the most effective drug. Since it acts on all components of the reentrant circuit and has Na^+ channel blocking effects, β-adrenoreceptor blocking effects, K^+ channel blocking effects, and Ca^{++} channel blocking effects, it is difficult to determine which vulnerable parameter is specifically attacked.

Drug Treatment of Atrial Fibrillation in the Wolff-Parkinson-White Syndrome

In patients with overt preexcitation and atrial fibrillation, digitalis and verapamil may cause a life-threatening situation by increasing the ventricular rate to such an extent that a rhythm resembling ventricular fibrillation ensues. The electrophysiologic mechanisms include:

1. shortening of the refractory period of the accessory pathway by digitalis (Wellens and Durrer, 1973);
2. increased atrioventricular nodal blockade of atrial impulses, resulting in a decrease in the number of ventricular impulses that retrogradely penetrate the accessory pathway, thereby blocking anterograde impulses via that pathway (Falk, 1992); and
3. hypotension due to vasodilatation and negative inotropic effects of calcium channel blockers, leading to enhanced sympathetic activity that shortens the refractory period of the accessory pathway (Wellens et al, 1982a).

Therefore, digitalis and calcium channel blocking agents should be avoided in patients with paroxysmal atrial fibrillation or flutter.

Prophylactic drug treatment should be aimed at prolonging the anterograde refractory period of the accessory pathway. Amiodarone is the most successful drug in these patients, not only because it reduces the ventricular rate during atrial fibrillation, but also because it may prevent the occurrence of atrial fibrillation. Other drugs with similar effects are sodium channel blockers such as flecainide and propafenone.

Chapter 8

Catecholamine-Dependent Tachycardias

In Ch. 7, we used the Wolff-Parkinson-White Syndrome as a prototypical example of an arrhythmogenic mechanism that can be considered in light of critical components and vulnerable parameters. In this chapter, we refer to a heterogeneous group of arrhythmias referred to as catecholamine-dependent tachycardias. They provide another example of how the understanding of a vulnerable parameter can aid in applying a pathophysiologic approach to therapy. Moreover, this category of arrhythmias makes a strong case for the use of target-specific drugs in the identification of mechanisms. It is for this reason that more space is devoted to catecholamine-dependent tachycardias than their clinical incidence might warrant.

Diagnosis

The diagnosis of catecholamine-dependent tachycardias is usually considered in the presence of exercise- or stress-induced monomorphic ventricular tachycardia, occurring in subjects in whom the presence of ischemic heart disease has been ruled out. The only criterion almost uniformly required to confirm the diagnosis is sensitivity of the arrhythmia to β-adrenergic blockade, be it the interruption of an ongoing ventricular tachycardia or the prevention of arrhythmia

From *Antiarrhythmic Therapy: A Pathophysiologic Approach* edited by Members of the Sicilian Gambit © 1994, Futura Publishing Co., Inc., Armonk, NY.

recurrence. Less uniformly applied criteria include: reproducible induction by exercise testing, reversible induction by isoproterenol infusion, and a QRS morphology indicative of left bundle branch block with right axis deviation.

Consistent with these diagnostic guidelines, catecholamine-dependent tachycardias have been referred to commonly as exercise-induced tachycardias (Vlay, 1987; Sung et al, 1983; Wu et al, 1981; Woelfel et al, 1985; Coumel et al, 1982; Palileo et al, 1982; Lerman et al, 1986), nonischemic ventricular arrhythmias (Coumel et al, 1982), and right ventricular tachycardia (Vlay, 1987; Palileo et al, 1982; Buxton et al, 1983). Catecholamine-dependent tachycardia and exercise-induced tachycardia are frequently used as synonyms. Although catecholamine-dependent tachycardias may frequently present during physical activity, the two entities should not be confused and the former should be diagnosed by more specific criteria. In fact, it is deemed advisable to restrict the term catecholamine-dependent tachycardias to tachyarrhythmias for which catecholamine challenge appears to be the main causative factor and constitutes a reproducible method of induction.

Isoproterenol infusion, even if ineffective alone, may facilitate the induction of ventricular tachycardia by premature electrical stimulation (Olshansky and Martin, 1987; Reddy and Gettes, 1979). In this case, catecholamines might act by shortening local refractoriness, thus allowing premature stimulation with shorter coupling intervals. Therefore, such an effect should be interpreted as true catecholamine sensitivity of the induced arrhythmia only if the same coupling intervals for stimulation are used before and during isoproterenol infusion. When this criterion is fulfilled, isoproterenol facilitation of extrastimulus inducibility predicts long-term efficacy of β-blocking therapy (Olshansky and Martin, 1987), suggesting that the underlying mechanism may be operative also in spontaneous arrhythmias.

The term "catecholamine-dependent tachycardias" is very useful clinically because it describes a subset of arrhythmias for which antiadrenergic therapy may represent a very effective remedy. In the terminology proposed by the Sicilian Gambit, the diagnosis of catecholamine-dependent tachycardias already identifies a target for therapy, i.e., adrenergic receptors, that, while independent of the electrophysiologic mechanism underlying the arrhythmia, indicate specific vulnerability.

Relevance of Substrate

Catecholamine-dependent tachycardias have been divided into two types (Vlay, 1987). Type 1 includes all catecholamine-dependent tachycardias occurring in the absence of myocardial ischemia, and either in the absence or in the presence of other heart diseases (types 1A and 1B, respectively). Type 2 refers to catecholamine-induced arrhythmias whose appearance is related to the occurrence of myocardial ischemia.

In the presence of ischemic heart disease, catecholamine challenge may cause acute myocardial ischemia. This can often, but not always, be detected by symptoms or electrocardiogram changes. Acute myocardial ischemia, per se, constitutes a substrate for the genesis of arrhythmias according to mechanisms potentially different from those directly promoted by catecholamines. Thus, the exclusion of patients affected by ischemic heart disease from the diagnosis of catecholamine-dependent tachycardias is well suited to the purpose of restricting the number of mechanisms potentially involved in each clinical arrhythmia. With few exceptions (e.g., Lerman, 1993), this attitude is expressed by most authors.

Whether catecholamine-dependent tachycardias occurring in otherwise normal hearts should be distinguished from those complicating chronic heart diseases other than ischemic heart disease is questionable. Patients affected by cardiomyopathies or mitral valve prolapse are generally included in clinical reports on catecholamine-dependent tachycardias (Vlay, 1987). This position may be justified by the assumption that catecholamine challenge should not acutely alter the pathologic substrate of the arrhythmia in these conditions. This idea is supported by the absence of obvious differences between subjects with normal and abnormal hearts in the electrocardiographic patterns of catecholamine-dependent tachycardias and in the response to electrophysiologic testing (Palileo et al, 1982; Sung et al, 1983; Lerman, 1993; Lerman et al, 1986). Moreover, the cellular abnormalities diffusely present in overt cardiomyopathies may initially be localized and escape detection, but still contribute to arrhythmogenesis, in apparently normal hearts. Thus, the number of mechanisms potentially involved in catecholamine-dependent arrhythmogenesis should not be increased if chronic heart diseases other than ischemic heart disease are included in the diagnosis of these arrhythmias.

According to these considerations, we suggest redefining cate-

cholamine-dependent tachycardias as arrhythmias induced by catecholamine challenge in subjects without ischemic heart disease.
Hence, all the information on clinical catecholamine-dependent tachycardias to be discussed refers only to cases that meet the criteria im-
plicit in this definition.

Supraventricular Arrhythmias

The term catecholamine-dependent tachycardias usually refers to
ventricular arrhythmias, although the possibility of clinical atrial and
atrioventricular junctional arrhythmias with adrenergic etiology has
also been considered. Moreover, signs of enhanced sympathetic activity consistently precede a subset of clinical atrial fibrillation; in these
cases, the arrhythmia may be reproduced by catecholamine infusion
and prevented by β-adrenergic blockade (Coumel, 1992).

Induction of supraventricular arrhythmias by catecholamines has
been demonstrated in normal isolated atrial preparations and in situ
hearts (Wit and Rosen, 1992; Malfatto et al, 1988). The site of origin
of these arrhythmias is circumscribed to the coronary sinus area,
where both enhanced automaticity and triggered activity can be induced by catecholamine superfusion. Thus, it is possible to postulate
the existence of a category of supraventricular arrhythmias strictly
dependent on adrenergic activation. However, the link between clinical "adrenergic" atrial fibrillation and experimental catecholamine-
dependent atrial arrhythmias is elusive. This is mainly due to the fact
that while nonreentrant mechanisms have been clearly identified for
the latter, it is questionable whether mechanisms other than reentry
may support the fast, sustained activity peculiar to atrial fibrillation.
The possibility that catecholamine-dependent focal activity (either
triggered or automatic) may initiate ectopy, later perpetuated by reentry, should be considered. This hypothesis could be tested by assess-
ing the efficacy of antiadrenergic interventions in interrupting, rather
than in preventing, episodes of "adrenergic" atrial fibrillation.

In the identification of the arrhythmogenic mechanism, the response to adenosine- or muscarinic-receptor stimulation is less in-
formative in supraventricular than in ventricular arrhythmias. Indeed,
both these receptors activate similar K^+ currents ($I_{K(ACh)}$ for muscarinic and $I_{K(Ado)}$ for adenosine) (Pappano and Mubagwa, 1992; Kurachi
et al, 1986), which induce modifications of the electrical properties of

the atrial cell membrane independent of cyclic AMP generation, and likely to affect all the arrhythmogenic mechanisms to some extent.

Therefore, the definition of catecholamine-dependent supraventricular arrhythmias may be clinically useful because it implies adrenergic receptors as a potential therapeutic target, but cannot be used to define mechanism-specific targets.

Arrhythmogenic Mechanisms

The definition of catecholamine-dependent tachycardias identifies a therapeutic target (i.e., adrenergic receptors) that is independent of the electrophysiologic mechanism underlying the arrhythmia. Thus, one may ask what is the practical advantage of identifying the mechanisms of clinical catecholamine-dependent tachycardias. In some cases, the therapeutic strategy for catecholamine-dependent tachycardias may actually be based on the simple notion of their potential sensitivity to β-adrenergic blockade. However, the identification of mechanism-specific targets should be pursued whenever possible, because it may provide the rationale for alternative therapies when β-blockade fails, or the desired degree of adrenergic blockage cannot be practically achieved. Moreover, identification of the relationship between the response to therapy and the arrhythmogenic mechanisms of clinical ventricular tachycardias is essential to the advancement of our knowledge of the pathophysiology of arrhythmias in humans.

In the following discussion, we will address two questions: (1) which of the known arrhythmogenic mechanisms may be more sensitive to adrenergic modulation, and (2) does the definition of catecholamine-dependent tachycardias provided above help in identifying arrhythmogenic mechanisms?

Adrenergic Modulation of Arrhythmogenic Mechanisms

Automaticity

Sinus node and Purkinje myocytes express a hyperpolarization activated inward current (I_f), with different activation thresholds in the two tissues (DiFrancesco and Zaza, 1992). I_f fully accounts for normal automaticity in Purkinje fibers and is probably the main pace-making current in the sinus node (DiFrancesco, 1985; DiFrancesco, 1991). Enhancement of this current is also responsible for the chrono-tropic effect of catecholamines in both tissues (DiFrancesco and Zaza, 1992). In Purkinje fibers, the maximum rate of normal automaticity is limited by overdrive suppression, a phenomenon dependent on Na^+/K^+ pump activation by Na^+ influx (Gilmour and Zipes, 1986; Vassalle, 1970). Since overdrive suppression is minimal in the Ca^{2+}-dependent action potentials of the sinus node, ectopic rate is generally overridden by sinus rate. Catecholamine enhancement of normal automaticity in subsidiary pacemaking regions is more likely to account for repetitive ectopic rhythms when diastolic membrane potential is slightly depolarized (between -80 and -70 mV). In this range, diastolic potential would be closer to the action potential threshold, but, under adrenergic stimulation, still negative enough to activate the pacemaker current (Gilmour and Zipes, 1986).

In the presence of the electrotonic influence of normally polarized surrounding tissue, membrane depolarization beyond -70 mV inhibits pacemaker activity of Purkinje fibers. When depolarized to potentials more positive than about -50 mV, both Purkinje fibers and ventricular muscle become automatic (Pappano and Carmeliet, 1979; Rosenthal and Ferrier, 1983). The threshold for activation of the hyper-polarization-activated pacemaker current is not reached at such positive diastolic potentials; in this condition, automatic firing, referred to as "abnormal automaticity," can be supported by deactivation of outward K^+ currents, superimposed on inward Ca^{2+} and Na^+-dependent currents (Gilmour and Zipes, 1986). Due to inactivation of I_{Na} at depolarized potentials, abnormal automaticity is rather insensitive to overdrive suppression and can generate rhythms at rates well exceeding the sinoatrial one. Thus, abnormal automaticity is a likely mechanism for catecholamine-dependent tachycardias in the presence of partially depolarized fibers.

Both normal and abnormal automaticity are highly sensitive to catecholamines (Gilmour and Zipes, 1986). Indeed, I_f and I_{Ca-L} are strongly enhanced by β_1-adrenergic stimulation, mainly through cyclic AMP-dependent mechanisms (DiFrancesco and Zaza, 1992; DiFrancesco and Tortora, 1991; Hartzell, 1988). α_1-adrenergic receptors may also contribute to adrenergic modulation of Purkinje fiber normal automaticity (Rosen et al, 1977). The chronotropic effects of α-receptor agonists vary from negative to positive depending on the availability of a specific regulatory G-protein (Rosen et al, 1988) and on the function of the Na^+/K^+ pump (Shah et al, 1988; Zaza et al, 1990). If intracellular signaling processes are altered, or the Na^+/K^+ pump is down-regulated by membrane depolarization (reduced Na^+ influx), the positive chronotropic effect might prevail. However, the extent to which this may contribute to the overall chronotropic effects of catecholamines is still undefined.

As reviewed in Ch. 4, automatic activity, both normal and abnormal, cannot be induced by programmed stimulation, can often be overdriven by pacing, but resumes immediately after its termination (Wit and Rosen, 1992). Noninducibility by programmed stimulation protocols is the feature most frequently used to define an arrhythmia as automatic.

Triggered Activity

Triggered activity may be based on early or delayed afterdepolarizations. Both these types of membrane potential oscillations are enhanced by adrenergic stimulation (Wit and Rosen, 1992). Thus, whatever its origin, triggering is a putative mechanism for arrhythmias specifically induced by catecholamines. Early afterdepolarizations are favored by bradycardia, while delayed afterdepolarizations are enhanced by tachycardia. In the presence of a normal chronotropic response to catecholamines, delayed afterdepolarization-induced triggered activity is a more likely mechanism of catecholamine-dependent tachycardias, even if the role of early afterdepolarizations cannot be excluded.

The amplitude of delayed afterdepolarizations is influenced by diastolic membrane potential: it is maximal between $-75\,mV$ and -80 mV, and decreases at more positive potentials (Wit and Rosen, 1992). Thus, at variance with abnormal automaticity, delayed afterdepolarization-dependent triggered activity can support catecholamine-induced arrhythmogenesis in normal or slightly depolarized tissues.

Most of the effects of catecholamines potentially involved in the genesis of delayed afterdepolarizations are mediated by the β_1-receptor subtype. The observation that β_1-receptor blockade is sometimes inadequate to prevent catecholamine-dependent tachycardias leads one to consider the possible involvement of α_1-adrenergic receptors (Kimura et al, 1984).

At variance with automaticity, triggered rhythms can be both induced and terminated by programmed stimulation and pacing (see Ch. 4 and Wit and Rosen, 1992). Delayed afterdepolarization-dependent triggered arrhythmias are more easily induced by rapid pacing than by single extrastimuli; the initial rate of the ectopic rhythm is generally proportional to the rate of the pacing used for induction (overdrive enhancement). An existing triggered rhythm may be either accelerated or interrupted by pacing, but it cannot be overdriven and resume after the end of stimulation.

Reentry

Because of its greater tendency to self-perpetuation, reentry is the arrhythmogenic mechanism most likely involved in repetitive ectopic activity. However, it is not clear whether a reentrant circuit may be primarily induced by catecholamines, particularly in normal hearts, where cell dysfunction or well-defined anatomic substrates are probably absent.

Adrenergic stimulation, although inducing microreentry in infarcted epicardium (Zuanetti et al, 1990), tends to improve conduction, even in ischemic or infarcted myocardium (Janse et al, 1985; Zuanetti et al, 1990). These effects should oppose rather than favor reentry. On the other hand, catecholamines might act by enhancing automatic or triggered ectopic activity that, in the presence of a suitable anatomic substrate, might initiate reentrant circuits. Catecholamine-induced shortening of repolarization may cause reentry by initiating conduction through an otherwise refractory accessory pathway. This may explain some adrenergic supraventricular tachycardias, but does not account for the typical catecholamine-dependent tachycardias ensuing in otherwise normal ventricles.

Reentrant arrhythmias can generally be induced and interrupted by premature stimuli. The coupling intervals of the stimulated premature beat and of the first spontaneous beat of the tachycardia are usually inversely related. Reentrant circuits can be entrained (Waldo et al, 1984), i.e., their rate can be driven by fast pacing, and returns to the original value on abrupt cessation of pacing or on slowing of the pacing rate below the intrinsic rate of the rhythm. The demonstration of transient entrainment is strongly suggestive of reentry (Rosen, 1986) and, if associated with several other related features (progressive fusion of ventricular complexes, etc.), can be considered as conclusive evidence for this mechanism (Waldo et al, 1984). However, entrainment can be achieved only in circuits with a significant excitable gap; therefore, the absence of entrainment does not rule out the reentrant nature of an arrhythmia.

Arrhythmogenic Mechanisms of Clinical Catecholamine-Dependent Tachycardias

The assessment of the mechanism of a clinical arrhythmia relies on the analysis of its response to drugs and stimulation protocols.

Pharmacologic response is a limited tool in discriminating among arrhythmogenic mechanisms, because most drugs have multiple effects, and also because there is some nonspecificity of the response of each mechanism to drugs. Although the information available is still incomplete, a notable exception to this statement may be represented by the response of the arrhythmia to adenosine or to substances that increase tissue adenosine concentrations (e.g., dipyridamole). Both adenosine and muscarinic agonists interfere with the electrophysiologic effects of adrenergic stimulation mediated by an increase in intracellular cyclic AMP concentration. Since these effects include most catecholamine actions potentially involved in arrhythmogenesis, muscarinic and adenosine receptor stimulation should antagonize all the effects of β-adrenergic activation on ventricular arrhythmias. However, sensitivity to adenosine or muscarinic agonists is specific for catecholamine-dependent tachycardias having a response to pacing protocols suggestive of triggered activity (Lerman, 1993). The reasons for such specificity are not obvious. A potential explanation (Lerman, 1993) is based on the observation that adenosine fails to antagonize the electrophysiologic effects of catecholamines in depolarized Purkinje fibers (Rosen et al, 1983) and ventricular myocytes (Isenberg and Belardinelli, 1984). Thus, arrhythmogenic mechanisms supported by membrane depolarization, such as abnormal automaticity, might be less sensitive to adenosine. The weakness of this interpretation is that it does not account for the failure of vagal maneuvers to inhibit catecholamine-dependent tachycardias based on enhanced automaticity (Lerman, 1993). It should also be considered that both adenosine and dipyridamole are vasodilators and, particularly in the presence of coronary stenosis, they might suppress or facilitate arrhythmias through changes in blood supply. Although potentially useful in the clinical setting, the selectivity of adenosine (or dipyrida-mole) for triggered activity needs to be confirmed in larger series.

Experimental studies, which await clinical confirmation, suggest that flunarizine (Vos et al, 1990) and the combined response to lido-caine and ethmozine (Ilvento et al, 1982) may also discriminate be-tween automatic and triggered arrhythmogenic mechanisms.

The reliability of electrophysiologic testing in discriminating among arrhythmogenic mechanisms has been discussed in detail else-where (Rosen, 1986). If all the entrainment criteria (Waldo et al, 1984) are tested and fulfilled, a positive diagnosis of reentry can be reason-ably made. However, in the majority of clinical reports on catechol-amine-dependent tachycardias, such a diagnosis is based on the in-duction and termination of the arrhythmia by premature stimulation, and the presence of entrainment is seldom tested. An arrhythmia that cannot be induced or terminated by premature stimulation is usually attributed to enhanced automaticity, whereas the diagnosis of trig-gered activity is based on the presence of overdrive enhancement. While keeping in mind the limitations of these criteria, a review of the literature may help in identifying whether typical catecholamine-dependent tachycardias share common patterns of response to stimu-lation protocols suggestive of specific mechanisms. The following dis-cussion is based on the meta-analysis of seven studies (Palileo et al, 1992; Wu et al, 1981; Sung et al, 1983; Buxton et al, 1983; Coelho et al, 1986; Lerman et al, 1986; Lerman, 1993), from which we selected 40 cases strictly matching the definition of catecholamine-dependent tachycardias given in this chapter. In 23 of these patients (58%), the arrhythmia was not inducible by electrical stimulation, consistent with enhanced automaticity. Among inducible subjects, eight (47%) had a pattern of response consistent with triggered activity, while in the remaining nine cases, the response was either equivocal or compatible with reentry. Thus, mechanisms other than reentry can be interpreted as responsible for almost 80% of the cases of catecholamine-dependent tachycardias analyzed. This is in sharp contrast with the pattern of response suggestive of reentry found in idiopathic ventricular tachy-cardias unrelated to adrenergic activation (Ohe et al, 1988) and in the large majority of those complicating ischemic heart disease. Thus, if appropriately defined, the category of catecholamine-dependent tachy-cardias seems adequate to identify a group of arrhythmias in which nonreentrant mechanisms are involved in an unusually high propor-tion of cases. However, we are still left with two possibilities, enhanced automaticity and triggered activity, implying partially different therapeutic targets. We are also concerned with the limitations inherent in the electrophysiologic diagnosis of mechanisms of these arrhythmias.

These problems have been addressed by Lerman in a recent study (1993) that deserves to be discussed in detail for two reasons: firstly, the electrophysiologic diagnosis of the arrhythmogenic mechanism was made according to rather strict criteria (including the presence of entrainment) and, secondly, pharmacologic and electrophysiologic characterizations of the arrhythmia were closely matched. This study showed that suppression of exercise-induced ventricular tachycardia by dipyridamole, edrophonium, or vagal maneuvers identified arrhythmias induced by isoproterenol in otherwise normal hearts, which had a pattern of response to electrical stimulation suggestive of triggered activity. Arrhythmias identified as "automatic," although induced by isoproterenol, were not suppressed by dipyridamole or cholinergic interventions. Reentrant arrhythmias, found almost exclusively in subjects with organic heart disease, were similarly insensitive to adenosine- or muscarinic-receptor stimulation. A correlation between adenosine sensitivity, nonreentrant mechanism, and absence of organic heart disease was found also in a previous study on exercise-induced ventricular tachycardias (Lerman et al, 1986). The results of these studies suggest the following. Exercise-induced ventricular tachycardias may be based on either of the three arrhythmogenic mechanisms; however, isoproterenol-induced ventricular tachycardias, sensitive to muscarinic stimulation and/or dipyridamole, should largely represent delayed afterdepolarization-dependent triggered activity. This arrhythmogenic mechanism would prevail in otherwise normal hearts. Based on this interpretation, sensitivity to dipyridamole (or adenosine) can tentatively be used to identify catecholamine-dependent tachycardias with a triggered origin. The mechanisms that may account for the ability of adenosine to discriminate between automatic and triggered rhythms have been discussed above.

Critical Components and Vulnerable Parameters

Figure 1 shows the sequence of cellular events leading from activation of β_1-adrenergic receptors to the facilitation of delayed afterde-

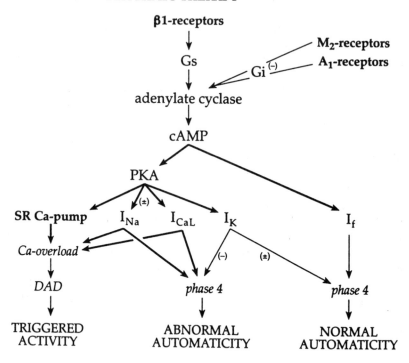

Figure 1. *Critical components in β_1-receptor modulation of the arrhythmogenic mechanisms most likely involved in the genesis of catecholamine-dependent tachycardias. Vulnerable parameters are represented in italics and targets of drug action are shown in bold. Unless specified, lines connecting steps indicate stimulation of the step downstream; thinner lines refer to actions that should not contribute to the proarrhythmic effect of catecholamines (for explanations, see text). Muscarinic M_2-receptors and adenosine A_1-receptors have been represented here as negative modulators of β_1-receptor pathway. Notice that these are mechanism-specific targets, even if the figure may suggest the contrary (see text). SR: sarcoplasmic reticulum; $(-)$: inhibition; $(\pm)$: variable effects; G_s and G_i: excitatory and inhibitory GTP regulatory proteins; PKA: protein kinase A; DAD: delayed afterdepolarizations.*

polarizations and automaticity, the arrhythmogenic mechanisms most likely involved in catecholamine-dependent tachycardias. Critical components for the genesis of these arrhythmias include all the steps of the sequence. As outlined in Figure 1, some of them are common to all catecholamine-dependent tachycardias, while some are specific for an individual arrhythmogenic mechanism.

Ca^{2+} overload and delayed afterdepolarizations may be identified as the vulnerable parameters for dipyridamole-sensitive tachycardias, while phase 4 depolarization is the vulnerable parameter for dipyridamole-insensitive tachycardias.

Targets

As already discussed, catecholamine-dependent tachycardias are a unique category of arrhythmias in terms of target identification. Indeed, the definition of catecholamine dependence implies that adrenergic receptors are a general, mechanism-independent target for the pharmacologic treatment of these arrhythmias. In fact, the target here is a modulator of several mechanisms. The evidence reported so far suggests that β_1-adrenergic receptors are responsible for arrhythmogenesis in catecholamine-dependent tachycardias, and that their effects are mediated by the adenylate cyclase system. Thus, beside B_1-adrenergic receptors (to be blocked), other receptors inhibiting the adenylate cyclase pathway may act as targets (to be stimulated). Among those well characterized and already exploited clinically are muscarinic M_2 and adenosine A_1-receptors. Peptidergic receptors with inhibitory effects on adenylate cyclase, such as the somatostatin receptor (Wharton and Gulbenkina, 1987), are also potentially interesting, largely unexplored, targets.

In the treatment of catecholamine-dependent tachycardias, β_1-adrenergic receptors can be used as targets independently of the arrhythmogenic mechanism involved. On the other hand, according to the evidence presented by Lerman's group (Lerman et al, 1986; Lerman, 1993), adenosine A_1- and muscarinic M_2-receptors might be considered as targets only for catecholamine-dependent tachycardias based on triggered activity.

As shown in Figure 1, ion channels may be mechanism-specific targets or may interfere with multiple mechanisms. A well-known mechanism by which catecholamines induce cellular overload of Ca^{2+} is the stimulation of Ca^{2+} influx through the dihydropyridine-sensitive channel (I_{Ca-L}). Nonetheless, β_1-receptor agonists also increase the rate of Ca^{2+} uptake by the sarcoplasmic reticulum (Kirchberger et al, 1974; Tada et al, 1974; Lindemann et al, 1983). Since this process competes with Ca^{2+} extrusion from the cell by the Na^+/Ca^{2+} exchanger (Bers, 1993), catecholamine challenge might increase the proportion of Ca^{2+} that is retained by the cell after each contraction. This action might contribute to catecholamine-induced Ca^{2+} overload. Thus, the Ca^{2+} pump of the sarcoplasmic reticulum, as well as the Ca^{2+} release channel (ryanodine receptor), are potential targets for modulating the cytoplasmic Ca^{2+} oscillations responsible for delayed afterdepolarizations. However, since the effects of their modulation are complex and incompletely defined, these proteins can be considered as therapeutic targets only in perspective. Intracellular Ca^{2+} oscillations may cause delayed afterdepolarizations either through transient increases in the Na^+/Ca^{2+} exchanger current, or by activating a Ca^{2+}-dependent nonselective inward current (I_{NS}) (Wit and Rosen, 1992). The Na^+/Ca^{2+} exchanger is an unlikely target for pharmacologic prevention of delayed afterdepolarizations because its inhibition would accelerate the Ca^{2+} accumulation process. Blockers of I_{NS} are not currently available.

It has been observed that delayed afterdepolarization-dependent triggered activity can be inhibited, although not uniformly, by Na^+ channel blockers (Wit and Rosen, 1992). These agents may act by shortening action potential duration and by increasing the Na^+ gradient driving the Na^+/Ca^{2+} exchanger; both these actions reduce intracellular Ca^{2+}. Moreover, Na^+ channels provide the depolarizing current required to convert delayed afterdepolarizations or phase 4 depolarization in propagated triggered or automatic activity. β_1-receptor agonists stimulate I_{Na} at negative membrane potentials and inhibit I_{Na} at more positive ones (Schubert et al, 1990; Matsuda et al, 1992; Ono et al, 1993). Thus, the role of I_{Na} in catecholamine-dependent arrhythmias would depend on the membrane potential at which arrhythmias are generated.

Among the currents enhanced by adrenergic stimulation, I_{Ca-L} is the one that contributes most significantly to phase 4 depolarization in partially depolarized cells; thus, I_{Ca-L} can be considered as the primary target for the treatment of arrhythmias resulting from abnormal automaticity.

Particularly in Purkinje fibers, adrenergic stimulation of normal automaticity should occur mainly through a β_1-adrenergic mediated increase in the pacemaker current I_f (DiFrancesco and Zaza, 1992). Indeed, due to their positive thresholds (-60 mV to -50 mV and -40 mV to -30 mV for I_{Ca-T} and I_{Ca-L}, respectively, in Purkinje myocytes) (Hirano et al, 1989; Tseng and Boyden, 1989), Ca^{2+} currents should activate only in the terminal portion of phase 4 depolarization. I_{Ca-T} has been reported to contribute to automaticity in the sinoatrial node (Hagiwara et al, 1988); however, this current is not affected by β-receptor agonists and may be variably modulated by α-adrenergic receptors (Tseng and Boyden, 1989).

β_1-receptor agonists increase the delayed rectifier current (I_K) (Harvey and Hume, 1989; Duchatelle-Gourdon et al, 1989; Connors and Terrar, 1990) and α_1-receptor agonists inhibit it (Apkon and Nerbonne, 1988). Abnormal automaticity should be inhibited by an increase in I_K. The consequences of I_K modulation on normal automaticity depend on the balance between the hyperpolarizing effect of this current (which would reduce automaticity), the shortening of action potential duration, and changes in other diastolic currents resulting from membrane hyperpolarization (e.g., increased I_f, leading to increased automaticity). The unpredictability of the effects of I_K modulation makes this current a poor target for the therapy of catecholamine-dependent tachycardias.

Abnormal automaticity can be suppressed also by reversing membrane depolarization through activation of outward background currents. Those that can be modulated pharmacologically include $I_{K(ATP)}$ (de Weille, 1992) and, largely limited to atrial tissues, $I_{K(ACh)}$ and $I_{K(Ado)}$ (Pappano and Mubagwa, 1992). Thus, even if unaffected by adrenergic stimulation, these currents may be considered targets for the treatment of catecholamine-dependent tachycardias.

In summary, the treatment of catecholamine-dependent tachycardias may aim at the following general and mechanism-specific targets (the list also includes targets, not accessible at present, that deserve future evaluation):

Common to all catecholamine-dependent tachycardias (mechanism independent): β_1-adrenergic receptors, I_{Ca-L} channels, Na^+ channels (all to be inhibited).

Specific for dipyridamole-sensitive catecholamine-dependent tachycardias (triggered): A_1-adenosine receptors and M_2-muscarinic receptors (to be stimulated); ryanodine receptors and sarcoplasmic reticulum Ca-ATPase (potentially useful, requiring evaluation).

Specific for dipyridamole-insensitive catecholamine-dependent tachycardias (automatic): $I_{K(ATP)}$ channels (to be activated); $I_{K(ACh)}$ and $I_{K(Ado)}$ (to be activated, limited to supraventricular arrhythmias).

Therapy

The therapeutic choice is based on the availability of agents as specific as possible for the targets identified and suitable for use in individual cases. If the mechanism underlying the arrhythmia has been sufficiently defined, the first choice should be an intervention specific for that mechanism. This would limit side effects and, in the case of a success, would provide more information on the pathophysiology of the arrhythmia. The failure of a mechanism-specific intervention may be due either to an erroneous identification of the mechanism or to inadequate action of the drug on the target (low dosage, unfavorable drug metabolism or distribution, etc.). By definition, adrenergic stimulation is an important trigger in all catecholamine-dependent tachycardias. Thus, an "adequate" degree of β-adrenergic blockade should suppress these arrhythmias in all cases. However, side effects, drug metabolism, and such local phenomena as receptor up-regulation may prevent achievement of the adequate degree of receptor antagonism. In this case, the association of β-blockade with an intervention directed to other membrane targets may prove successful. The higher the specificity of the added intervention for the mechanism of the arrhythmia, the better the chance to achieve desired results without side effects. Targets, specific for dipyridamole-sensitive arrhythmias, include membrane receptors to be stimulated. As a general rule, persistent receptor stimulation leads to desensitization of the response that may take from minutes to weeks, depending on the cellular process involved. Thus, therapeutic interventions involving receptor stimulation (dipyridamole, adenosine, cholinergic agonists, etc.), although useful in the acute treatment of symptomatic catecholamine-dependent tachycardias, may be deceptive in the long-term prevention of these arrhythmias.

Flunarizine, a drug used in the treatment of vascular diseases, is a promising intervention specific for dipyridamole-sensitive catecholamine-dependent tachycardias; however, its efficacy, only recently suggested by experimental studies, needs to be confirmed and tested in the clinical setting.

To summarize, the therapeutic interventions identified according to general and mechanism-specific targets are as follows:

Common to all catecholamine-dependent tachycardias (mechanism independent): β_1-adrenergic blockers, Ca^{2+} antagonists, Na^+ channel blockers.

Specific for dipyridamole-sensitive catecholamine-dependent tachycardias (triggered): adenosine, dipyridamole, edrophonium or muscarinic agonists (all for acute therapy), flunarizine (potentially useful chronically, but still to be evaluated).

Specific for dipyridamole-insensitive catecholamine-dependent tachycardias (automatic): $I_{K(ATP)}$ openers; adenosine and muscarinic agonists (only for acute therapy of supraventricular arrhythmias).

Conclusions

If defined using strict criteria, the term catecholamine-dependent tachycardias identifies clinical arrhythmias with rather homogeneous mechanisms. The limited evidence available so far suggests that the mechanism involved in individual clinical arrhythmias may be diagnosed with reasonable accuracy by pharmacologic means (dipyrida-

---

Table 1

Diagnostic Flowchart for Patients with Suspected Catecholamine-Dependent Tachycardias

---

We propose that each patient with a presumptive diagnosis of catecholamine-dependent tachycardia should be submitted to as many as possible (ideally all) of the following procedures:

1. Tests adequate to exclude ischemic heart disease and the idiopathic long QT syndrome.
2. Study of the inducibility of the clinical arrhythmia by catecholamine infusion. Norepinephrine would best reproduce the effects of neural activation (and, indeed, a role for α-adrenergic receptors in the genesis of catecholamine-dependent tachycardias cannot be ruled out). However, the resulting increase in blood pressure and baroreceptor responses would evoke vagal activity, potentially limiting adrenergic effects on the heart. Thus, epinephrine or isoproterenol are probably preferable for testing adrenergic inducibility.
3. Test inducibility by exercise stress testing to identify a rate threshold for the appearance of the arrhythmia.
4. Test arrhythmia suppression by: β-blockers, dipyridamole, edrophonium, and flunarizine.
5. Invasive electrophysiologic testing including: induction and termination by premature stimuli; induction and termination by rapid pacing; and tests for the presence of entrainment.

mole sensitivity, etc.) only. This important hypothesis needs to be further tested in the clinical setting. Parallel pharmacologic and electrophysiologic diagnosis of the mechanism should still be performed in all cases of catecholamine-dependent tachycardias for this purpose. The immediate benefit deriving from the identification of mechanism-specific targets is still partly limited by the availability of adequate pharmacologic tools. However, promising selective therapeutic interventions have been recently identified, which cannot be tested and used to their full potential without acquiring information on the pathophysiology of clinical catecholamine-dependent tachycardias.

Catecholamine-dependent tachycardias are a relatively infrequent arrhythmia; thus, information on a significant number of cases can be obtained only by pooling data from different studies. The reliability of such a process depends on the uniformity of criteria and diagnostic procedures used by various authors. Table 1 is a proposed flowchart for the work-up of the patient with catecholamine-dependent tachycardias that provides information on many of the open questions relating to this disease entity.

SECTION III

Specific Cardiac Arrhythmias

The preceding chapters have considered selected arrhythmias while highlighting the pathophysiologic approach recommended by the Gambit. The chapters in Section III deal with commonly occurring cardiac arrhythmias and follow an approach not dissimilar to that already employed by the clinician, adding, wherever possible, a consideration of the strengths and weaknesses of the Gambit in helping with consideration of arrhythmia mechanisms and management.

Chapter 9

Supraventricular Tachycardias

Before planning a treatment strategy for the patient with a supraventricular tachycardia, the physician must accurately diagnose the arrhythmia. Several approaches exist to effect this activity (Zipes, 1992). The method used here is advocated because it is predicated on simple electrocardiographic observations available to the clinician who has a 12-lead recording of the tachycardia. The 12-lead electrocardiogram recorded during the supraventricular tachycardia therefore becomes a critical tool for the physician and, consequently, comprehensive attempts should be made to obtain this piece of diagnostic information.

Differential Diagnosis of Supraventricular Tachycardias Based on RP-PR Relationships

The supraventricular tachycardias can be divided into those tachycardias that have a short RP-long PR interval and those that have a long RP-short PR interval. By that differentiation we mean that during the tachycardia, the P wave is located in the first 50% of the cardiac cycle following the QRS complex (short RP) or it is located in the second 50% of the cardiac cycle (long RP). In the former category

From *Antiarrhythmic Therapy: A Pathophysiologic Approach* edited by Members of the Sicilian Gambit © 1994, Futura Publishing Co., Inc., Armonk, NY.

are included typical atrioventricular nodal reentry tachycardia and orthodromic atrioventricular reciprocating tachycardia. In the latter group are atrial tachycardias, sinus nodal reentry and inappropriate sinus tachycardia, atypical atrioventricular nodal reentry, and the permanent form of atrioventricular junctional reciprocating tachycardia. At times, Ebstein's anomaly having an accessory pathway with a long conduction time can create an orthodromic atrioventricular reciprocating tachycardia with a long RP interval. Certain exceptions to this classification can exist. For example, an uncommon presentation of atrioventricular nodal reentry can exhibit a retrograde P wave located midway between QRS complexes during tachycardia. In some forms of antedromic atrioventricular reciprocating tachycardia, the retrograde P wave can also be located midway between QRS complexes. These issues will be discussed under the individual tachycardias.

Short RP Interval Tachycardias

Atrioventricular Nodal Reentrant Tachycardia

In its usual form, the mechanism of atrioventricular nodal reentrant tachycardia involves reentry with anterograde conduction over a slow pathway and retrograde conduction over a fast pathway (Rosen et al, 1972; Jackman et al, 1992; Mitrani et al, 1992; Janse et al, 1993; Jazayeri et al, 1993; McGuire et al, 1993; Ward and Garratt, 1993). Although considerable electrophysiologic data support the presence of two pathways (Figs. 1 and 2), their anatomic presence and location are unsettled (Ho et al, 1993; Racker, 1993). Data obtained from ablation studies during which either the slow or fast pathway can be ablated selectively (Jackman et al, 1992; Gursoy et al, 1993; Kay et al, 1993; Mitrani et al, 1992) demonstrate that the atrial insertion of these pathways is into separate parts of the atrium, and suggest that the slow pathway is located in the posterior portion of the atrioventricular nodal region; it represents the posterior atrial input to the compact portion of the atrioventricular node. The fast pathway is located anterosuperiorly and represents the anterior approach to the compact portion of the atrioventricular node. Importantly, the location of these pathways indicates that the atrium, or a portion of it, comprises an obligatory portion of the reentrant loop sustaining the tachycardia.

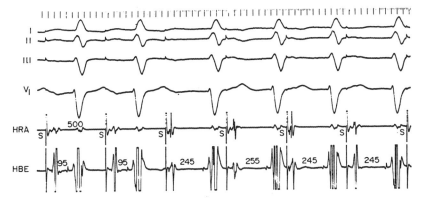

Figure 1. *Demonstration of dual atrioventricular nodal pathways. Constant high right atrial pacing at a cycle length of 500 ms results in an atrio-Hisian interval of 95 ms. Following the third atrial stimulus, the atrio-Hisian interval suddenly "jumps" to 245 ms and remains in that range due to anterograde block over the fast atrioventricular nodal pathway and conduction then occurs over the slow atrioventricular nodal pathway. HRA: high right atrial electrogram; HBE: His bundle electrogram; Leads I, II, III, and V₁: scalar electrocardiograms.*

The critical components of the atrioventricular nodal reentrant tachycardia pathway are defined by those structures necessary for completion of the reentrant loop. Typically, the impulse travels anterogradely from the atrium over the slow pathway to the final common pathway (that may be in the distal part of the atrioventricular node or initial portion of the His bundle) where it can then "turn around" and retrogradely enter the fast pathway and return to the atrium. After activating the atrium, the impulse then reenters the slow pathway and continues in this circular or reentrant fashion (Fig. 3). Activation of the His bundle and perhaps the very distal portion of the atrioventricular node (distal to the final common pathway) is not necessary for initiation or maintenance of the atrioventricular nodal reentry tachycardia (Fig. 3).

Clinical electrophysiologic data from pharmacologic probes suggest that slow channel-dependent tissue makes up the slow pathway, while the fast pathway that is used for retrograde conduction during the atrioventricular nodal reentry tachycardia (and may not necessarily be the same atrioventricular nodal pathway that is used for anterograde conduction during normal sinus rhythm) may have fast chan-

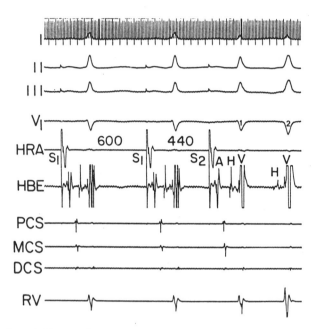

Figure 2. Two QRS complexes in response to a single atrial premature complex demonstrating dual atrioventricular nodal pathways. Following a basic train of S_1 stimuli at 600 ms, an S_2 at 440 ms is introduced. The first QRS complex in response to S_2 occurs with a short (95 ms) atrio-Hisian (AH) interval due to anterograde conduction over the fast atrioventricular nodal pathway. The first QRS complex is labeled number 1 (in lead V_1). The second QRS complex in response to the S_2 stimulus (labeled number 2) occurs with a long atrio-Hisian interval (430 ms) due to anterograde conduction over the slow atrioventricular nodal pathway. HRA: high right atrial electrogram; HBE: His bundle electrogram; PCS: proximal coronary sinus electrogram recording; MCS: midcoronary sinus electrogram; DCS: distal coronary sinus electrogram recording; RV: right ventricular apex electrogram recording; A: low right atrial electrogram; H: His bundle electrogram; V: ventricular electrogram. Reproduced with permission from Zipes DP: Specific arrhythmias: Diagnosis and treatment. In Braunwald E (ed): Heart Disease: A Textbook of Cardiovascular Medicine. Fourth edition. Philadelphia, PA: WB Saunders Co, 1992, p. 689.

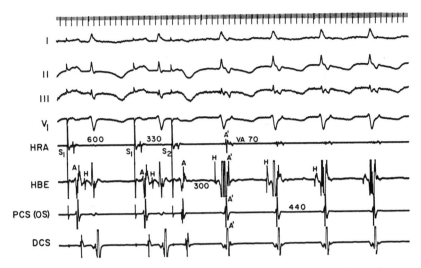

Figure 3. *Precipitation of atrioventricular nodal reentrant tachycardia. Following high right atrial pacing at a basic cycle length of 600 ms (S_1), a premature atrial stimulus (S_2) is introduced at a cycle length of 330 ms. The atrio-Hisian (AH) interval lengthens to 300 ms due to anterograde conduction over the slow atrioventricular nodal pathway and returns retrogradely to activate the atrium (A') and initiate atrioventricular nodal reentral tachycardia at a cycle length of 440 ms. The ventriculoatrial (VA) interval in the high right atrial recording of 70 ms is too short to be explained by conduction over an accessory pathway. The first retrograde P wave may actually be a fusion atrial complex because of the relatively early activation in the high right atrial electrogram (HRA) lead.*

nel-dependent cells. The ionic current responsible for depolarization of cells in the slow channel-dependent slow pathway is $I_{Ca\text{-}L}$, and I_{Na} is responsible for the atrium and probably the retrogradely conducting fast pathway (Hartzell and Duchatelle-Gourdon, 1993). I_K is the predominant ionic current responsible for repolarization in both cell types (Joho, 1993). These channels represent the potential targets of drug interventions.

Anterograde conduction over the slow pathway represents the vulnerable parameter of the reentrant circuit that is most likely and most safely interrupted pharmacologically. To accomplish acute termination of atrioventricular nodal reentrant tachycardia, M2 receptor activation, usually achieved by reflex vagal stimulation via a Valsalva maneuver or carotid sinus massage, is effected. As pharmacologic alternatives, calcium channel blocking drugs, e.g., verapamil and diltiazem, and purinergic (A_1) receptor agonists, e.g., adenosine, can be administered intravenously to produce transient anterograde block in the slow pathway. The response of the effector pathway to the effects of adenosine and M_2 receptor stimulation, which cause suppression of the Ca^{2+} current, is identical; the same result is obtained using Ca^{2+} channel blockers. In some instances, β-adrenoceptor blockade with a short-acting drug like esmolol, or M_2 activation and/or Na/K pump inhibition with a cardiac glycoside, can be tried when the initial approaches fail (Zipes, 1992).

Prevention of recurrences includes long-term administration of the types of drugs noted above, as well as with drugs that affect the fast channel-dependent cells in the reentry pathway. These latter drugs act by Na channel blockade and/or by I_K blockade and, in one instance (amiodarone), also by antiadrenergic and slow channel blocking actions. Drugs slowing conduction and prolonging refractoriness in the atrium and the retrogradely conducting fast pathway include quinidine, procainide, and disopyramide. Drugs slowing conduction and prolonging refractoriness in the atrium, fast pathway, and slow pathway include flecainide, propafenone, sotalol (also a β-blocker), and amiodarone. In general, drugs that affect the slow calcium channel are tried first and, if found ineffective, given singly or in combination, the other drugs are then considered.

The drugs that affect fast channel-dependent tissue can have important proarrhythmic potential and it is often worthwhile to consider radiofrequency catheter modification of atrioventricular nodal conduction to totally eliminate atrioventricular nodal reentrant tachycardia prior to instituting therapy with these agents. Further, in many patients who do not wish to take *any* drugs long term, who do not tolerate the drugs because of side effects, or in whom drugs produce incomplete control of the atrioventricular nodal reentrant tachycardia, radiofrequency ablation should be considered as an early option. Increasingly, this form of therapy is being offered as an initial choice for patients with symptomatic atrioventricular nodal reentrant tachycardia since a part of the pathway extrinsic to the atrioventricular node can be safely and reproducibly ablated, successfully eliminating atrioventricular nodal reentrant tachycardia in about 95% of patients (Jackman et al, 1992; Gursoy et al, 1993; Kay et al, 1993; Mitrani et al, 1992).

Premature atrial or ventricular depolarizations are the events initiating atrioventricular nodal reentrant tachycardia in many individuals and, in some instances, suppression of this triggering mechanism may be warranted. Since the electrophysiologic basis of these premature complexes is not clearly established, and can probably be due to reentry, normal/abnormal automaticity, or afterdepolarizations, the ionic currents involved include those noted above plus I_f, I_{Ca-T}, and the various K currents. The drugs listed above would still be the agents chosen, however.

Wolff-Parkinson-White Syndrome

This tachycardia has been detailed in Ch. 7.

Atriofascicular Tachycardias

Substantial electrophysiologic data support the existence of a right-sided atrioventricular communication that has properties different from the usual accessory pathway responsible for the typical atrioventricular reciprocating tachycardia, noted above (Gallagher et al, 1981; Leitch et al, 1990; Benditt, 1990). The atriofascicular accessory pathway bypasses the atrioventricular node, joining the atrium to the distal part of the right bundle branch (less commonly to the ventricular myocardium at the tricuspid annulus when it is called an atrioventricular pathway). The pathway only conducts anterogradely and demonstrates considerable conduction delay during normal sinus rhythm that is increased by premature atrial stimulation or rapid atrial pacing, behaving almost like an atrioventricular node. This pathway does not seem to be part of an atrioventricular nodal structure and, parenthetically, may have been what was originally reported by Kent as a "right lateral bundle" (Kent, 1914). Proof of its independent atrial origin and atrioventricular connection is found in the observation that atrial stimulation during tachycardia fails to preexcite atrial tissue located near the atrioventricular node and recorded in the His bundle, while at the same time preexciting the His bundle and advancing the tachycardia, and the fact that the accessory pathways can be ablated at sites far removed from the atrioventricular node (Haissaguerre et al, 1990; Klein et al, 1993). The tachycardia is antedromic, with critical components formed by anterograde conduction over the atriofascicular accessory pathway and retrograde conduction over the right bundle

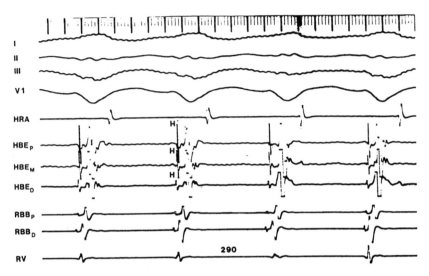

Figure 4. *Recordings from a patient with an atriofascicular accessory pathway. During reciprocating tachycardia using the atriofascicular fiber for anterograde conduction and the His-Purkinje system for retrograde conduction, activation of the distal His bundle precedes that of the proximal His bundle. Note that His-Purkinje activation is retrograde, beginning with the distal right bundle branch, and that activation of the ventricular myocardium at the right ventricular apex is early. HRA: high right atrial electrogram; HBE_P: proximal His bundle electrogram; HBE_M: middle His bundle electrogram; HBE_D: distal His bundle electrogram; RBB_P: proximal right bundle branch; RBB_D: distal right bundle branch; RV: right ventricular apex electrogram recording. Reproduced with permission from Klein LS, Hackett FK, Zipes DP, et al: Radiofrequency catheter ablation of Mahaim fibers at the tricuspid annulus. Circulation 1993; 87:738–747. Copyright 1993 American Heart Association.*

branch to the His bundle and atrioventricular node, and then back to the atrium (Fig. 4).

The approach is as discussed above for atrioventricular reciprocating tachycardia, with the exception that the accessory connection can also be blocked in some patients by drugs such as adenosine, calcium blockers, and β-blockers that do not affect the usual Wolff-Parkinson-White accessory pathway. This observation would suggest that the accessory pathway in these patients has slow channel-dependent tissue. Radiofrequency ablation is a very effective choice.

Long RP Interval Tachycardias

Sinus Node Reentry

The electrophysiologic basis of sinus node reentry is thought to be reentry within the sinus node, between the sinus node and contiguous atrium, or within the atrium located very close to the sinus node (Zipes, 1992). Which one or more of these possibilities exist has not been clearly established, and conceivably could vary from patient to patient. Since the actual pathways of the tachycardia are not known, the critical components of the tachycardia circuit cannot be established with any certainty, but are probably comprised of Ca-dependent slow channel tissue in the sinus node and Na-dependent fast channel tissue in the atrium. Depending on the pathways of the tachycardia, the ionic currents could include both fast- and slow channel-dependent components. Despite these uncertainties, therapeutic approaches are those outlined for atrioventricular nodal reentrant tachycardia above.

Inappropriate Sinus Tachycardia

There exist a group of patients who have a persistent sinus tachycardia that is inappropriately fast for their physical activity level. Minimal physical exertion accelerates the sinus rates still further. Carotid sinus massage slows the sinus rate slightly but it quickly speeds back to its former rate. Adenosine also produces gradual sinus slowing and then speeding as the drug effects wear off. Thus, the rhythm behaves as an automatic focus, and probably represents an acceleration of normal automaticity. In some, but not all, patients, the problem arises after cardiac surgery for atrioventricular nodal reentrant tachycardia or atrioventricular reciprocating tachycardia. In others, it occurs after radiofrequency ablation delivered to the posterior portion of the atrioventricular node for elimination of conduction in the slow atrioventricular nodal pathway or over a posteroseptal accessory pathway (Kocovic et al, 1992). One may speculate that it represents loss of the vagal innervation that normally restrains sinus node automaticity.

The critical component of the tachycardia is the sinus node and the ionic current involved may be I_{Ca-L} or other ionic components of the sinus node pacemaker such as I_f. Clinically, the most useful drugs generally are the β-adrenoceptor blockers and the calcium channel blockers.

Atrial Tachycardia

The electrophysiologic mechanisms responsible for most atrial tachycardias are not yet known and could be reentry, normal/abnormal automaticity, or afterdepolarizations (Garson et al, 1990). In patients with digitalis-induced atrial tachycardia, delayed afterdepolarizations may be operative. Thus, the critical component of the substrate is the atrium, but the ionic targets will vary, depending on alterations in the substrate and the inciting cause. Drugs most likely to be effective are the Na channel blockers, sometimes the Ca channel blockers, and occasionally β-adrenoceptor blockers. Often, slowing the ventricular rate, as with atrial flutter/fibrillation, is all that can be done reasonably and safely. For atrial tachycardias not due to reversible causes, such as digitalis toxicity, radiofrequency ablation is effective in eliminating the tachycardia in 50% to 75% of patients (Kay et al, 1993). Recurrences can result after an apparently successful ablation in 10% to 20% of patients, however.

Permanent Form of Atrioventricular Junctional Reciprocating Tachycardia

This supraventricular tachycardia results from conduction over a slowly conducting accessory pathway and is more properly considered as a variant of the Wolff-Parkinson-White syndrome discussed in Ch. 7. However, because it is a long RP tachycardia, it will be discussed in this section.

The permanent form of junctional reciprocating tachycardia (Coumel et al, 1967) is a reentrant tachycardia characterized by antero-grade conduction over the normal atrioventricular node-His bundle axis and retrograde conduction over the accessory pathway (Zipes, 1992). The accessory pathway conducts very slowly and, therefore, the impulse propagating retrogradely reaches the atrium after considerable delay, inscribing the retrograde P wave in the second half of the cardiac cycle. Thus, the critical components of the circuit are atrium, anterograde conduction over the atrioventricular node-His bundle-ventricle, and then retrograde conduction over the accessory pathway and back to the atrium. Slow conduction in this type of accessory pathway is thought to be due to an anatomically tortuous route taken by the accessory pathway and not slow channel-dependent activation. Nevertheless, slow conduction in the accessory pathway can be blocked in some patients by adenosine or verapamil and improved with isoproterenol, suggesting that propagation over this accessory pathway in some instances might be slow channel dependent.

The tachycardia is usually present 80% to 90% of the time and, therefore, brief interruption, as described for acute termination of atrioventricular nodal reentrant tachycardia and atrioventricular reciprocating tachycardia, is only transiently successful. Long-term drug prevention of permanent junctional reciprocating tachycardia can be targeted against Ca-dependent conduction in the atrioventricular node (and possibly the accessory pathway) with the drugs outlined Ch. 5, Figure 1 or Na-dependent conduction in the accessory pathway with Na channel blockers. Drugs such as amiodarone, sotalol, flecainide, and propafenone can affect conduction in both structures. In many patients, probably the majority, radiofrequency ablation of the accessory pathway is the preferred treatment. Success of this therapy reflects the recognition of a different vulnerable parameter. Finally, some patients can have multiple accessory pathways (Shih et al, in press).

Atypical Atrioventricular Nodal Reentry

The mechanism responsible for atypical atrioventricular nodal reentrant tachycardia is reentry, as it is for the usual form of atrioventricular nodal reentrant tachycardia discussed earlier. However, in atypical atrioventricular nodal reentrant tachycardia, the impulse travels in a direction opposite to that of typical atrioventricular nodal reentrant tachycardia, i.e., anterogradely over the fast atrioventricular nodal pathway and retrogradely over the slow atrioventricular nodal pathway, causing the retrograde P wave to be inscribed in the second half of the cardiac cycle. Some evidence suggests that an occasional patient can have multiple atrioventricular nodal pathways and have tachycardia sustained by reentry over two slow pathways, so-called slow-slow atrioventricular nodal reentrant tachycardia. The retrograde P wave may be midcycle in this tachycardia. The vulnerable parameters and approach to therapy for atypical atrioventricular nodal reentrant tachycardia are as outlined for typical atrioventricular nodal reentrant tachycardia.

Chapter 10

Atrial Flutter and Atrial Fibrillation:
Mechanisms

Atrial flutter is defined as a rapid (rate ≥ 240 beats/min), very regular atrial rhythm found in paroxysmal or chronic persistent forms (Wells et al, 1979). Classical or Type I atrial flutter occurs at rates from 240 beats/min to 340 beats/min, and Type II atrial flutter at rates greater than 340 beats/min (Wells et al, 1979). Atrial fibrillation is a rapid (rate >250 beats/min and usually in the range of 380 to 450 beats/min), irregular atrial rhythm (Wells et al, 1978). The classical definitions and observations concerning both arrhythmias are electrocardiographic (Katz and Pick, 1956). Despite the major effort expended in studying these rhythms electrocardiographically, surprisingly little is known about either the mechanism of onset or the mechanism of maintenance of either arrhythmia in patients. It is anticipated that recent advances in cardiac activation mapping techniques will permit studies in patients that should provide critical data to unravel these mechanisms. However, at present, we are left largely to extrapolating from studies in experimental models (principally animal models, although computer models, too, have been studied). Until recently, most such models have been of atrial flutter, as reliable models of atrial fibrillation have been difficult to create.

From *Antiarrhythmic Therapy: A Pathophysiologic Approach* edited by Members of the Sicilian Gambit © 1994, Futura Publishing Co., Inc., Armonk, NY.

Type I Atrial Flutter

Mechanisms, Critical Components, and Vulnerable Parameters of the Ongoing Tachycardia

It is widely accepted that classical (Type I) atrial flutter in patients is due to reentry, with the reentrant circuit being confined to the right atrium (Waldo, 1987). Based on a series of catheter electrode mapping studies beginning in the late 1950s by Puech and colleagues (Puech, 1956; Puech et al, 1970) and continuing to the present, it is thought by some that the atrial flutter reentrant circuit travels cranially up the intraatrial septum on the right side, goes up the truncus intercavarum, then turns caudally in the crista terminalis, and then travels around the inferior vena cava to turn back up (cranially) the interatrial septum (Fig. 1). In this circuit, the central area of block in part consists of the

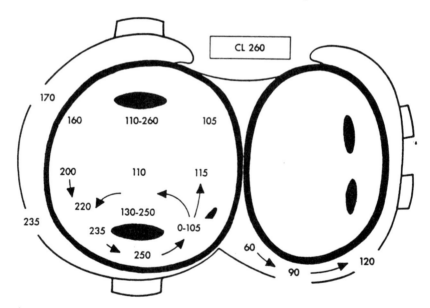

Figure 1. *Activation map of the typical reentrant circuit in patients with classical (Type I) atrial flutter. The arrows indicate the general direction of the circulating reentrant wavefront. See text for discussion. Reproduced with permission from Cosio FG: Endocardial mapping of atrial flutter. In Touboul P, Waldo AL (eds): Atrial Arrhythmias. St. Louis, MO: Mosby Year Book, 1990, pp. 229–240.*

orifice of the inferior vena cava and an area of functional block between the inferior vena caval orifice and the truncus intercavarum. Also, at least one area of slow conduction, thought to be functional, exists inferiorly and posteriorly in this circuit in an area bounded by the tricuspid valve orifice, the coronary sinus, and perhaps the inferior vena cava (Cosio, 1990; Cosio et al, 1993). The precise location and actual extent of this area of slow conduction is uncertain. Of note, no animal model with this reentrant circuit has been described, although based on sequential site mapping of a very few sites, Sir Thomas Lewis and colleagues (1920) concluded that the reentrant wavefront in induced atrial flutter in a normal canine heart sometimes coursed around the anatomic obstacles of both the superior vena caval and inferior vena caval orifices.

Most recently, it has been suggested that the atrial reentrant circuit for atrial flutter in some patients may be the tricuspid valve ring (Waldo, 1987). That such a reentrant circuit should be possible comes from the studies of Frame and colleagues (Frame et al, 1986 and 1987) in the canine heart, which showed that following creation of a "Y" lesion in the right atrial free wall (Fig. 2), atrial flutter due to reentry around the tricuspid ring can be initiated and sustained (Fig. 3). This model clearly has an anatomic obstacle, the tricuspid valve orifice, around which the reentrant wavefront circulates; but of note, conduction velocity around the tricuspid ring is uniform; i.e., there is no described area of slow conduction. Clinical counterparts for this atrial flutter mechanism have been suggested for patients undergoing surgical correction of congenital cardiac abnormalities in which a Mustard, Senning, or Fontan procedure was performed (Waldo, 1987). Atrial flutter following these procedures is well described (Flinn et al, 1984; Bink-Boelkens et al, 1983), and the surgical incisions in the right atrium mimic in part the "Y" lesion used to create the tricuspid ring reentry model of atrial flutter in the canine heart. Whether reentry around the tricuspid ring occurs in patients in the apparent absence of overtly large lesions in the right atrial free wall, i.e., whether tricuspid ring reentry is a major mechanism of atrial flutter in patients, is an important question that, at present, is unanswered. In this regard, it is noteworthy that Lewis et al (1920) proposed that atrial flutter could be due to reentry around the mitral valve annulus in their canine model. This latter conclusion, too, suffers from the considerable limitations of the small number of sites mapped sequentially.

Finally, with regard to lesions created in the atria to facilitate

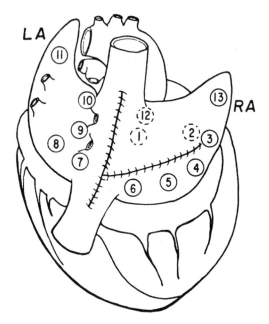

Figure 2. *This diagram of the heart viewed from the right posterior oblique projection shows the location of the Y-shaped lesion to create the model of Frame et al (1986 and 1987). The intercaval lesion extends from the superior vena cava to the inferior vena cava, and another lesion extends from the intercaval lesion across the right atrium towards the right atrial appendage. Each number indicates the position of a bipolar pair of electrodes. LA: left atrial appendage; RA: right atrial appendage. Reproduced with permission from Frame LH, Page RL, Hoffman BF: Atrial reentry around an anatomic barrier with a partially refractory excitable gap. A canine model of atrial flutter. Circ Res 1986; 58:495–511. Copyright 1986 American Heart Association.*

induction and maintenance of atrial flutter, it is clear that if a lesion includes a long enough obstacle, either as an extension of an anatomic obstacle like the superior vena cava, as shown by Rosenblueth and Garcia Ramos (1947) and later confirmed by Kimura and colleagues (1954), or as a "freestanding" lesion in the right atrium, as shown by several groups (Boineau et al, 1980; Inoue et al, 1981; Shimizu et al, 1991a; Feld et al, 1992; Yamashita et al, 1992), atrial flutter can be induced. While much can and has been learned from such models, it is probable that this mechanism represents an infrequent mechanism of atrial flutter in patients.

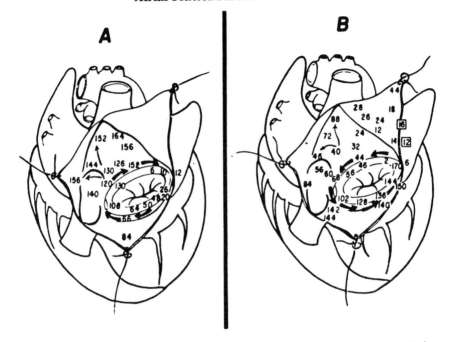

Figure 3. *Endocardial activation times recorded at the right atrium during atrial flutter while the heart is on total cardiopulmonary bypass. Panel A shows a clockwise activation sequence around the ring of the tricuspid valve orifice. Panel B shows a counterclockwise activation sequence around the ring of the tricuspid valve orifice. Reproduced with permission from Frame LH, Page RL, Hoffman BF: Atrial reentry around an anatomic barrier with a partially refractory excitable gap. A canine model of atrial flutter. Circ Res 1986; 58:495–511. Copyright 1986 American Heart Association.*

There are several other animal models of atrial flutter with uncertain, but likely, clinical counterparts. Boyden and Hoffman (1981) have developed a canine right atrial enlargement model of atrial flutter by banding the pulmonary artery and creating tricuspid regurgitation. These animals are left to recover and, after a period of eight to 12 weeks, atrial flutter due to reentry in the right atrial free wall can be induced easily and reliably. It might be expected that this model has a clinical counterpart in patients with tricuspid regurgitation or chronic obstructive pulmonary disease, both of which are well appreciated to be associated with an important incidence of atrial flutter (and atrial fibrillation as well). In this model, the central area of block around which the reentrant wavefront circulates is functional, as are areas of slow conduction in the reentrant circuit (Boyden, 1988). Of note, in vitro microelectrode studies of atrial tissues from this model have failed to demonstrate abnormal transmembrane resting or action potentials to explain the vulnerability of the atria in this model to atrial flutter (Boyden et al, 1982).

Yet another relevant model is that of atrial flutter induced by sterile pericarditis in dogs (Pagé et al, 1986). This model is based on the high incidence of atrial flutter in patients following open heart surgery and the fact that the incidence of atrial flutter (and atrial fibrillation) in these patients follows the time course of the sterile pericarditis that occurs as a result of the surgery. In the canine sterile pericarditis model, atrial flutter is due to reentry in the right atrial free wall. Importantly, the reentrant circuit is functionally determined, has a fully excitable gap, and appears to be of the anisotropic reentrant type (Shimizu et al, 1991b and 1991c; Niwano et al, in press). No study has yet shown that atrial flutter in patients following open heart surgery is due to the same mechanism as shown in this canine model. If atrial flutter in patients does occur due to reentry in the right atrial free wall, it is unclear whether this location of this reentrant circuit is limited to patients with pericarditis.

Two other canine models of atrial flutter due to reentry are of note. Allessie and colleagues (1984) infused acetylcholine into the atria of a Langendorff-perfused preparation, and were able to initiate atrial flutter caused by a single reentrant circuit that was shown to be present circulating either around one of the atrial appendages or circulating inferiorly in the left or right atrium (Fig. 4). Importantly, atrial flutter in this model was of a very short cycle length, usually ≤100 milliseconds, causing Allessie et al (1984) to suggest that this might represent a Type II atrial flutter. Finally, a canine mitral regurgitation model of atrial flutter has been presented (Cox et al, 1991), although more detailed mapping data are required before the nature of the atrial flutter can be stated. Nevertheless, it does appear that functionally determined reentry in the right atrium, and probably in the right atrial free wall, is present in this model.

The final model to be discussed is atrial flutter secondary to exposure to aconitine at a localized atrial site. These studies, first done by Scherf and colleagues (1947, 1949, and 1958) and repeated by others (Kimura et al, 1954; Brown and Acheson, 1952), demonstrated that

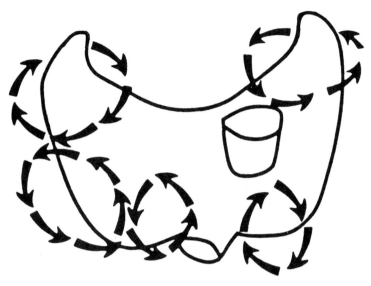

Figure 4. *Demonstration of the location and direction of circus movement in six different examples of atrial flutter induced by Allessie and colleagues in a canine acetylcholine infusion model of atrial flutter. Reproduced with permission from Allessie MA, Lammers WJEP, Bonke FIM, Hollen J: Intraatrial reentry as a mechanism for atrial flutter induced by acetylcholine in rapid pacing in the dog. Circulation 1984; 70:123–135. Copyright 1984 American Heart Association.*

an arrhythmia electrocardiographically similar to atrial flutter could be induced by a single focus firing rapidly. As summarized recently (Cranefield and Aronson, 1988), only in recent years has it become apparent that aconitine causes early afterdepolarizations in Purkinje fibers and ventricular tissue. However, limited studies of rabbit atria (Goto et al, 1967; Azuma et al, 1969) did not find early afterdepolarizations, but did find an increased rate, suggesting enhanced phase 4 depolarization. Realistically, while aconitine clearly is not a substance found in the atria of patients, it does demonstrate that a single focus firing rapidly (automatic, triggered, or microreentrant) might be responsible for atrial flutter. This idea must be tempered by the fact that radiofrequency ablation has successfully terminated/prevented atrial flutter in patients via lesions placed in the region of the coronary sinus or between the inferior vena cava and tricuspid ring. The success of such ablation is consistent with reentry, as proposed by Mines (1914). Nevertheless, there may be more than one mechanism for the clinical rhythm we call atrial flutter.

How does this information tie into the Sicilian Gambit approach to treatment of atrial flutter? For ongoing atrial flutter, it is important to establish that the rhythm is due to reentry. One way to identify reentry is to confirm the presence of a reentrant circuit during atrial activation mapping. Although simultaneous multisite mapping (difficult to do) is preferable, to date, in patients, this has generally meant some form of sequential site atrial mapping. Unfortunately, this, too, is presently quite difficult to do in patients. Furthermore, even with simultaneous multisite mapping, there must be a sufficient number of electrode recording sites to achieve the resolution needed to identify and localize the reentrant circuit. Finally, we must again remember the admonition of Mines (1914) that simply demonstrating a probable reentrant circuit is not sufficient in and of itself to confirm a reentrant mechanism. Rather, it must be demonstrated that a lesion properly placed in the reentrant circuit terminates the rhythm and prevents its reinduction.

The most practical and reliable method to identify reentry in patients is to demonstrate entrainment during rapid pacing (Waldo et al, 1977; Waldo et al, 1983; Waldo et al, 1984; Okumura et al, 1985; Okumura et al, 1987; Henthorn et al, 1988; Waldecker et al, 1993; Shimizu et al, 1991b; Waldo and Wit, 1994). If during and following rapid pacing any of four established criteria (Table 1) are demonstrated, a reentrant mechanism is established, as these criteria can be explained only on the basis of reentry. Unfortunately, this technique may be limited because entrainment of a tachyarrhythmia may occur, but may be concealed, i.e., none of the entrainment criteria may be demonstrated (Okumura, et al, 1985; Waldo and Henthorn, 1989; Waldo and Wit, 1994). Formerly, the ability to initiate or terminate a tachycardia with either premature beats or rapid pacing was thought to be sufficient to identify a reentrant mechanism (Waldo, 1987). However, it is now clear that these responses to pacing also are consistent with a triggered mechanism (Moak and Rosen, 1984; Johnson et al, 1986; Wit et al, 1981; Waldo and Wit, 1994). Because the great majority of clinically important tachyarrhythmias are due to reentry, many still use the simple initiation or termination of a tachycardia by pacing as an indication of reentry, recognizing the inherent limitations described above.

Table 1
Criteria to Establish the Presence of Transient Entrainment

1. The demonstration of constant fusion beats in the electrocardiogram during the period of rapid pacing at a constant rate, except for the last captured beat, which is entrained but not fused (i.e., the last entrained beat demonstrates the electrocardiogram morphology of the spontaneous tachycardia).
2. The demonstration of progressive fusion; i.e., constant fusion beats in the electrocardiogram during rapid pacing at any constant rate, but different degrees of constant fusion at different rapid rates.
3. The demonstration that interruption of the tachycardia is associated with localized conduction block to a site(s) for one beat, followed by subsequent activation of that site(s) from a different direction, manifested by a change in morphology of the electrogram at the blocked site(s), and with a shorter conduction time.
4. The demonstration of a change in conduction time and electrogram morphology at one recording site when pacing from another site at two different constant pacing rates, each of which is faster than the spontaneous rate of the tachycardia but fails to interrupt it (electrogram equivalent of progressive fusion).

Having established or assumed that reentry is present, the Sicilian Gambit approach to therapy requires that the critical components of the reentrant circuit be considered and their potential vulnerability to therapeutic intervention also be considered. The critical components of reentrant circuits include: a wavelength; a path length; a central area of block (anatomic, functional, or a combination) around which the reentrant wavefront circulates; one or more areas of slow conduction (except perhaps as in the tricuspid ring reentrant model); and an excitable gap (without which headtail interaction of the circulating reentrant wavefront would terminate reentrant excitation) which may be fully or partially excitable. These critical components of the reentrant circuit are not equally vulnerable to an ultimate drug intervention to terminate ongoing atrial flutter. For a long time, it has been known that when the wavelength of reentrant excitation exceeds the path length, reentrant excitation ceases (Waldo and Wit, 1994). Therefore, the excitable gap has been considered a vulnerable parameter. A drug that prolongs refractoriness without affecting conduction velocity should increase the wavelength until it equals or exceeds the path length and extinguishes the reentrant excitation. However, in most reentrant circuits, conduction velocity is not uniform, and the properties of refractoriness and conduction usually vary nonuniformly (Spinelli and Hoffman, 1989; Niwano et al, 1993 and in press; Waldecker et al, 1993). Furthermore, in the canine pericarditis model, drugs with markedly different effects on refractoriness and conduction velocity such as quinidine (Okumura and Waldo, 1987), flecainide (Scalabrini et al, 1986), moricizine (Ortiz et al, 1994), N-acetylprocainamide (Okumura et al, 1987), and ouabain (Nozaki et al, 1989) all have been shown to interrupt flutter by causing block of the circulating reentrant wavefront in an area of slow conduction. This occurs after an initial prolongation of cycle length caused by slowing of conduction in an area of slow conduction. Thus, for this model, the notion that manipulating the wavelength will interrupt atrial flutter does not seem to hold. More recent studies (Niwano et al, 1993 and in press; Ortiz et al, 1994) strongly point to a failure of the safety factor for conduction localized to an area of slow conduction in the reentrant circuit as the explanation rather than the traditional wavelength concepts.

The same is true for the tricuspid ring reentry model of atrial flutter. In this model, several mechanisms of interruption of reentry have been described (Spinelli and Hoffman, 1989; Boyden and Graziano, 1993a and 1993b; Pinto et al, 1993), but none is in accord with the traditional concept of how drug manipulation of the wavelength would compromise (i.e., eliminate) the excitable gap. Thus, in this model, interruption of reentrant excitation can occur either as the result of reflection induced by drug therapy, which eliminates the excitable gap (Fig. 5), or because of slowing of conduction due to drug administration that either breaks down lateral boundaries and permits short circuiting and elimination of the excitable gap (Fig. 6), or initiates cycle length oscillation so that a critical long-short cycle eliminates the excitable gap (Frame and Simson, 1988) or decreases the safety factor for conduction.

Antiarrhythmic drug therapy has been studied using simultaneous, multisite mapping techniques in a right atrial free wall crush lesion model (Feld et al, 1992). In this model, sotalol interrupted the atrial flutter at a pivot point in the reentrant circuit. Surprisingly, no area of slow conduction was described for this model. However, we suspect that areas of relatively slow conduction are present at the pivot points for two reasons. First, studies in a cryolesion model of atrial flutter (Shimizu et al, 1991a) in which electrograms were recorded from 190 electrodes in the vicinity of the reentrant circuit, also described in the cardiac sterile pericarditis model, showed slow

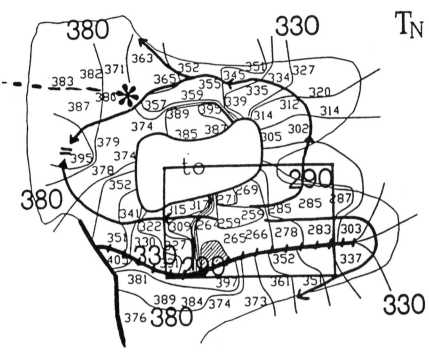

Figure 5. *Right atrial endocardial activation map of beat T_n showing termination of atrial flutter in the tricuspid ring reentry canine model following administration of flecainide. Each number represents activation time at a pair of recording electrodes. The diagram shows the right atrium opened along the intercaval lesion and along the superior portion of the atrium to the tip of the appendage. The location of the Y-shaped lesion along the intercaval area and across the anterior wall of the right atrium is indicated by the thick solid and hatched lines. In this example, termination results because of a form of reflection (return reexcitation) of the activation wavefront that occurred during the previous beat (not shown). This became possible because of changes in conduction (marked slowing and unidirectional block) in the reentrant circuit as a result of flecainide administration. to: tricuspid orifice. Modified with permission from Pinto JMB, Graziano JN, Boyden PA: Endocardial mapping of reentry around an anatomical barrier in the canine right atrium: Observations during the action of the class IC agent, flecainide. J Cardiovasc Electrophysiol 1993; 4:672–685.*

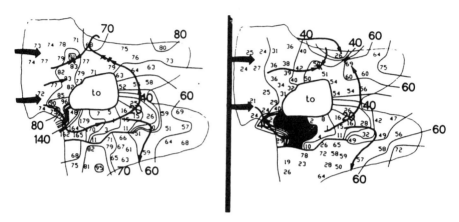

Figure 6. *Right atrial endocardial activation maps of the last two beats (left and right panels) of atrial flutter in the tricuspid ring reentry canine model following administration of d-sotalol. Other aspects of the diagram are the same as shown in Figure 5. In this example, termination occurs because of slowing of conduction associated with failure of lateral boundaries following administration of d-sotalol. This permitted the large, broad excitatory wavefront (large broad arrows) first to reset the atrial flutter (left panel) and then terminate it (right panel). Modified with permission from Boyden PA, Graziano JN: Multiple modes of termination of re-entrant excitation around an anatomic barrier in the canine atrium during the action of d-sotalol. Eur Heart J 1993; 14(suppl H):41–49.*

conduction at the cryolesion pivot points of the reentrant circuit. Because in both the cryolesion and crush lesion models the length of the atrial lesion is the critical factor for induction and maintenance of atrial flutter, and the lengths of the lesions were quite similar, it is reasonable to predict that areas of slow conduction might be present at the pivot points in the crush lesion model, too. Second, the study of Feld and Shahandeh-Rad (1992) only used simultaneous recordings from 56 electrodes, significantly decreasing the resolution of the resulting activation map (Dillon et al, 1988).

In sum, during atrial flutter in experimental models, an area of slow conduction in the reentrant circuit is a vulnerable parameter; slowing of conduction in the reentrant circuit to permit short circuiting is another vulnerable parameter; and provocation or exaggeration of cycle length alternans that permits either short circuiting because of breakdown of lateral boundaries or head-tail interaction of the reentrant wavefront is still another vulnerable parameter.

No studies similar to those in animal models have been performed yet in patients. Hence, it seems obvious that

1. appropriate studies during atrial flutter in patients are required;
2. vulnerable parameters may be different depending on whether the reentrant circuit is completely functional or partly anatomic and partly functional;
3. conduction in functionally determined areas of slow conduction must be better understood, ultimately at the molecular level (channels, receptors, etc.), so that targets ripe for drug therapy can be selected; and
4. consideration must be given to the possibility that atrial flutter might be due to a single focus firing rapidly (as suggested by Scherf et al, 1947, 1949, and 1958; Brown and Acheson, 1952; Kimura et al, 1954).

Mechanisms, Critical Components, and Vulnerable Parameters of the Onset of the Tachycardia

Although the prevention of atrial flutter is an important reason for initiating drug therapy, the onset of flutter in patients has not been thoroughly studied. However, there are data that indicate that atrial flutter in patients develops after a transitional period of variable duration of atrial fibrillation. These data come principally from studies of the spontaneous onset of atrial flutter in patients following open heart surgery (Waldo and Cooper, preliminary data) and of induced atrial flutter in patients during clinical cardiac electrophysiologic studies during cardiac catheterization (Watson and Josephson, 1980). These observations are consistent with the onset of atrial flutter in all experimental models, beginning with studies in the laboratory of Sir Thomas Lewis (Lewis et al, 1920), in which atrial flutter was induced by a period (usually brief) of very rapid atrial pacing. Mapping studies in the canine sterile pericarditis model of the pacing-induced onset of atrial flutter using an eight-beat train followed by one or two premature beats or very rapid atrial pacing have shown that for atrial flutter to evolve, conditions in the atrial tissue substrate have to develop (because they are not inherently already present) during the transitional rhythm (atrial fibrillation) that results ultimately in the development of slow conduction, unidirectional block, and an obstacle (functional block in this model) around which the reentrant wavefront can circulate (Shimizu et al, 1991c) (Figs. 7 and 8). Also critical is the development of a long enough central area of block to permit stable atrial flutter to evolve (Shimizu et al, 1991c; Ortiz et al, 1994). To the extent that these data can be extrapolated to patients, more detailed knowl-

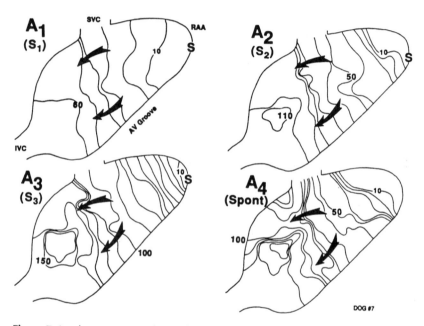

Figure 7. *Isochronous maps during the onset of atrial flutter in the canine pericarditis model induced by an eight-beat drive train (S₁) followed by two premature beats (S₂ and S₃, respectively 300/130/80 ms) delivered from the right atrial appendage (RAA) at site S. Isochrones are displayed at 10-ms intervals. Arrows indicate the direction of the main activation wavefront. Beats A₁, A₂, and A₃ represent isochronous maps corresponding to S₁, S₂, and S₃, respectively. Beat A₁ (S₁) was the last driven beat at a cycle length of 300 ms. Beat A₂ (S₂) was the first premature beat. Beat A₃ (S₃) was the second premature beat. In beats A₂ and A₃, radial activation preceded from the pacing site, and crowding of 10 ms isochrones developed in some areas. In beat A₄, the first spontaneous (Spont) beat, the earliest activated area was close to the pacing site. SVC: superior vena cava; IVC: inferior vena cava; AV: atrioventricular. Reproduced with permission from Shimizu A, Nozaki A, Rudy Y, Waldo AL: Onset of induced atrial flutter in the canine pericarditis model. J Am Coll Cardiol 1991; 17:1223–1234.*

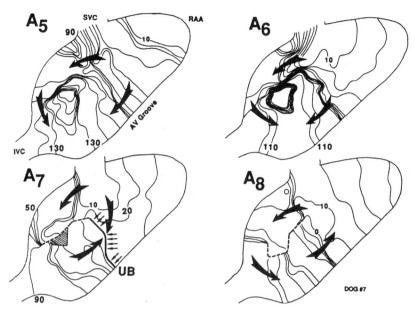

Figure 8. *Continuation of the sequence of activation from Figure 7. Beats A5 to A8 represent subsequent spontaneous beats. Beats A5 and A6 showed development of the areas of slow conduction along the sulcus terminalis and in the pectinate muscle region. With beat A7, unidirectional block (UB) (solid thick black line) of the inferior wavefront occurred at the pectinate muscle region in the area of slow conduction. Then, the nonblocked superior activation wavefront conducted around a line of functional block (dashed lines) and through an area of slow conduction close to the inferior vena cava to conduct through the areas of unidirectional block from the opposite direction. The shaded area represents an area of localized block. Beat A8 was the first spontaneous atrial flutter beat, which traveled counterclockwise around an area of functional block (dashed line) at a cycle length of 152 ms. Abbreviations identical to Figure 7. Reproduced with permission from Shimizu A, Nozaki A, Rudy Y, Waldo AL: Onset of induced atrial flutter in the canine pericarditis model. J Am Coll Cardiol 1991;17:1223–1234.*

edge is needed to explain what occurs to permit the functional development of localized regions of slow conduction, unidirectional block, and a line of block. Only after we have such information can drug therapy directed at appropriate targets be selected. Obviously, factors contributing to the initiation and termination of atrial flutter may be quite similar or quite different.

Type II Atrial Flutter

To date, there have been very few studies of Type II atrial flutter. As a result, identification of critical components and vulnerable parameters is difficult. This rhythm in patients is very rapid (>340 beats/min, range 340 to 430 beats/min) (Fig. 9), and it cannot be interrupted with rapid atrial pacing (Wells et al, 1979; Waldo and MacLean, 1980). It is unclear if there is an experimental counterpart, although Allessie et al (1984) suggested that the atrial flutter in their canine acetylcholine model might be such a counterpart because of its very short cycle length. Atrial flutter in the latter model is thought to be due to leading circle type reentry (Allessie et al, 1973, 1976 and 1977). If this were to be the mechanism of clinical Type II atrial flutter, then the excitable

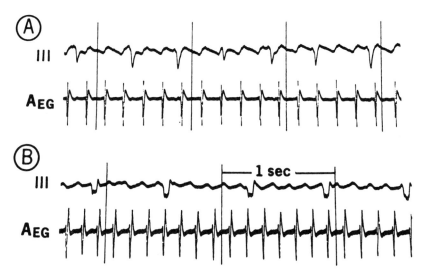

Figure 9. *A and B. Both demonstrate the simultaneous recording of electrocardiogram lead III and a bipolar atrial electrogram (A_{EG}) during Type I atrial flutter with an atrial rate of 296 beats/min (usual rate range 240 to 340 beats/min) (A) and Type II atrial flutter and a rate of 420 beats/min (usual range 380 to 430 beats/min) (B). In each example, note the constant beat-to-beat cycle length, polarity, morphology, and amplitude of recorded atrial electrogram signal characteristic of atrial flutter. Modified with permission from Wells JL Jr, MacLean WAH, James TN, Waldo AL: Characterization of atrial flutter. Studies in man after open heart surgery using fixed atrial electrodes. Circulation 1979; 60:665. Copyright 1979 American Heart Association.*

gap of the reentrant circuit would be very short, and the effective refractory period would be expected to be the vulnerable parameter.

It appears that the mechanisms for this very rapid form of atrial flutter also may contribute to atrial fibrillation. Recently, Waldo and Cooper (preliminary data) have obtained evidence in patients following open heart surgery that suggests that Type II atrial flutter with a very short cycle length can drive the atria at a rate so rapid that the remainder of the atria cannot follow with 1:1 activation. The result is atrial fibrillation. This notion is also consistent with the recent work of Schuessler et al (1992), demonstrating a stable figure of eight reentrant circuit of very short cycle length in the inferior right atrial free wall of an in vitro canine atrial preparation superfused with acetylcholine. In this example, the cycle length of the reentrant circuit was so short that the rest of the atrial tissue could not follow with 1:1 activation, resulting in what reasonably could be called atrial fibrillation.

Atrial Fibrillation

This arrhythmia has been recognized for some nine decades, and it is a clinically common and important tachycardia. Yet, surprisingly little is known about its mechanism. Just as for atrial flutter, this is in part due to the difficulty in mapping the sequence of atrial activation during this arrhythmia in patients, and in part due to limitations in the few available animal models.

Probably the first reliable animal model of atrial fibrillation was the aconitine model of Scherf and colleagues (Scherf, 1947, 1949, and 1953). Atrial fibrillation in this model is due to the placement of aconitine on an atrial site that then fires so rapidly that the rest of the atrial tissue cannot follow with 1:1 activation. Instead, the rapid rate produces an irregular but rapid response that, in turn, generates heterogeneities in conduction and refractoriness in the atrial tissue. With the isolation or cooling of the aconitine focus, the atrial fibrillation almost always stops (Scherf et al, 1947, 1949, and 1958; Kimura et al, 1954; Moe and Abildskov, 1959). The concept that a focus, constant or moving, that generates a very rapid rate due to any mechanism (automaticity, early or delayed afterdepolarizations, reentry, or pacing) may be responsible for the initiation and maintenance of atrial fibrillation clearly is not new. However, only recently has additional evidence been generated from studies in animal models and even patients to indicate that this concept may be operative.

Until recently, it had been assumed that atrial fibrillation was due to random reentry of multiple, simultaneously circulating reentrant wavelets. This latter theory was proposed by Moe and Abildskov (1959), and was demonstrated to be operative in a computer model of atrial fibrillation (Moe et al, 1964). Then, in the last decade, Allessie and colleagues (1982 and 1984) infused acetylcholine into an isolated, Langendorff-perfused canine atrial model and, using simultaneous multisite mapping techniques, demonstrated that atrial fibrillation was due to several (≥5) simultaneously circulating random reentrant wavelets of the leading circle type. It is suspected, but as yet not demonstrated, that chronic atrial fibrillation is most often due to this mechanism. However, initial mapping studies in the sterile pericarditis atrial fibrillation model (Ortiz et al, 1993 and 1994), which appears to be a model of paroxysmal fibrillation, have suggested that atrial fibrillation may be due to one or two unstable reentrant circuits that generate very short cycle lengths while meandering across the right atrial free wall, briefly disappearing and then reforming. Those cycle lengths are so short that the rest of the atrial tissue cannot follow with 1:1 activation. This induces atrial fibrillation, which is maintained by the same mechanism, and which terminates when the unstable reentrant circuit disappears and fails to reform. Although it is not established that this sequence of events occurs in patients, Cox et al (1991) have provided some intraoperative electrophysiologic mapping evidence consistent with that notion. Thus, it seems reasonable to propose a continuum of mechanisms from one or occasionally two reentrant circuits of very short cycle lengths largely responsible for paroxysmal atrial fibrillation to multiple reentrant wavelets simultaneously circulating during chronic atrial fibrillation.

Additionally, the electrophysiologic properties of the atria can vary over time as a result of the continuous rapid rates generated during atrial fibrillation. These properties must be characterized in greater detail. For instance, the recent studies of atrial fibrillation in goats by Wijffels and colleagues (1993) have shown that following return to sinus rhythm after several days of atrial fibrillation, the atrial effective refractory period is dramatically shortened to <100 milliseconds, just as occurs during pacing-induced atrial fibrillation during infusion of acetylcholine in Langendorff-perfused canine hearts (Allessie et al, 1982 and 1985). Thus, in chronic atrial fibrillation, a very short atrial effective refractory period may be a critical component for the maintenance of fibrillation and, therefore, may be a vulnerable parameter for antiarrhythmic drug therapy. In sum, all these models appear to be important and relevant for understanding atrial fibrillation in patients. As we learn more about atrial fibrillation from these models, it will help us greatly to understand atrial fibrillation in patients. Furthermore, there is a need to study this arrhythmia systematically in patients to provide more information about the critical components and vulnerable parameters that support its onset and maintenance.

Nevertheless, there are some aspects of atrial fibrillation that presently lend themselves to a Sicilian Gambit approach to prevention and treatment of atrial fibrillation. For example, there is a category of patients in whom the atrial fibrillation is vagally mediated (Coumel, 1992). In such patients, a critical component is the increased vagal tone with its, in this case, adverse effects on the atria (assumed to be the resulting short action potential duration and short effective refractory period). For such patients, antiarrhythmic drugs that are parasympatholytic may be indicated because of the critical role of vagal tone. Also, there are some forms of atrial fibrillation that, although rare, are adrenergically mediated (Coumel, 1992). In such instances, a critical component is endogenous catecholamine, the vulnerable parameters are the β-receptors in the atria, and the drug therapy is a β-adrenergic blocker.

In sum, for most instances of atrial fibrillation in patients, we appear to be on the verge of obtaining a critical understanding of the mechanism(s) responsible for paroxysmal and chronic fibrillation. This ultimately must be translated into an understanding of the molecular mechanisms responsible, which then will permit identification of targets and of the most appropriate drug therapy.

Chapter 11

Atrial Flutter and Atrial Fibrillation:
Treatment

Management of Atrial Flutter

The discussion below will deal with classical (Type I) atrial flutter. Treatment of Type II atrial flutter has not been well characterized, and it does not appear to be a common, stable, or chronic rhythm. When recognized, it probably should be treated much as one would treat atrial fibrillation. Overall, the treatment of Type I atrial flutter is little different than that for atrial fibrillation with the exception that atrial flutter can be treated with rapid atrial pacing, whereas atrial fibrillation cannot.

Acute Treatment of Atrial Flutter

When the diagnosis of classical (Type I) atrial flutter is established, three options are available to restore sinus rhythm: one, administer antiarrhythmic drug therapy; two, initiate direct current cardioversion; or three, initiate rapid atrial pacing to interrupt atrial flutter. In large measure, the treatment depends on the clinical status of the patient. The preferred option for interrupting atrial flutter is either direct current cardioversion or rapid atrial pacing. Antiarrhythmic drug therapy usually only slows the atrial flutter rate. However,

From *Antiarrhythmic Therapy: A Pathophysiologic Approach* edited by Members of the Sicilian Gambit © 1994, Futura Publishing Co., Inc., Armonk, NY.

drug therapy may be initiated prior to performing either direct current cardioversion or rapid atrial pacing in order to:

1. slow the ventricular response rate (with either a β-adrenergic blocker, a calcium channel blocker, or digoxin);
2. enhance the efficacy of rapid atrial pacing in restoring sinus rhythm (use of quinidine, procainamide, or disopyramide) (Olshansky et al, 1988; Camm et al, 1980);
3. enhance the likelihood that sinus rhythm will be sustained following effective direct current cardioversion (use of quinidine, procainamide, disopyramide, flecainide, propafenone, sotalol, or amiodarone).

In the first instance, the vulnerable parameter is the atrioventricular nodal action potential, with all three pharmacologic interventions contributing to suppression of calcium-dependent action potentials. In the second and third instances, the effective drugs have, in common, sodium channel blocking effects, and therapy is largely empirical.

For many years, the standard initial treatment of atrial flutter was the aggressive administration of a digitalis preparation, usually intravenously, until the arrhythmia either converted to atrial fibrillation with a slow ventricular response rate or converted to sinus rhythm. This mode of therapy is still acceptable, but is not generally the treatment of choice (Waldo and MacLean, 1980). Whenever rapid control of the ventricular response rate to atrial flutter is desirable, this can readily be accomplished by administering either an intravenous calcium channel blocking agent (e.g., verapamil or diltiazem) or an intravenous β-blocking agent (e.g., esmolol). Administering an antiarrhythmic drug intravenously to convert atrial flutter to sinus rhythm is not recommended because the currently available intravenous antiarrhythmic drugs usually will only slow the atrial flutter rate without interrupting the arrhythmia. There are exceptions to this statement, however (e.g., see Hellestrand, 1988).

Rapid Atrial Pacing or Direct Current Cardioversion as Acute Therapy

Selection of acute therapy for atrial flutter with either direct current cardioversion or atrial pacing will depend on the clinical presenta-

tion of the patient and both the clinical availability and ease of application either of these techniques. Since direct current cardioversion requires administration of an anesthetic agent, this may be undesirable
in some patients. Such individuals are best treated with rapid atrial
pacing to interrupt atrial flutter or with agents to slow the ventricular
response rate. For the patient who develops atrial flutter following
open heart surgery, use of temporary atrial epicardial wire electrodes
to perform rapid atrial pacing and restore sinus rhythm is the treatment of choice (Figs. 1 and 2) (Waldo and MacLean, 1980; Waldo et
al, 1977).

As indicated above, when atrial pacing is performed following
initiation of therapy with procainamide, disopyramide, or quinidine,
there is a very high incidence of successful conversion of atrial flutter
to sinus rhythm without any period of atrial fibrillation (Olshansky

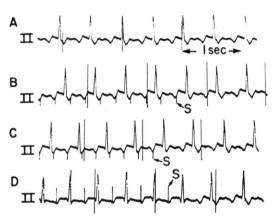

Figure 1. *Electrocardiogram lead II recorded from a patient with classical (Type
I) atrial flutter (atrial cycle length of 264 ms) (Panel A) and at the end of 30 s of
rapid atrial pacing from a high right atrial site at a cycle length of 254 ms (Panel
B), at a cycle length of 242 ms (Panel C), and at a cycle length of 232 ms (Panel
D). The atrial flutter was transiently entrained at each pacing rate. Note that when
comparing the morphology of the atrial complexes during atrial pacing at each
cycle length, especially comparing the atrial complexes during atrial pacing in
Panel D with those in Panels A and B, progressive fusion has occurred. S: stimulus
artifact. Time lines are at 1 s intervals. Modified with permission from Waldo AL,
MacLean WAH, Karp RB, Kouchoukos NT, James TN: Entrainment and interruption of atrial flutter with atrial pacing: Studies in man following open heart surgery.
Circulation 1977; 56:737–745. Copyright 1977 American Heart Association.*

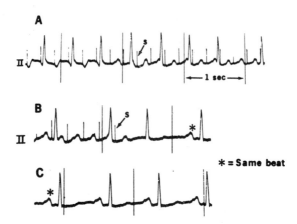

Figure 2. Panel A: Electrocardiogram lead II recorded in the same patient as in Figure 1 during high right atrial pacing from the same site at a cycle length of 224 ms. Note that with the seventh atrial beat in this tracing, and after 22 s of atrial pacing at a constant rate, the atrial complexes suddenly became positive. Panel B: Electrocardiogram lead II recorded at the termination of atrial pacing in the same patient. Note that with abrupt termination of pacing, sinus rhythm occurs. Panel C: The first beat in this panel (asterisk) is identical with the last beat in Panel B (asterisk). S: stimulus artifact. Time lines are at 1 s intervals. Modified with permission from Waldo AL, MacLean WAH, Karp RB, Kouchoukos NT, James TN: Entrainment and interruption of atrial flutter with atrial pacing: Studies in man following open heart surgery. Circulation 1977; 56:737–745. Copyright 1977 American Heart Association.

et al, 1988; Camm et al, 1980). Therefore, when using rapid atrial pacing, administration of one of these agents is recommended. For those patients in whom classical (Type I) atrial flutter recurs despite its successful interruption by rapid atrial pacing, continuous rapid atrial pacing to precipitate and sustain atrial fibrillation may be indicated on a temporary basis in selected patients (Fig. 3) until pharmacologic control of atrial flutter is achieved (Waldo and MacLean, 1980; Waldo et al, 1976).

Direct current cardioversion of atrial flutter to sinus rhythm has a very high likelihood of success. Because 100 J is virtually always successful and virtually never harmful, it should be considered as the initial shock, although as little as 25 J may be effective. The high degree of success with 100 J shocks avoids the need for delivery of a second shock should the first be unsuccessful.

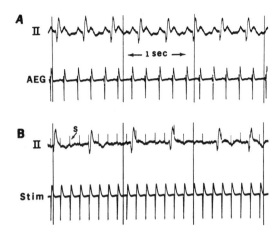

Figure 3. *Panel A demonstrates electrocardiogram lead II recorded simultaneously with a bipolar atrial electrogram during Type I atrial flutter at a rate of 320 beats/min with 2:1 atrioventricular conduction, producing a ventricular rate of 160 beats/min. In this post-open heart surgical patient, the atrial flutter was interrupted successfully on several occasions with rapid atrial pacing. However, the atrial flutter recurred each time. Therefore, as shown in Panel B, continuous rapid atrial pacing at 450 beats/min was initiated. Pacing at this rate precipitated and sustained atrial fibrillation, and was associated with a slowing of the ventricular rate to about 120 beats/min. Digoxin was then administered to slow the ventricular rate still further. Continuous rapid atrial pacing to sustain atrial fibrillation for control of ventricular rate was required for 26 hours in this patient (longer than usual) while antiarrhythmic drug therapy (digoxin and quinidine) was administered. When rapid atrial pacing was finally terminated, atrial fibrillation spontaneously converted to sinus rhythm within several minutes. S: stimulus artifact. Time lines are at 1 s intervals. Modified with permission from Waldo AL, MacLean WAH, Karp RB, Kouchoukos NT, James TN: Continuous rapid atrial pacing to control recurrent or sustained supraventricular tachycardias following open heart surgery. Circulation 1976; 54:245–250. Copyright 1976 American Heart Association.*

Chronic Treatment of Atrial Flutter

For a long time, standard, empirical treatment consisted of administration of quinidine, procainamide, or disopyramide in an effort to prevent recurrence. However, recent studies indicate that flecainide and propafenone are as effective, if not more effective, than the above agents (Anderson et al, 1989; Pritchett et al, 1991). Because of the potential for serious adverse effects (presumably proarrhythmic ventricular tachyarrhythmia) of the drugs used in The Cardiac Arrhythmia Suppression Trial I (CAST I) (The Cardiac Arrhythmia Suppression Trial Investigators, 1989), it is widely acknowledged that flecainide and propafenone should not be given to treat atrial flutter in the presence of underlying ischemic heart disease. However, because of their efficacy, these agents should be considered for long-term suppression of atrial flutter in the absence of structural heart disease. Moricizine also may be effective in the long-term suppression of atrial flutter (Waldo, in press), as may amiodarone and sotalol (Gosselink et al, 1992; Reimold et al, 1993).

It may be quite difficult to suppress atrial flutter completely with drug therapy of any sort. In fact, based on available long-term data, there appears to be a limited ability to maintain sinus rhythm without occasional-to-frequent recurrence of atrial flutter, even when multiple agents are used (NHLBI Working Group, 1993). Thus, when considering drug efficacy, an important measure should be the frequency of recurrences of atrial flutter rather than a single recurrent episode. For instance, recurrence only one time per year probably should be considered quite good therapy.

Permanent Antitachycardia Pacemakers

In selected patients, consideration should be given to implantation of a permanent antitachycardia pacemaker to treat recurrent atrial flutter. Although the published series of patients with these devices has been small, it nevertheless has been shown to be effective in interrupting recurrent atrial flutter (via block of the orthodromic wavefront of the pacing impulse in an area of slow conduction in the atrial flutter reentrant circuit) with return to sinus rhythm (Barold et al, 1987; Goicolea et al, 1992). Thus, in properly selected patients, the ability to interrupt atrial flutter promptly whenever it recurs should provide safe and effective treatment. Since precipitation of atrial fibrillation is always a potential problem when using any form of pacing to treat atrial flutter, placement of a permanent antitachycardia pacemaker to treat atrial flutter should be avoided if episodes of atrial fibrillation are clinically unacceptable. To decrease the likelihood of inadvertent precipitation of atrial fibrillation, chronic use of an antiarrhythmic drug may be desirable (Olshansky et al, 1988; Camm et al, 1980). Also, chronic antiarrhythmic drug therapy may be required to decrease the incidence of recurrent atrial flutter.

Catheter Ablation Therapy

Catheter ablation techniques involve the application of destructive energy, presently either radiofrequency energy or a direct current shock from a cardioverter-defibrillator, delivered to selected portions of the heart via an electrode catheter. Two types of catheter ablation have been used for the treatment of chronic or recurrent atrial flutter. Both are directed at vulnerable parameters, but of different sorts. One is His bundle ablation to create high degree atrioventricular block (generally third degree atrioventricular block), thereby eliminating the rapid ventricular response rates to atrial flutter (Scheinman, 1989). For patients in whom antiarrhythmic drug therapy is not tolerated or in whom atrial flutter with a rapid and clinically unacceptable ventricular response rate recurs despite antiarrhythmic drug therapy, catheter ablation to produce third degree atrioventricular block or a high degree of atrioventricular block provides a successful form of therapy without the need for further antiarrhythmic drugs. Such patients are then treated with a standard permanent pacemaker system.

A second type of catheter ablation therapy is still investigational, but seeks to destroy a vulnerable region of the atrial flutter reentrant circuit. This technique involves first mapping the atria during atrial flutter to identify a critical area of slow conduction in the reentrant circuit. When the area is identified, ablative energy can be delivered through the catheter electrode to this area to destroy it. An initial small series of patients treated with this technique has been reported (Saoudi et al, 1990; Feld et al, 1992). Also, ablation of a critical isthmus between the inferior vena cava and the tricuspid valve may prove efficacious (Cosio et al, 1993). A wider experience is required to understand its short- and long-term efficacy rates and potential adverse experience rate before this technique can be recommended as routine therapy. Also, a greater understanding of the mechanism of atrial flutter, particularly the reliable identification of a critical (and ablatable) portion of the atrial flutter reentrant circuit, should greatly enhance the applicability of this technique. Early follow-up suggests that, in some patients, recurrent atrial fibrillation may replace recurrent atrial flutter (Touboul et al, 1992).

For patients with atrial flutter in the presence of an accessory atrioventricular connection (Wolff-Parkinson-White syndrome), especially with a history of 1:1 conduction of atrial flutter impulses to the ventricles via the accessory atrioventricular connection, catheter ablation, usually using radiofrequency energy, of the accessory atrioventricular connection is the treatment of choice. Furthermore, there is a high, though clearly not absolute, likelihood that, with successful ablation of the accessory atrioventricular connection, the atrial flutter will no longer recur (Waldo et al, 1988).

It seems well established that classical (Type I) atrial flutter is due to reentrant excitation in the right atrium. It is usually easily diagnosed. Acute treatment consists of obtaining rapid control of the ventricular response rate and restoring sinus rhythm, although precipitation of atrial fibrillation may, on occasion, be useful. Chronic treatment consists of using antiarrhythmic drug therapy to suppress recurrent atrial flutter episodes, recognizing that occasional recurrences are the norm. Use of an antitachycardia pacemaker also may provide useful therapy in selected patients. Surgical techniques may provide a cure for atrial flutter, but catheter ablation techniques may provide the best hope of cure.

Management of Atrial Fibrillation

Atrial fibrillation is the most common sustained arrhythmia seen in clinical practice. In the Framingham study, the incidence is estimated to be 2% to 4% of the general population above 65 years of age (Kannel et al, 1982). The incidence is even higher in patients with underlying heart disease (Kulbertus, 1991). Atrial fibrillation may be associated with hemodynamic impairment, occasionally disabling symptoms, and a decrease in life expectancy. In advanced heart failure, atrial fibrillation is common and was found to be a marker for increased risk of death (Middlekauff et al, 1991). The most important concern with atrial fibrillation relates to its embolic manifestations that, in 75% of instances, are complicated by cerebrovascular accidents (Cabin et al, 1990; Rawles, 1992).

Atrial fibrillation is generally subdivided into two forms: paroxysmal atrial fibrillation and established or chronic atrial fibrillation. Chronic atrial fibrillation may be the end result of paroxysmal fibrillation in about 30% of the latter. However, in most patients, the arrhythmia presents as chronic fibrillation. As there is no universal definition of chronic atrial fibrillation, the definition used here is fibrillation lasting more than one month.

Conversion of Atrial Fibrillation to Sinus Rhythm

Conversion to sinus rhythm represents the ideal endpoint of therapy for chronic atrial fibrillation, as this should restore normal hemodynamics with the restoration of the normal atrioventricular activation sequence. The result would be a slower heart rate and, likely, a decreased risk of emboli. Conversion to sinus rhythm may be accomplished either pharmacologically or electrically.

Pharmacologic treatment (Table 1) dates back over 200 years, although the modern era commenced in 1918 when Frey (1918) used quinidine to terminate atrial fibrillation of recent onset. Today, quinidine is less used for this indication as its safety has been questioned based on reported cases of sudden death (Coplen et al, 1990; Cramer, 1968). A number of other antiarrhythmic agents have been given orally for this indication, including procainamide, disopyramide, and oral amiodarone. However, there is no control trial demonstrating the safety and efficacy of such use, and amiodarone is not approved for this indication. More recently, oral flecainide or propafenone has been used in atrial fibrillation of recent onset in order to restore sinus rhythm (Capucci et al, 1992; Capucci et al, 1990). Success rates as high

---

Table 1

Pharmacologic Conversion of Chronic Atrial Fibrillation to Sinus Rhythm

---

Mechanism of Arrhythmia: random reentry

Vulnerable Parameter: atrial refractory period

Therapeutic Choice: increase atrial refractoriness; increase the wavelength

Targets: Na channels or K channels (I_K)

Drugs: Na channel blockers; K channel blockers*

---

* See text regarding channel blockers.

as 91% were recently reported (Capucci et al, 1992) with a single oral dose of 300 mg of flecainide. This was significantly higher than the success rates with placebo (48%) during an observation period of eight hours. In other reports (Goy et al, 1988; Suttorp et al, 1990), the success rates with flecainide ranged between 67% and 95%. Studies with oral propafenone (600 mg as a single dose) showed success rates as high as 81% at 12 hours, which was significantly better than placebo (33%) or the combination of oral quinidine and intravenous digoxin (50%) (Capucci et al, 1990).

Pharmacologic conversion of atrial fibrillation of recent onset or prolonged episodes of paroxysmal atrial fibrillation is routinely attempted in hospital practice using intravenous injection of an antiarrhythmic agent. Intravenous digoxin (0.5–1 mg in the absence of ongoing digitalis therapy) is commonly used, although the efficacy of the drug and the mechanism of action are still uncertain. Furthermore, controlled studies have suggested that the conversion rate to sinus rhythm is no better than with placebo (Falk et al, 1987; Falk and Leavitt, 1991), although the effect of digoxin to slow the ventricular response during atrial fibrillation is unquestioned. Intravenous amiodarone 5 mg/kg over 10 to 30 minutes followed by an infusion of 500 mg over 24 hours has been reported to be associated with a high success rate (Faniel and Schoenfeld, 1983; Halpern et al, 1980), although there is no controlled study.

Newer antiarrhythmic agents have been used for this indication. Intravenous flecainide (1.5 mg/kg), intravenous propafenone (2 mg/kg), and intravenous cibenzoline (1.5 mg/kg) have been reported to be successful in recent onset atrial fibrillation with a wide range of good results related at least in part to differences in the patient population (Suttorp et al, 1989; Lacombe et al, 1988). In established atrial fibrillation, the results are less impressive than in paroxysmal or recent onset atrial fibrillation. Comparing intravenous propafenone (2 mg/kg) and intravenous flecainide over 10 minutes in atrial fibrillation of less than six months' duration, Suttorp et al (1989) found a better result (18 of 20 patients or 90%) with flecainide than with propafenone (11 of 20 patients or 55%). Pharmacologic conversion with Na channel blockers carries the risk of converting atrial fibrillation to atrial flutter and ventricular proarrhythmia as the slowing of atrial rate may allow 1:1 propagation through the atrioventricular node. This phenomenon may be facilitated by the anticholinergic action of certain Na channel blockers like quinidine and disopyramide.

Mechanism of Pharmacologic Conversion

Recent work by Allessie et al (1990) has supported the hypothesis that atrial fibrillation is related to a reentry mechanism. They made simultaneous recordings from 192 sites and showed that five or more reentrant circuits are present in an experimental model of atrial fibrillation. Allessie et al (1990) made use of the concept of wavelength; that is, the product of effective refractory period and conduction velocity. For an electrical impulse to propagate around an area of block and induce a reentrant circuit, slow conduction should be present to allow the fibers located ahead of the area of block to recover and to become excitable again. A short refractory period will facilitate propagation of another action potential. A critical wavelength is required for atrial fibrillation induction or perpetuation. If the wavelength is short, a greater number of reentry pathways can be maintained. Therefore, one of the therapeutic choices may be to prolong atrial refractoriness. Although the mechanism of pharmacologic termination of atrial fibrillation is not known, one may speculate from the work of Allessie et al (1990) that, if in an atrium of given size, the wavelength exceeds the given space, and/or there is less than the minimum number of required wavefronts, fibrillation will terminate. Such extrapolation seems appropriate to understand the effects of antiarrhythmic agents.

Therapeutic Strategies

In terms of concepts put forward by the Sicilian Gambit (The Task Force, 1991; Schwartz and Zaza, 1992), the vulnerable parameter for atrial fibrillation termination would be the atrial refractory period. Based on the work of Allessie et al (1990), prolongation of refractory period may be the endpoint. One may speculate that a significant increase in the atrial refractory period might result in prolongation of wavelength and termination of atrial fibrillation. Some Na channel blocking agents that also prolong refractoriness, such as quinidine, procainamide, and disopyramide, may prolong wavelength and terminate atrial fibrillation in this fashion. Given that Na channel blockers that tend to slow conduction will decrease wavelength, the balance between the prolongation of repolarization and the slowing of conduction with any Na channel blocker is critical. Other Na channel blockers such as lidocaine and mexiletine have been shown clinically to be without significant effect on atrial fibrillation possibly because they neither prolong refractoriness nor have an important effect on conduction (Katzung et al, 1985). An increase in atrial refractoriness may be obtained by targeting the K channel using amiodarone or sotalol. The mechanism of action of amiodarone is complex as it induces Na, K, and Ca channel block and noncompetitive β-adrenergic block. Sotalol not only increases atrial refractoriness via its K channel blocking action, but is a β-blocking agent as well.

Electrical Conversion

Pharmacologic conversion is essentially used in patients with atrial fibrillation of recent onset. Should it fail, or in cases of longstanding or chronic atrial fibrillation, the method of choice is delivery of an external shock (precordial or transthoracic). A technique of internal defibrillation that is useful in patients who failed both external and pharmacologic conversion has also been reported (Lévy et al, 1992).

Prevention of Recurrences

Following pharmacologic or electrical cardioversion, recurrences of atrial fibrillation are common, and only 25% of patients taking placebo are in sinus rhythm at one year versus 50% of patients when quinidine is administered (Coplen et al, 1990). Therefore, pharmacologic therapy is needed to prevent recurrences of atrial fibrillation.

Therapeutic Strategy (Table 2)

Induction of atrial fibrillation may be precipitated by premature atrial depolarizations or, less commonly, by premature ventricular depolarizations through appropriately timed retrograde conduction to the atria, or by changes in heart rate related to increases in sympathetic or parasympathetic tone. To date, only a limited number of cases of vagally-induced fibrillation have been reported (Coumel et al, 1978). To prevent recurrences of atrial fibrillation, one may choose to suppress the trigger mechanism of premature atrial depolarizations and premature ventricular depolarizations or to modify the atrial sub-

Table 2
Prevention of Recurrences of Atrial Fibrillation Following Conversion to Sinus Rhythm

Mechanism of Arrythmia: random reentry	
Vulnerable Parameters: atrial refractoriness; sympathetic tone	
Therapeutic Choice:	1. increase atrial refractoriness 2. decrease sympathetic tone 3. decrease vagal tone
Targets:	1. Na channels and/or K channels 2. β-adrenergic receptors 3. muscarinic receptors
Drugs:	1. Na and K channel blockers 2. β-antagonists 3. vagolytic agents

strate by modifying atrial refractoriness, which may be another vulnerable parameter. An increase in atrial refractoriness may be achieved by Na channel blockers, such as quinidine, procainamide, disopyramide, propafenone, or flecainide, which prolong inactivation of Na channels, or by antiarrhythmic agents whose major electrophysiologic effect is to prolong action potential duration and refractoriness, such as amiodarone or sotalol. In selected cases of catecholamine-induced atrial fibrillation, the therapeutic option may be to decrease sympathetic tone. The target in this particular situation is constituted by β-adrenergic receptors and the logical antiarrhythmic agent is a β-blocking agent.

Clinical Use of Antiarrhythmic Agents

Quinidine is the antiarrhythmic agent with the most widespread application in prevention of atrial fibrillation recurrences. A recent meta-analysis (Coplen et al, 1990) has shown that 50% of patients taking quinidine were in sinus rhythm at one year versus 25% of controls. However, the mortality in the quinidine group was 2.9% versus 0.8% in the placebo group, suggesting that proarrhythmia may

194 • ANTIARRHYTHMIC THERAPY

be responsible for the excess mortality. This was echoed by a report derived from the Stroke Prevention in Atrial Fibrillation study (Flaker et al, 1992) showing that the mortality in patients with atrial fibrillation and having a history of congestive heart failure was 4.7 times higher during antiarrhythmic therapy than in patients not taking antiarrhythmic agents. However, there was a better outcome during antiarrhythmic therapy in those patients without heart failure. These studies highlight the importance of a patient's overall cardiovascular status in determining the outcome of drug therapy.

Disopyramide is as effective as quinidine in preventing recurrences following cardioversion of atrial fibrillation (Lloyd et al, 1984), but long-term safety remains to be evaluated. Propafenone reportedly prevented recurrences of atrial fibrillation in about 40% of patients at six months and intolerable side effects were observed in only 5% of patients (Antmann et al, 1990), but studies of long-term outcome are needed. Flecainide is associated with a high rate of maintenance of sinus rhythm (58%) at six months.

Whether K channel blockers are safer than Na channel blockers in the prevention of recurrences of atrial fibrillation is not established. A recent study has shown that sotalol is as effective as quinidine, and better tolerated (Juul-Moller et al, 1990). At one year, 52% of patients were in sinus rhythm in the sotalol group versus 48% in the quinidine group. Recent reports (Lévy et al, 1992; Lundstrom and Ryden, 1990) have shown that low dose amiodarone treatment is effective (38% to 65% in sinus rhythm) and associated with very few side effects at one year. However, there have been no controlled or comparative studies particularly regarding the long-term mortality with amiodarone or its long-term safety in atrial fibrillation. Therefore, except for selected indications, amiodarone is not recommended as a first line drug for preventing recurrences of atrial fibrillation. As suggested by Feld (1990), knowledge about the prevention of arrhythmia recurrences with antiarrhythmic agents needs to be reevaluated in light of long-term safety. Moreover, regardless of the drug used, atrial fibrillation tends to recur in at least 50% of patients (NHLBI Working Group, 1993).

Control of Ventricular Response

In chronic or established atrial fibrillation, two endpoints of therapy when conversion is not indicated or fails are to control patients' symptoms and to improve cardiac function. These may be achieved by slowing ventricular rate.

Therapeutic Strategies

A convenient vulnerable parameter for achieving control of ventricular rate is the atrioventricular nodal action potential. To facilitate block of atrioventricular nodal conduction, the target is the L-type calcium channel (Table 3). Calcium channel blockers such as verapamil and diltiazem are appropriate drugs. These agents both slow atrioventricular nodal conduction and prolong the nodal effective refractory period.

Conduction through the atrioventricular node may also be slowed and refractoriness prolonged through another target, i.e., β-adrenergic receptors. The appropriate drugs are β-adrenergic blockers that control ventricular rate both at rest and during exercise. The prototype, propranolol, has been extensively studied for this indication. The drawbacks of β-adrenergic blockers are their negative inotropic effects and their contraindications in conditions such as bronchial asthma or peptic ulcer.

Digoxin is still, in most centers, the first line drug in patients having atrial fibrillation with a rapid ventricular response and/or congestive heart failure. Digoxin has a direct effect, as well as an indirect effect mediated by the vagus. Digoxin exerts its direct effects on the atria and the atrioventricular node, and in the atria, tends to increase the refractory period. However, the vagotonic actions of digitalis appear to be of far greater importance than its direct actions in the setting of atrial fibrillation. The vagotonic action results in ap-

---

Table 3
Chronic Atrial Fibrillation: Control of Ventricular Rate

Vulnerable parameter: atrioventricular nodal (Ca-dependent) refractoriness and propagation

Target: I_{Ca-L}

Drugs: Calcium channel blockers, e.g., verapamil, diltiazem.

Alternatives: β-adrenergic blockers; digitalis

---

parent sensitization to the effects of acetylcholine. This, in turn, induces the slowing of atrioventricular nodal conduction, and the prolongation of the atrioventricular nodal refractory period. The effect on the atrioventricular node represents the major action of digoxin relied on by the clinician to slow the ventricular rate in atrial fibrillation. Finally, digoxin's positive inotropic effect makes it the drug of choice in patients with atrial fibrillation associated with heart failure.

Clinical use of drugs

The prototype calcium channel blocker used is verapamil, which has been administered for more than two decades to slow the ventricular rate in chronic atrial fibrillation (Lundstrom and Ryden, 1990). However, verapamil is not effective in restoring sinus rhythm. Control of the ventricular response in atrial fibrillation is observed both at rest and during exercise. Diltiazem has also been shown to be effective in controlling ventricular rate in chronic atrial fibrillation.

β-Adrenergic receptor blockers are also useful in controlling heart rate both at rest and during exercise (Atwood et al, 1987). The β-blocking agents associated with bradycardia such as propranolol and nadolol seem to be more effective than β-blocking agents with intrinsic sympathetic activity such as acebutolol or pindolol.

Digoxin was the first agent to be used for slowing the ventricular response in patients with atrial fibrillation. However, there have been a few studies showing that ventricular rate is consistently reduced during exercise (Redfors, 1971). Digoxin is of particular value in patients with atrial fibrillation associated with heart failure or in patients with depressed left ventricular function.

In patients in whom the ventricular response may not be controlled by pharmacologic agents, alone or in combination, radiofrequency modification or ablation of the His bundle may be recommended (Kay et al, 1988; Scheinman, 1989; Kuck et al, 1991). Finally, oral anticoagulant therapy is indicated in patients at risk of embolic complications.

Chapter 12

Ventricular Extrasystoles:
Prevention and Treatment

In this chapter, we review the presentation and mechanisms of ventricular extrasystoles and consider how successfully the approach suggested by the Sicilian Gambit can be applied to these arrhythmias.

Presentation of Ventricular Extrasystoles

Historically, several terms have been used synonymously: ventricular extrasystole, premature ventricular contraction, premature ventricular depolarization, and premature ventricular beat. Schamroth (1987) discussed the limitations of the various terms. The original term "extrasystole" was first used by Engelmann (1896); it has subsequently been used by a number of authorities. The extrasystole quickly was associated with a very specific property, namely, fixed coupling of the premature beat to the preceding sinus beat. Therefore, Schamroth (1987) defined a ventricular extrasystole as an "impulse that arises prematurely in an ectopic ventricular focus and is fixedly coupled to the preceding beat." He preferred to use the term "impulse" for the extrasystole, not "beat" or "contraction," because it is

From *Antiarrhythmic Therapy: A Pathophysiologic Approach* edited by Members of the Sicilian Gambit © 1994, Futura Publishing Co., Inc., Armonk, NY.

primarily an electrical event, whereas contraction is the secondary event following electrical activation. Furthermore, a premature ventricular "contraction" can also occur as a manifest ventricular parasystolic discharge, a ventricular capture beat, a reciprocal beat of ventricular or atrioventricular junctional origin, a conducted atrial or atrioventricular junctional extrasystole, or a relatively early beat during atrial fibrillation. For instance, the use of the term "premature junctional contraction" would require that the atrioventricular junction itself contracts, and does so in isolation. Thus, there seem to be some arguments to favor the use of the term "ventricular extrasystole," defined as a primary electrical event.

Schamroth (1987) has critically analyzed ectopic ventricular rhythms manifested either as ventricular parasystole or ventricular extrasystoles. Ventricular extrasystoles, being premature by definition, exhibit the following features (Schamroth, 1987), as discussed below.

1. Constancy of the extrasystolic coupling intervals. Ventricular extrasystoles are characterized by fixed or constant coupling intervals that indicate that the extrasystoles are in some way dependent on the preceding beat. The two prevailing concepts that Schamroth (1987) proposed to explain this relationship are the reentry theory and the theory of ectopic enhancement.
2. The phenomenon of concealed ventricular extrasystoles. This is explained on the basis of a persistent and continuous (e.g., bigeminal) rhythm that may be present, but with some ventricular extrasystoles remaining localized to the ectopic focus without invading the surrounding myocardium.

Ventricular extrasystoles may occur as isolated though recurring events that may either lack any prognostic significance (i.e., in the setting of an otherwise normal heart) or represent markers of electrical instability. In other settings, they may concur with more complex arrhythmias such as ventricular couplets or nonsustained or sustained ventricular tachycardia. In addition, they may exhibit different electrocardiographic characteristics such as uniform versus multiform morphology. Depending on the clinical circumstances, the underlying mechanisms may vary, and even morphologically identical ventricular extrasystoles may have different underlying mechanisms. In many instances, it is not possible to draw a distinct line separating single or repetitive ventricular extrasystoles and ventricular tachycardia (which will be discussed in Ch. 13).

Mechanisms of Ventricular Extrasystoles

The mechanism of a given ventricular extrasystole frequently remains conjectural and is not amenable to experimental or clinical evaluation. Therefore, in many instances, only a probable or even only a hypothetical mechanism can be provided that must then serve for subsequent identification of probable critical components and a vulnerable parameter to target for intervention. Due to these uncertainties about the mechanisms of this frequently occurring arrhythmia, which does not require antiarrhythmic treatment in most instances, the response of a given arrhythmia to an intervention may provide feedback concerning its probable mechanism. This is only the case, however, if the intervention is highly specific.

Reentry

The idea that reentry may induce isolated ventricular extrasystoles is based on the assumption that a localized area of refractoriness and slow conduction exists within an arrhythmogenic substrate. The sinus impulse may initially not penetrate this site but may approach the site from another direction when it has regained excitability. This concept was offered by De Boer (1921). Therefore, the same sinus impulse would cause two ventricular activations, i.e., the sinus beat and the following extrasystole. This can only be explained by a combination of complex pathophysiologic circumstances incorporating unidirectional block and slow conduction within some part of the myocardium. This process allows sufficient time for recovery of excitability in adjacent tissue and its invasion by the slowly conducted impulse, thus causing the extrasystole.

Schamroth (1987) considered several arguments against reentry, as discussed below. If ventricular extrasystoles were due to reentry, he felt that there should be marked changes in coupling intervals due to varying refractoriness as a function of the preceding cycle length or changes in sympathetic tone. In addition, the sometimes extremely long extrasystolic coupling interval would require very slow conduction or complex entrance and/or exit block that is unlikely to be present consistently, especially in otherwise healthy hearts. Despite these arguments, the theory that the event underlying an extrasystole is based on some type of reentry has been argued for many years (Schamroth, 1987).

Reflection

Reflection represents a specific conduction abnormality where an impulse propagating into a depressed segment of tissue may be delayed for a sufficiently long interval to permit refractoriness at a proximal site to terminate. As a result, the impulse can travel back along the same pathway (Moe et al, 1977). Experimental demonstration of the phenomenon confirmed a hypothesis proposed by Schamroth and Marriott (1961).

Reflection has been demonstrated in a three-compartment tissue bath where the middle segment, which is only a few millimeters long, is depressed by sucrose or by a high K^+ solution (Antzelevitch et al, 1980). An impulse originating in the proximal compartment may elicit a response in the distal compartment, but with great delay, as the result of electrotonic transmission through the inexcitable middle segment. When the delay is great enough, and proximal elements have repolarized, retrograde electrotonic current flow from the distal element may reexcite the proximal tissue. For reflection to occur, only a small amount of tissue need be involved. Whereas the length of a reentrant wave in ischemic tissue may be as long as 6 to 8 cm, reflection may occur in areas only a few millimeters in length. Indeed, arrhythmias arising from reflection may be indistinguishable from those due to reentry.

Abnormal Automaticity (Parasystole and Modulated Parasystole)

Parasystolic rhythms are characterized by varying coupling intervals between the ectopic (parasystolic) complexes and the dominant (sinus) rhythm. However, there is a common, minimal time interval among manifest interectopic intervals (the longer intervals being multiples of this minimum interval). Moreover, fusion complexes are often seen.

Parasystole has been attributed to the function of a regularly discharging pacemaker site that has developed phase 4 depolarization. In the simplest cases, its activity appears to be unperturbed by the dominant sinus rhythm as the result of entry block. Thus, it produces a depolarization whenever the myocardium is excitable.

In fact, the dominant cardiac rhythm may modulate the parasystolic focus to accelerate or to slow its rate (modulated parasystole) (Antzelevitch et al, 1982). It was in this sense that Schamroth and Marriott (1961) hypothesized ventricular extrasystoles to be the expression of electrotonic interactions between the sinus impulse and an ectopic ventricular focus that was protected from the sinus impulse. Protection was attributed to lowering of resting membrane potential with resulting refractoriness and local block. A sinus impulse arriving at a blocked region might then influence the discharge of an ectopic pacemaker beyond the site of block (Schamroth, 1966).

Early and Delayed Afterdepolarizations

The mechanisms for early and delayed afterdepolarizations are reviewed in Ch. 4.

Early afterdepolarizations occurring at high levels of membrane potential give rise to bradycardia-dependent tachyarrhythmias that can be suppressed by overdrive stimulation similar to that which occurs with automatic rhythms (Damiano and Rosen, 1984). However, arrhythmias triggered by early afterdepolarizations at low levels of membrane potential are far less subject to overdrive suppression (Damiano and Rosen, 1984). The ionic currents responsible for the upstroke of the action potential during triggered activity caused by early afterdepolarizations are influenced by the membrane potential at which the action potential occurs. During the plateau phase and early phase 3, when most sodium channels are still inactivated, the L-type calcium current probably plays the major role. During late phase 3, where there is partial reactivation of the fast sodium channels, upstrokes are most probably caused by the fast inward sodium current.

Delayed afterdepolarizations follow attainment of full repolarization. They are not a variant of the pacemaker potential, but represent a distinct ionic event. Although different types of delayed afterdepolarizations depend on different mechanisms, they have in common the occurrence of an overload of intracellular free calcium for their induction (Cranefield and Aronson, 1988; Wit and Rosen, 1992). To serve also as an explanation for nonsustained ventricular tachycardia, afterdepolarizations would have to be repetitive, which is indeed the case (Wit and Rosen, 1992).

Heart Rate and Innervation

Isolated extrasystoles are frequently rate dependent as can be studied by comparing the cycle length of sinus beats followed or not followed by an extrasystole. A "window" of cardiac rates can thus be identified with a lower and an upper rate limit for appearance of ventricular extrasystoles (Coumel et al, 1987). Coumel et al (1987) hypothesized that the more the arrhythmia is sensitive to sympathetic drive, the less the amount of adrenergic stimulation necessary and, hence, the less apparent the change in sinus rate preceding the occurrence of extrasystoles. This is referred to as the "adrenergic paradox."

Mechanisms of Nonsustained Ventricular Tachycardia

The lack of information that we have with regard to isolated extrasystoles is even greater when the mechanisms of repetitive extrasystoles or even nonsustained ventricular tachycardia are considered. Indeed, any form of abnormal impulse initiation or propagation may contribute here. Although it is easily conceivable that a given mechanism may be repetitive, it is uncertain whether the mechanism for the first premature excitation is the same as for the next one. Alternatively, one mechanism may set the stage for another to occur. For instance, a single extrasystole resulting from a delayed afterdepolarization may set the stage for reentry.

Selection of the Vulnerable Parameter(s) and of the Targets

The Sicilian Gambit (1991) has proposed the concept of the vulnerable parameter as the electrophysiologic variable most responsive to an intervention. It has also emphasized the importance of targets that must be influenced to achieve a desired change in the vulnerable parameter. However, in light of our limited knowledge of the mechanisms underlying clinically occurring ventricular extrasystoles and runs of nonsustained ventricular tachycardia, any suggestion as to the vulnerable parameters and the targets for drug action on these arrhythmias must remain speculative. Furthermore, the vulnerable parameter may change rapidly in complex situations such as acute myocardial ischemia or myocardial infarction.

The tools available to assess the underlying mechanism of an arrhythmia in the clinical setting are pacing and programmed electrical stimulation, recording of ventricular late potentials, recording of monophasic action potentials, and the observation of the effects of drugs that are specific in suppressing a given arrhythmogenic mechanism. Programmed stimulation has been used extensively to differentiate among reentry, abnormal automaticity, and triggered activity (Wit and Rosen, 1992; Josephson and Gottlieb, 1990). Monophasic action potentials have been used to differentiate between early and delayed afterdepolarizations (Hariman and Gough, 1990).

The potential vulnerable parameters of ventricular extrasystoles and nonsustained ventricular tachycardia and the therapeutic targets are outlined below.

Ventricular Extrasystoles Based on Enhanced Abnormal Automaticity

To suppress abnormal automaticity, the vulnerable parameters are the maximal diastolic potential, which should be hyperpolarized, or phase 4 depolarization, which should be decreased.

Ventricular Extrasystoles Based on Triggered Activity

When early afterdepolarizations are the underlying mechanism, the action potential duration should be shortened or the regenerative activity that leads to the early afterdepolarization should be suppressed. Delayed afterdepolarizations would require reduction in calcium overload and/or in the inward current that generates the afterdepolarization.

Ventricular Extrasystoles Based on Reentry

We can consider two types of reentry: that based on sodium channels in which there is impaired conduction and in which there is a long excitable gap and that in which conduction encroaches on refractoriness, with a presumably short excitable gap. In the former case, excitability and conduction can be decreased by impairing sodium channel conductance; in the latter case, the refractory period can be prolonged by I_K block. However, the specific type of reentry is not often identifiable in the clinical setting, rendering targeted therapy difficult.

The Use of Drug Response to Identify Mechanisms of Arrhythmias

Given the great difficulties in differentiating among the various mechanisms of ventricular extrasystoles, it is tempting to draw conclusions on pathophysiology based on the efficacy of specific antiarrhythmic drugs in suppressing them.

One such drug is flunarizine, a calcium antagonist that does not influence normal and abnormal automaticity, but is effective in suppressing digitalis-induced arrhythmias in the dog and guinea pig heart (Gorgels et al, 1990; Jonkman et al, 1986). It is effective in suppressing delayed afterdepolarizations and has been proposed to be target selective (Gorgels et al, 1990 and 1993). However, the study by Gorgels et al (1993) does not include any comparison with conventional antiarrhythmic drugs in the same patient population.

Application of the Sicilian Gambit to Specific Clinical Settings

The problem with the approach described above is that it assumes knowledge of the mechanism where, clinically, such knowledge often does not exist. In this section, an attempt is made to apply the Sicilian Gambit approach to specific clinical conditions, and to consider the probable mechanisms, the critical components and vulnerable parameters, the targets for antiarrhythmic drug action, and the interventions and clinical results. The arrhythmias delineated include those appearing in both the normal heart and during acute ischemia and infarction.

The Normal Heart

Clinical Presentation

Ventricular extrasystoles are increasingly identified in patients with apparently normal hearts. In many textbooks, these extrasystoles are described as

1. having a left bundle branch block morphology;
2. manifesting a less pronounced prolongation in QRS duration than occurs in the setting of organic heart disease;
3. occurring after the T wave; and
4. rarely or never being repetitive.

They may occur in isolation, bigeminally, or in more complex sequences. They may also follow the rules of parasystole.

Probable Mechanisms

Some clinical observations may help to elucidate the mechanisms of ventricular extrasystoles, although any of the arguments brought forward must remain speculative. Ventricular extrasystoles frequently occur at rest and at relatively low (albeit normal) heart rates. This would suggest increased automaticity, probably originating from the His-Purkinje system or, alternatively, bradycardia-dependent triggered automaticity due to early afterdepolarizations. In other instances, the occurrence of extrasystoles is clearly related to increased catecholamine levels, which might be compatible with enhanced automaticity or triggered activity. Hypokalemia or hypomagnesemia may aggravate the situation, but their role as single provoking factors is controversial. On the other hand, it is highly unlikely that ventricular extrasystoles in normal hearts are reentrant since there are presumably no regional inhomogeneities in conduction and refractoriness that would be sufficiently large to sustain reentry (Adhar et al, 1983; Brugada et al, 1983; Hamer et al, 1984).

Critical Components and Vulnerable Parameters

Accepting enhanced automaticity or triggered activity as probable underlying mechanisms, a logical approach would be to decrease phase 4 depolarization or hyperpolarize the maximum diastolic potential for automatic rhythms; or decrease Ca^{2+} overload or decrease inward current for triggered rhythms. An alternative approach would be to block conduction exiting the "focus" (exit block).

Targets

To achieve a decrease in phase 4 depolarization in the Purkinje system, the ion currents I_f or I_{Ca-T} should be blocked, or I_{K1} should be increased. To suppress delayed afterdepolarizations, Ca^{2+} entry blockers may be used, as may local anesthetics like lidocaine that block inward Na^+ currents associated with these oscillations.

Interventions and Clinical Results

Possible interventions include β-adrenergic antagonists to reduce phase 4 depolarization for the administration of sodium channel blocking agents. Both approaches are highly effective in a substantial proportion of patients, although none is fully effective in all. β-Adrenergic blockade is especially useful if increased adrenergic tone is the presumptive mechanism. Sodium channel blocking agents, especially those with slow recovery characteristics of sodium channel blockade without major effects on other channels (e.g., flecainide or ethmozine), have proven to be remarkably effective, although they have a high potential for proarrhythmia as part of their spectrum. Also, amiodarone is considered a very effective agent, although it is not clear whether this is by virtue of its antiadrenergic properties, its relatively weak sodium channel blocking activity, or its strong potassium channel blocking activity. It should not be considered as a first line choice due to its extracardiac side effects.

It is to be stressed that asymptomatic ventricular extrasystoles in a normal heart require no antiarrhythmic therapy, and that even in the presence of arrhythmia-related symptoms, the potential risks of therapy must be considered carefully. Under appropriate circumstances, interventions such as the administration of potassium and/or magnesium are clearly preferred to ion channel blocking agents. However, evaluating the clinical efficacy of manipulations in potassium and magnesium is difficult, and based more on anecdotal than on well-controlled studies.

Ischemia and Infarction

Clinical Presentation

Almost all patients with acute myocardial infarction, especially if seen early after onset of symptoms, exhibit some type of arrhythmia that may range from isolated ventricular extrasystoles to nonsustained and sustained ventricular tachycardia, ventricular fibrillation, and accelerated idioventricular rhythms. During the early phase, nonsustained ventricular tachycardia frequently is polymorphic and tends to stop spontaneously or to degenerate into ventricular fibrillation. In addition, other arrhythmias such as sinus bradycardia or atrial fibrillation may occur (O'Doherty et al, 1983). In this setting, ventricular extrasystoles are a ubiquitous finding. A comprehensive description of the ventricular arrhythmias of acute ischemia and infarction and their underlying electrophysiologic mechanisms has recently been provided by Wit and Janse (1993) and is reviewed in Ch. 4.

Critical Components, Vulnerable Parameters, and Targets for Drug Action

Depending on the presumed mechanism of early ischemia-induced ventricular arrhythmias, different approaches might be considered. In the case of reentrant excitation, regional inhomogeneities in conduction and/or refractoriness should be the most responsive parameters that can be affected, either by further decreasing conduction velocity to the degree of complete block or by normalizing conduction to the degree that no regional slow propagation persists. The latter might best be achieved by restoring blood flow as early as possible by thrombolytic therapy or by revascularization using percutaneous transluminal coronary angioplasty. This would also affect the abnormalities in regional activation and the inhomogeneities in refractory periods. On the other hand, using sodium channel blocking drugs to decrease conduction velocity until block occurs is an apparently effective measure, especially when one considers that abnormal tissue may be more responsive than normal tissue to the effect of an antiarrhythmic drug (especially if the drug binds to channels in their inactivated state). However, such therapy heightens the risk of inducing abnormalities in conduction in areas that do not yet exhibit significant abnormalities. This may provide the basis of proarrhythmia.

Proarrhythmia is, in fact, a major concern in the setting of acute ischemia. Conduction abnormalities are accentuated in the presence of drugs that normally do not affect conduction (Patterson et al, 1982). Similarly, drugs like flecainide exert a more pronounced effect on conduction parameters in the presence of abnormal tissue (Cooper et al, 1989; Kou et al, 1987; Lederman et al, 1989; Lubinski et al, 1992). The poor outcome of patients taking flecainide and encainide in the Cardiac Arrhythmia Suppression Trial I study (Akhtar et al, 1990; Echt et al, 1991a) has been attributed to intervening ischemic episodes, although this interpretation remains speculative.

Catecholamines play a significant role during the early phase of ischemia. The mechanisms of the potentially beneficial effects of β-blockers in the setting of acute ischemia are still controversial. They may act by reducing the degree of ischemia, thereby improving conduction, or by reversing catecholamine-stimulated activity.

Ventricular arrhythmias induced by delayed afterdepolarizations might respond to calcium antagonists. Indeed, the arrhythmias associated with the early stages of myocardial ischemia may be suppressed by calcium blockers (Clusin et al, 1982). However, in vivo, the potentially beneficial effects of such drugs may be offset by their vasodilating capacity and a subsequent increase in sympathetic tone.

Subacute and chronic infarction may start as early as one to two days after onset of the infarct and may last permanently, with a continuing risk of life-threatening ventricular arrhythmias. The arrhythmias may present as isolated or as more complex forms of ventricular extrasystoles, including nonsustained runs. Their time course and their prognostic significance in the subacute or chronic phase of myocardial infarction have been well documented. These arrhythmias manifest power to predict prognosis after myocardial infarction independently of the extent of left ventricular dysfunction (Kostis et al, 1987; Roberts et al, 1975; Moss et al, 1987).

Patients may also develop episodes of sustained monomorphic or pleomorphic ventricular tachycardia (see Ch. 13), which has attracted considerable clinical interest. This has culminated in methods to identify the structures involved in the genesis of these arrhythmias and to ablate them either surgically or by catheter techniques.

Interventions and Clinical Results

The classical interventions for suppressing extrasystoles include the use of sodium channel blocking drugs. This approach has been highly effective, especially with the use of drugs like flecainide or encainide. However, despite suppression of ventricular extrasystoles, the result has not been a decrease in mortality but, rather often, a worsening of prognosis (Echt et al, 1991a). Meta-analyses of randomized controlled trials using antiarrhythmic agents that block sodium channel conductance have shown that the treatment effect was much more likely to be adverse than beneficial. In contrast to these studies, the pooled results of major secondary prevention trials using β-blocking agents have demonstrated a significant reduction in the sudden death rate by an average of 24% during observation periods between nine and 36 months (Pratt and Roberts, 1983; Yusuf et al, 1985). In the β-blocker trials, however, patients with contraindications for this type of drug, such as overt congestive heart failure or chronic obstructive lung disease, were excluded. The role of antiarrhythmic drugs that prolong refractoriness with no or only modest effects on conduction, like d-sotalol or amiodarone, remains to be settled, although, especially with regard to amiodarone, the results of recent trials are encouraging (Ceremuzynski et al, 1992; Pfisterer et al, 1992 and 1993; Burkart et al, 1990). In fact, the Basel Antiarrhythmic Study of Infarct Survival (BASIS), a prospective, controlled, randomized trial using low dose amiodarone as an antiarrhythmic agent, could demonstrate a 60% reduction in sudden death rate and a 74% reduction in the incidence of arrhythmic events during the first year after myocardial infarction (Pfisterer et al, 1992 and 1993; Burkart et al, 1990).

Conclusions

Given the diverse etiologies of ventricular extrasystoles as well as their intermittent nature, it is difficult to be specific about mechanisms, critical components, and vulnerable parameters. It is clear, however, that a variety of targets has been identified, with the result of therapy including a high risk of proarrhythmia, especially when Na^+ channel blockers are used. With regard to the many still unresolved issues, ventricular extrasystoles should presently be treated only if severely symptomatic, but not with the aim to prevent the occurrence of sustained ventricular tachyarrhythmias. A therapeutic attempt with β-blockers without intrinsic sympathomimetic activity seems advisable.

Chapter 13

Ventricular
Tachycardia

Viewed in terms of either electrocardiographic diagnosis, clinical expression, pathophysiologic mechanisms, or therapeutic targets, the ventricular tachyarrhythmias are a heterogeneous group of arrhythmias. Accordingly, the ability to apply Sicilian Gambit logic to this category of arrhythmias is a complex function, involving consideration of multiple interactive factors including both electrophysiologic and more general pathophysiologic mechanisms.

Definitions

The historic definition of ventricular tachycardia as three or more consecutive ventricular impulses at an effective rate of greater than 100 impulses/min, without respect to specific QRS morphology patterns, is obsolete. Both the determination of clinical relevance and of therapeutic targets are now specific for subtypes of the ventricular tachycardia group (Myerburg et al, 1994). Ventricular tachycardia is best defined in terms of both its duration and its QRS morphology pattern. Duration is commonly categorized as *"sustained"* (>30 seconds of continuous ventricular impulses) versus *"nonsustained"* (three impulses up to 30 seconds), the latter being subgrouped by some into salvos (three to five impulses) and nonsustained tachycardias (six impulses up to 30 seconds) (Myerburg et al, 1984). The latter distinc-

From *Antiarrhythmic Therapy: A Pathophysiologic Approach* edited by Members of the Sicilian Gambit © 1994, Futura Publishing Co., Inc., Armonk, NY.

tion is based on limited data suggesting increased risk of nonsustained episodes lasting six impulses or longer (Glicksman et al, 1988). QRS morphology is characterized as uniform patterns known as monomorphic ventricular tachycardia or polymorphic ventricular tachycardia in which QRS complexes vary from impulse to impulse. The categorical separation of sustained and nonsustained, and monomorphic and polymorphic, reflecting different clinical relevances and pathophysiologies, serves as a general basis for therapeutic distinctions.

Pathophysiology

Ventricular tachycardias generally occur in diseased hearts. The exceptions are of pathophysiologic interest and varying clinical relevance, but are of limited epidemiologic importance because of their very low incidence. In the United States and Europe, approximately 80% of life-threatening ventricular tachyarrhythmias are related to underlying atherosclerotic coronary artery disease, and another 10% to 15% are related to the various primary, nonischemic ventricular muscle disorders (the cardiomyopathies). The overwhelming majority thus have an underlying structural basis that has been the focus of experimental and clinical research in an attempt to define mechanisms and targets for therapy. The ultimate questions to which such studies are addressed are: why does a patient with an established abnormality develop ventricular tachycardia at any point in time, and why at a specific point in time?

The Conditioning Substrate

Among the 80% of patients whose life-threatening ventricular arrhythmias are associated with coronary artery disease, multiple mechanisms may contribute to the risk of arrhythmias, depending on clinical expression of the underlying disease and individual variations in expression. The conditioning substrate refers to the anatomic structural abnormalities that may be modified by transient functional changes (see below) (Myerburg et al, 1992a and 1993). The conditioning substrate may be present over different periods of time (long, as in healed myocardial infarction; short, as in acute myocardial infarction), and is generally considered to be responsible for establishing the anatomic basis for reentrant ventricular arrhythmias. The structure that can support a reentrant circuit incorporates anatomic and functional balances that, in addition to establishing the conditions for initiation and maintenance of the arrhythmia, also provides the opportunity for its termination by therapy targeted to its points of vulnerability. Unfortunately, coronary artery disease also is exemplified by very complex pathophysiology, making therapy targeted to one or two specific vulnerable parameters perplexing, if not impossible.

The pathophysiology of ventricular tachycardia in coronary heart disease includes elements of normal and abnormal conduction, interacting with nonuniform properties of refractoriness, in a heterogeneous matrix, all of which is inconstant over time. The temporal problem derives from both the fact that the substrate is continuously modified over time by transient functional factors such as ischemia, hemodynamic changes, and autonomic fluctuations (Myerburg et al, 1991, 1992a, and 1992b), and by the additional fact that the fundamental disease process continues to evolve longitudinally in time (Myerburg et al, 1993). Thus, while defined anatomy with definable pathophysiologic targets is a tempting model for the targeted use of Na^+ channel blocking drugs to modify conduction and K^+ channel blocking or activating drugs to modify refractoriness, present insights into clinical physiology are far too complex to allow application of these principles in any but a very general and superficial way. For the future, however, it is not without reason that new concepts and information may enhance our ability to target specific pharmacologic therapy.

The second most common cause of life-threatening ventricular arrhythmias, the cardiomyopathies, highlights both a physiologic dilemma more difficult than the coronary artery disease problem and an example of an extraordinarily specific vulnerable parameter. The former statement is supported by the fact that myopathic ventricles do not contain the specific anatomic pathways that are better definable in hearts having coronary artery disease, and that tachycardias are not commonly inducible in the clinical electrophysiology laboratory (Myerburg et al, 1994), suggesting that either the anatomy for supporting reentry is not present or that the functional factors are not constant over time. In contrast, the example of a very specific vulnerable parameter can be cited for ventricular tachycardia due to bundle branch reentry in nonischemic cardiomyopathies. This arrhythmia appears to use the right bundle branch and left bundle branch as limbs in a reentrant circuit and, therefore, therapy targeted to slowing conduction in a bundle branch (e.g., a Na^+ channel blocking drug) or prolonging refractoriness in His-Purkinje tissue (e.g., a K^+ channel blocking drug) could be viewed as examples of therapies targeted to specific vulnerable parameters. Since this arrhythmia is also amenable to catheter ablation of the right bundle branch, it serves primarily as an example of a uniquely vulnerable therapeutic parameter.

The role of ventricular hypertrophy has been gaining increasing appreciation both as a primary and an interactive structural risk factor for ventricular tachyarrhythmias. Epidemiologically, the presence of left ventricular hypertrophy has been recognized to contain powerful predictive value for sudden arrhythmic death (Cupples et al, 1992), both as an additive risk factor in the presence of coronary artery disease and as a primary risk factor. These statements are supported by clinical (Ginzton et al, 1989) and experimental (Cox et al, 1991) observations that hearts with healed myocardial infarctions consistently demonstrate areas of regional hypertrophy. Since hypertrophied myocytes have altered repolarization patterns, due at least in part to alterations in the kinetics of the delayed rectifier current (I_K) (Furukawa et al, in press) and an unusual susceptibility of that channel to ischemia and reperfusion (Furukawa et al, 1993), its anatomic presence may imply both a functional basis for arrhythmogenic associations and a rational target for defined therapy.

For ventricular tachycardias due to most other conditions, particularly those of focal origin such as the right ventricular outflow tract tachycardias, mechanisms and targets are even less well defined. Undoubtedly, some are due to mechanisms of altered automaticity, others may be due to focal reentry, and some may be generated by early or delayed afterdepolarizations, but the distinctions are difficult and targeted therapy remains problematic.

Transient Factors Controlling Risk and Expression of Ventricular Tachycardia

The anatomic substrate that conditions the heart to support a ventricular tachycardia, particularly a reentrant tachycardia, is susceptible to modification by a variety of transient pathophysiologic conditions, including ischemia, reperfusion, hemodynamic changes, metabolic state, autonomic conditions, and chemical substances (including antiarrhythmic drugs themselves) (Jackman et al, 1988; Myerburg et al, 1992b). These factors, in addition to altering function of the anatomic substrate, may also influence each other. Two implications derive from these statements:

1. modulating influences control the properties of the substrate and therefore become additional therapeutic targets themselves, and
2. their expression is discontinuous over time and thus can intermittently modify the influence of a drug on a vulnerable parameter.

Despite these limitations, the transient risk factors serve important and definable clinical targets, and provide additional insights into available parameters for targeting therapy.

It is generally accepted from clinical observations that transient myocardial ischemia constitutes a risk for cardiovascular events, including both myocardial infarction and sudden cardiac death. Associations between ischemia and initiation of nonsustained and sustained ventricular tachycardia are well described. Similar associations between healed myocardial infarction and ventricular arrhythmias are also described, but this example contains the feature of a defined anatomy establishing vulnerable parameter(s) present longitudinally in time (Myerburg et al, 1993) in addition to potential transient vulnerable parameters expressed cross-sectionally in time. The continuously present characteristics provide a Sicilian Gambit-based target for antiarrhythmic therapy, which is nonetheless still susceptible to modulation by transient ischemia or other factors. In this regard, an experimental observation on the effects of acute ischemia on arrhythmogenesis in hearts with prior myocardial infarction is relevant. In a model of graded reductions in coronary blood flow, it has been observed that lesser reductions in coronary flow were required to initiate spontaneous ventricular fibrillation and to electrically induce ventricular tachycardia in hearts with prior myocardial infarction, compared to those without prior infarction (Furukawa et al, 1991b). The implication of this observation, in addition to the general relationship between a potential ventricular tachyarrhythmia substrate and ischemia, is the possibility that moderate transient reductions of coronary blood flow, which may not be expressed clinically as ischemic symptoms, may modify vulnerable parameters, resulting in either their enhanced expression or a modification of their response to a specific therapeutic probe.

Reperfusion after a period of transient ischemia is arrhythmogenic via mechanisms that differ from those responsible for ischemic arrhythmias or their simple reversal. Accordingly, reperfusion may affect different vulnerable parameters than those identified and targeted during steady-state clinical conditions or in the presence of transient ischemia. Moreover, there is a time-dependent function for the generation of reperfusion arrhythmias (Manning and Hearse, 1984; Kimura et al, 1986a and 1986b). Short periods of ischemia—seconds to minutes—followed by reperfusion do not generate sustained reperfusion arrhythmias. Depending on the model studied, periods of ischemia lasting from 10 to 20 minutes have the highest probability of generating sustained reperfusion arrhythmias. Periods in excess of 30 minutes are unlikely to result in ventricular tachycardia or fibrillation on reperfusion.

At least two mechanisms may be responsible for reperfusion arrhythmias. A very early period of abrupt shortening of action potential durations in the periischemic zone may be associated with a reentrant mechanism for generation of ventricular fibrillation (Coronel et al, 1992). This is followed by a second mechanism within seconds to a minute or more, during which a Ca^{2+}-dependent triggered response pattern may occur, the latter having been observed in both multicellular (Kimura et al, 1986b; Priori et al, 1990) and isolated single cell (Furukawa et al, 1993) preparations. The implication of these observations is that several parameters specific to potentially fatal reperfusion arrhythmias may be targeted by therapy. These may include, but are not necessarily limited to, I_{to}, Na^+/K^+ exchange, $I_{K(ATP)}$, or a Na^+ activated K^+ channel for the very early reperfusion mechanism, or an I_K/I_{Ca} interaction for the triggered response pattern. The latter appears to be a blocked or blunted I_K, maintaining depolarization in the range of 0 to $-30mV$ and allowing reactivated I_{Ca} to oscillate across the cell membranes (Furukawa et al, 1993). For any of these mechanisms, the potential for specifically targeting a vulnerable parameter is theoretically possible in the susceptible individual.

Transient hemodynamic alterations may alter electrophysiology. In the isolated canine left ventricle, volume loading shortens refractory periods (Lab, 1982; Calkins et al, 1989) and establishes regional disparity of refractory periods in hearts with prior myocardial infarctions (Calkins et al, 1989). In humans, attempts to establish a relationship between systemic hemodynamic factors and inducibility of ventricular arrhythmias have been unsuccessful. However, studies to date have focused largely on the inability to reverse predetermined inducibility by reducing afterload on the ventricle (Carlson et al, 1989). Since inducibility at baseline suggests dominance of an established anatomic substrate, the more relevant design might be a test of the ability of increased preload or afterload to promote inducibility in the myopathic heart, which is not inducible into a tachyarrhythmia under baseline conditions. Transient fluctuations of hemodynamic status may be particularly relevant to the most confounding of clinical circumstances associated with ventricular tachyarrhythmias—nonischemic dilated cardiomyopathy. Because of the frequent inability to induce clinical ventricular tachycardia in such patients (with the exception of bundle branch reentry), and the limited evidence for a role for automatic mechanisms in such patients, the identification of (an) electrophysiologic vulnerable parameter(s) has been impossible. If an underlying hemodynamic triggering influence is identified and predictably manageable, it would provide the ability to determine both the hidden electrophysiologic targets and a hemodynamically determined target of therapy.

Metabolic and exogenous chemical factors influence cardiac electrophysiology. Acute hypoxemia, acidosis, and electrolyte imbalances each may contribute to transient electrophysiologic destabilization (Gettes, 1992; Multiple Risk Factor Intervention Trial Research Group, 1982; Packer, 1985). Among these, hypokalemia resulting from chronic diuretic therapy is best understood as a cause of the polymorphic ventricular tachycardia, torsades de pointes (Gettes, 1992; Multiple Risk Factor Intervention Trial Research Group, 1982), through an influence on a repolarizing K^+ channel. Drugs such as quinidine and sotalol may generate this same arrhythmia, at least in part by a K^+ channel blocking effect. Quinidine-induced torsades de pointes may be potentiated by hypokalemia. In addition, cocaine (Kimura et al, 1992) and terfenadine (Woosley et al, 1993) have been shown to block the delayed rectifier current (I_K) and may generate torsades de pointes. Thus, for patients manifesting this adverse effect, vulnerable parameters could include K^+ channel activation or control of the currents that induce torsades de pointes, presumably intracellular or transmembrane Ca^{2+} flux.

The central and autonomic nervous systems, neurohumors, and peripheral adrenoceptors exert important influences on both the substrate and other functional influences. Such influences may be exerted at either systemic or local cardiac levels. An example of systemic influences derives from recent observations on the use of measures of heart rate variability to estimate risk. Several studies have demonstrated that blunted heart rate variability, particularly when measured in the spectral components of frequency domain, identifies patients at risk for sudden death after myocardial infarction and can be subgrouped among patients who have coronary heart disease with and without life-threatening ventricular arrhythmias (Bigger et al, 1992; Huikuri et al, 1992; Kleiger et al, 1987). More recently, among patients who have both sustained and nonsustained episodes of tachycardias with uniform QRS morphology, it was observed that the blunted heart rate variability averaged over 24 hours had differential characteristics before sustained and nonsustained ventricular tachycardias (Huikuri et al, 1993). In the former case, heart rate variability remained blunted during the four 15-minute intervals prior to a ventricular tachycardia event, but for nonsustained episodes, heart rate variability increased abruptly during the final 15 minutes before the tachycardia. This suggests that autonomic fluctuations may not only be a marker of risk but, in addition, an active participant in modulation of risk. The protective effects of β-adrenoceptor blocking drugs for both sudden and total cardiovascular mortality in postmyocardial infarction patients further suggest an active role for modulation of risk by autonomic factors (Beta-blocker Heart Attack Trial Research Group, 1982; Pederson et al, 1985). Finally, at a local cardiac level, nonuniform β-adrenergic receptor distribution in the postmyocardial infarction patient (Kammerling et al, 1987) and reversal of "beneficial" drug effects by isoproterenol during programmed electrical stimulation studies support the concept that autonomic influences can alter critical components of a ventricular tachycardia mechanism.

Critical Components in the Clinical Expression of Ventricular Tachycardias

The determination of critical components in the pathophysiologic mechanisms of ventricular tachyarrhythmias is heavily dependent on the clinical setting. In the example of coronary artery disease, one can make the distinction between ventricular tachycardia occurring in the settings of acute myocardial infarction, transient ischemia, and healed myocardial infarction.

Available information in acute myocardial infarction suggests that reentry, normal and possibly abnormal automaticity, and triggered activity all may be operative at various stages of the process. During the early acute phase, reentry due to a major dispersion of refractoriness between epicardium and endocardium has been proposed (Kimura et al, 1986a). It has been considered that the epicardium is more susceptible to ischemia based on the more dramatic shortening of action potential duration in epicardial cells during acute ischemia. However, this appears to reflect primarily the enhanced sensitivity of one channel ($I_{K(ATP)}$) to the effects of ischemia in epicardium compared to endocardium (Furukawa et al, 1991a), while in a more general sense, the endocardium is more sensitive to the metabolic effects of ischemia. The electrophysiologic consequences of epicardial $I_{K(ATP)}$ sensitivity to ischemia may identify this channel as a critical component for ventricular tachycardia occurring during the acute phase of infarction. In contrast, in the presence of healed myocardial infarction, a stable physiology of endocardial and epicardial cells is thought to be present, but endocardium and epicardium appear to have different channel densities of I_K and I_{K1}; i.e., in epicardium: $I_K > I_{K1}$; endocardium: $I_{K1} > I_K$) (Furukawa et al, 1992), which may be relevant to the initiation of ventricular tachycardia under chronic conditions. In the 24-hour infarct, enhanced automaticity in the His-Purkinje system of the infarct zone may generate a slower, automatic ventricular tachycardia or accelerated idioventricular rhythm. Finally, during reperfusion of ischemic muscle during the early phase of the infarct, triggered activity generated from early afterdepolarizations may be expressed (Furukawa et al, 1993). Thus, in the single clinical setting of myocardial infarction, multiple mechanisms of arrhythmias each provide different critical components that can serve as specific vulnerable targets for therapy.

Therapeutic Targets

From a macrophysiologic perspective, therapeutic targets for prevention and treatment of ventricular tachycardia may be divided into three components:

1. suppression of triggering ventricular premature depolarizations;
2. alteration of the sustaining substrate;
3. blockade of the transient influences.

The first two involve direct insight into the electrophysiologic mechanisms of arrhythmias and the effects thereon of pharmacologic agents. The third category addresses ways in which electrophysiology may be modulated by a variety of confounding factors, and requires additional interventions to control the modulators.

To date, suppression of triggering ventricular premature depolarizations as a focus for therapy has been disappointing. While some drugs can achieve high-grade suppression of ventricular premature depolarizations, their effects on other components of vulnerability to sustained ventricular tachyarrhythmias may result in a net increase in risk, as demonstrated in the CAST data (Echt et al, 1991a). In contrast, antiarrhythmic drugs that alter the sustaining substrate for ventricular tachycardias may be identified and can be effective as long as the substrate remains stable. However, if the latter is altered by transient functional influences, a pharmacologic effect defined under baseline conditions may be modified. Therefore, control of transient functional influences has a potential role as a vulnerable parameter for therapy, as in β-blocker therapy after myocardial infarction. This approach is limited by the absence of a direct effect on abnormal cardiac electrophysiologic parameters. In conclusion, for the complex problem of ventricular tachyarrhythmias, a therapeutic approach based on vulnerable parameters is not monofactorial, except for a few infrequent specific cases. Thus, a Sicilian Gambit based strategy must take into account the presence and interactions of multiple simultaneous points of attack.

Consideration of Specific Ventricular Tachycardias Using the Sicilian Gambit Approach

Given the heterogeneity of ventricular tachycardias, it is not possible to review all variants here or to suggest a unifying pathophysiologic approach. Rather, we have selected two examples: the first is an infrequent but homogeneous entity that readily lends itself to the logic system recommended by the Sicilian Gambit. The second, tachycardias occurring during subacute and chronic phases of myocardial infarction, provides a heterogeneous group for comparison.

Idiopathic Left Ventricular Tachycardia

Clinical Presentation

In 1981, Belhassen et al (1981) described a unique form of ventricular tachycardia that is responsive to verapamil and occurs in young patients with structurally normal hearts. This has subsequently been observed by others (Ohe et al, 1988; German et al, 1983; Lin et al, 1983; Klein et al, 1984; Zipes et al, 1978; Ward et al, 1984; Kinoshita et al, 1992; Sakurai et al, 1990; DeLacey et al, 1992; Sethi et al, 1986; Vetter et al, 1981; Mont et al, 1992; Okumura et al, 1988). The patients typically present with recurrent sustained ventricular tachycardia of right bundle branch block configuration with left axis deviation.

Most studies do not report details on the presence or absence of nonsustained ventricular tachycardia in such patients. In the study by Lemery et al (1989), only one of 13 patients with ventricular tachycardia having a right bundle branch block pattern (suggesting left ventricular origin) presented with nonsustained episodes of tachycardia. The same group subsequently reported data on 60 patients with idiopathic ventricular tachycardia, of whom nine presented with a right bundle branch block configuration with either left axis or right axis deviation (Mont et al, 1992). Only two of the nine patients with left axis deviation presented with nonsustained ventricular tachycardia, whereas the proportion in those with right axis deviation was higher (six of nine patients). One of four patients with right bundle branch block ventricular tachycardia and left axis deviation presented with nonsustained episodes of ventricular tachycardia (Klein et al, 1984). Occasional cases with patients presenting with nonsustained or sustained but self-terminating ventricular tachycardias have been reported (Strasberg et al, 1986; DeLacey et al, 1992).

It is not known whether the morphology of any of these episodes of nonsustained ventricular tachycardia generally correspond to the one of the sustained episodes. Only Slama et al (1985) mention without presenting details that "the morphologic pattern of the sustained VT's is not exactly similar to that presented by the nonsustained forms."

Probable Mechanisms

Idiopathic left ventricular tachycardia is usually not related to physical activity and not provocable by exercise testing (Lin et al, 1983; Mont et al, 1992; Belhassen et al, 1984). Arrhythmia provocation by isoproterenol infusion has been reported in single cases but is rather unusual (DeLacey et al, 1992; Gaita et al, 1992; Miyajima et al, 1987). In contrast, ventricular tachycardia is frequently inducible by either programmed electrical stimulation using rapid atrial pacing (Ohe et al, 1988; Zipes et al, 1978; Mont et al, 1992), ventricular pacing (Ohe et al, 1988; German et al, 1983; Lin et al, 1983; Zipes et al, 1978; Belhassen et al, 1984), or ventricular extrastimulation (Ohe et al, 1988; German et al, 1983; Lin et al, 1983; Zipes et al, 1978; Mont et al, 1992; Okumura et al, 1988; Belhassen et al, 1984). In a considerable number of patients, a single ventricular extrastimulus can initiate the tachycardia (Slama et al, 1985; Ohe et al, 1988) with an inverse relationship between the coupling interval of the premature stimulus and the following interval to the first beat of ventricular tachycardia (Ohe et al, 1988; Lin et al, 1983; Mont et al, 1992). A frequent finding is an early retrograde His bundle deflection during ventricular tachycardia that, together with the relatively narrow QRS complex and the characteristic QRS configuration, suggests the Purkinje fiber network of the left posterior fascicle as a location of a microreentrant pathway (Ward et al, 1984). This location is further supported by the results of detailed endocardial mapping and of pacing interventions (Ohe et al, 1988; German et al, 1983; Ward et al, 1984; Sakurai et al, 1990; Okumura et al, 1988). In a small subset of patients with a right frontal plane axis, ventricular tachycardia originates from the anterior parts of the Purkinje network of the left fascicle (Ohe et al, 1988). Despite these findings, the mechanism of this type of tachycardia is still controversial. Both reentry and triggered activity have been postulated as possible mechanisms (Zipes et al, 1978; Sethi et al, 1986), whereas normal or abnormal automaticity appear to be unlikely. The inverse relationship between premature stimulus and subsequent tachycardia, the termination by programmed electrical stimulation, a correlation with the number of paced beats but not with the duration of pacing, and the finding of entrainment (though not consistently demonstrable) suggest reentry and involvement of an area of slow conduction (Ohe et al, 1988; Okumura et al, 1988).

Termination of ventricular tachycardia may occur spontaneously or as a result of pharmacologic or electrical intervention. Vagal maneuvers usually are ineffective (Slama et al, 1985). Many authors have reported uniformly successful termination of idiopathic left ventricular tachycardia by intravenous verapamil, which frequently suppresses reinduction of the tachycardia as well (Ohe et al, 1988; German et al, 1983; Lin et al, 1983; Sakurai et al, 1990; Sethi et al, 1986; Mont et al, 1992; Okumura et al, 1988; Belhassen et al, 1984). Intravenous ajmaline also terminated the tachycardia in the majority of patients in the one study where it was tested (Ohe et al, 1988). In contrast, β-blockers or lidocaine were rarely effective in terminating or preventing the tachycardia (Ohe et al, 1988; German et al, 1983; Lin et al, 1983).

Critical Components and Vulnerable Parameters

Assuming that reentry is the most probable mechanism, it would seem logical to suppress conduction in a presumed area of slow conduction (which has been demonstrated to be present during entrainment from the presumed site of origin of the tachycardia [Okumura et al, 1988]). However, it is still unclear whether there exists a long or a short excitable gap, although the difficulty in demonstrating entrainment from most sites of the right or left ventricle might suggest that, if at all, there is only a short excitable gap. In the latter case, prolongation of the refractory period should also be effective in terminating or preventing the tachycardia. Participation of a calcium channel mediated pathway within the reentrant circuit has been postulated (German et al, 1983) and would be consistent with the favorable response to verapamil.

Targets

The efficacy of verapamil, initially an empirical observation, suggests that interventions should be directed against slow channel-dependent reentry. This is most probably based on the calcium current, I_{Ca-L}.

Interventions and Clinical Results

During long-term treatment, oral verapamil prevented recurrences of sustained ventricular tachycardia in a considerable percentage of patients and improved symptoms by slowing the tachycardia rate and reducing the number of episodes in the remainder (Ohe et al, 1988; German et al, 1983). Drugs that prolonged repolarization were reportedly successful in about 50% of patients, whereas Na^+ channel blocking drugs and β-blockers were rarely effective (Mont et al, 1992). However, other authors reported successful therapy using β-blockers alone or in combination with Na^+ channel blockers (Gaita et al, 1992). Recurrences of ventricular tachycardia appear to be frequent despite antiarrhythmic treatment but are usually well tolerated. In a small number of patients in whom nonpharmacologic treatment was necessary for arrhythmia control, catheter ablation (DeLacey et al, 1992; Coggins et al, 1992; Smeets et al, 1993) or surgical ablation (Blakeman and Wilber, 1990; Lawrie et al, 1989) of the arrhythmogenic focus have been successfully performed.

The long-term prognosis of patients with idiopathic left ventricular tachycardia appears to be benign. Only occasional cases develop overt cardiomyopathy or die suddenly during long-term follow-up (Ohe et al, 1993; German et al, 1983).

Ventricular Tachycardias during the Subacute and Chronic Stages of Myocardial Infarction

Whether the isolated (or sometimes repetitive) ventricular extrasystoles occurring after myocardial infarction are in some way related to the site involved in the generation of sustained ventricular tachycardia or whether these extrasystoles are independent and originate remotely from the potential reentry circuit is a major issue. In the latter case, they might still originate from an area that is part of the infarct but might have mechanisms different from reentry or might even arise from normal myocardium.

If the morphology of the beat that initiates ventricular tachycardia is identical to that of the tachycardia, it can be hypothesized that the initiating beat may originate from the same area. This does not necessarily imply that their mechanisms are identical. However, if the morphology is totally different, the sites involved in the genesis of the initiating beat(s) and the subsequent tachycardia may well be remote.

This issue was addressed in several recent studies. Berger et al (1988) observed 16 episodes of spontaneously occurring sustained ventricular tachycardia in 16 patients. Eleven episodes began after a single ventricular premature depolarization, three episodes began after two ventricular premature depolarizations, and two episodes began after five ventricular premature depolarizations. In eight of the 11 episodes of spontaneous sustained ventricular tachycardia that began after a single premature depolarization, the morphology of the latter was similar to that of the tachycardia. In light of our current understanding of the mechanisms of sustained ventricular tachycardia, this suggests that concealed decremental slow conduction, reflected in the long coupling intervals of the initiating beats, may be responsible for the beat initiating sustained ventricular tachycardia. The coupling interval of the ventricular premature depolarization would then represent the conduction time of the previous sinus impulse through the area of slowed conduction and through the tachycardia circuit until the point of exit. If ventricular tachycardia starts after a premature beat with a QRS morphology different from that of the tachycardia, this could be due either to a different exit site for the premature beat or to the premature beat being unrelated to the reentrant circuit. Nevertheless, it would set the scene for reentry.

Berger et al (1988) found marked differences in the mode of spontaneous initiation of ventricular tachycardia and the mode of its induction during electrophysiologic study. The number of ventricular premature depolarizations necessary for spontaneous initiation tended to be less than the number of programmed extrastimuli necessary for tachycardia induction. Similarly, induction of ventricular tachycardia is much easier (requiring fewer extrastimuli and/or a lower basic drive rate) if programmed ventricular stimulation is performed from within the area of slow conduction rather than from the right ventricular apex (Borggrefe et al, 1988a; Borggrefe et al, 1988b). Stimulation from within the area of slow conduction might well correspond to the occurrence of ventricular premature depolarizations within the reentry circuit.

The mode of initiation of spontaneous sustained ventricular tachycardia was also studied by Greenberg et al (1990). They addressed the hypothesis that the initial beat of spontaneous ventricular tachycardia has a different origin than subsequent beats. Fifty patients having 227 runs of tachycardia were studied. In 70%, the morphologies of the first beats were identical or nearly identical to those of the subsequent beats. In 16%, the morphologies were not identical. In the remaining patients, the onset of ventricular tachycardia was heterogenous. The authors suggested that the first beat of ventricular tachycardia usually has the same mechanism and origin as subsequent beats and, therefore, is not a trigger beat. These findings are in contrast to observations by Weismüller et al (1992), who found that the morphology of ventricular salvos corresponded in only 16 of 37 instances to those of subsequent ventricular tachycardias.

Bardy and Olson (1990) studied the clinical characteristics of spontaneous onset, sustained ventricular tachycardia and ventricular fibrillation in 41 survivors of cardiac arrest. In only one of 12 patients with sustained monomorphic ventricular tachycardia were acute, ischemic ST-T changes found prior to tachycardia. In contrast, three of five patients with ventricular fibrillation experienced ischemia prior to fibrillation. In the majority of patients who manifested sustained monomorphic ventricular tachycardia during the monitoring period, the onset of ventricular tachycardia was not heralded by an identifiable ischemic, hemodynamic, autonomic, or rhythmic disturbance. No clear cause for ventricular tachycardia could be identified in 28 of 50 (56%) ventricular tachycardia episodes. In 19 of the latter 28 episodes, there was no identifiable cause for ventricular tachycardia whatsoever, including pauses, ventricular premature depolarizations, or R-on-T activation patterns. Ventricular tachycardia started immediately with a premature ventricular depolarization of which the morphology was completely identical to that of the subsequent tachycardia. In the other nine patients, ventricular tachycardia appeared to be pause dependent in its initiation. However, in some cases, abrupt changes in cycle length were also observed to be followed by similar intervals without initiation of tachycardia. In 24 of 50 episodes, the QRS morphology of the ventricular tachycardia was constant from the occurrence of the initiating ventricular premature depolarization through the entire duration of the arrhythmia. In another 24 episodes, sustained monomorphic ventricular tachycardia was preceded by up to 17 beats of a polymorphic ventricular tachycardia before it stabilized. Overall, there was a lack of any consistent pattern of arrhythmia onset. Not only were the mechanisms of arrhythmogenesis highly variable and often vague from patient to patient, but the mechanisms also varied within a patient who had more than one episode. Thus, one cannot naively expect to find a simplistic, uniform preventive approach to the problem of ventricular tachycardia.

To sum up, in the clinical setting, it is not clear whether, and perhaps unlikely, that ventricular extrasystoles and nonsustained ventricular tachycardia are based on the same mechanisms as sustained ventricular tachycardia. The available observations suggest that multiple mechanisms may underlie the same phenotype. In addition, it should be kept in mind that suppressing these frequently occurring spontaneous arrhythmias does not abolish the propensity to reentrant excitation, but may even create this propensity depending on the drugs used.

*Critical Components, Vulnerable
Parameters, and Targets*

Due to our ignorance concerning the mechanisms of these arrhythmias, there is little that a pathophysiologic approach offers to
their management at present. It has become convincingly clear that,
overall, suppression of ventricular extrasystoles is not paralleled by
a suppression of the propensity to (reentrant) ventricular tachycardia.
Theoretically, the same approach to suppressing ventricular extrasystoles as proposed in the normal heart (see Ch. 12) may be considered
in patients after myocardial infarction, provided that the same mechanisms underlie the ventricular extrasystoles (and nonsustained ventricular tachycardias). In the setting of reentry, therapeutic possibilities abound, including the further slowing of conduction until there
is bidirectional block, improvement in conduction velocity to abolish
unidirectional block and/or prolongation of refractoriness to cause en-
croachment of the circulating wavefront on refractoriness. Any of
these might be critical components in individual arrhythmias.

Chapter 14

Ventricular Fibrillation

Definition

Recognition of ventricular fibrillation initially was not as an electrophysiologic entity but as a mechanical process in which fibrillary contractions of the ventricular muscle produced no effective cardiac output. Only subsequently was the term applied to the corresponding surface electrocardiographic electrical activity. In classical electrocardiographic texts, ventricular fibrillation is described as a rapid, irregular, incoherent, or chaotic waveform. A "rate" definition of >250 or >300 beats/min may be applied when there is a clear waveform that intersects the isoelectric line, but "rate" cannot often be determined. It has long been held that ventricular fibrillation is a chaotic process, but research would support a variable degree of organization as reflected by spectral frequency analysis of the body surface electrocardiogram waveform (Clayton et al, in press). Although the subject of considerable controversy, there are examples purported to be of self-terminating ventricular fibrillation (Clayton et al, 1993). That this occurs suggests that ventricular fibrillation may indeed be an ordered process that may, on occasion, reach such a degree of organization as to self-terminate.

Probable Mechanisms

Ventricular fibrillation is generally regarded as being due to random reentry (Jalife et al, 1991; Surawicz, 1985; Zipes, 1975). The obser-

From *Antiarrhythmic Therapy: A Pathophysiologic Approach* edited by Members of the Sicilian Gambit © 1994, Futura Publishing Co., Inc., Armonk, NY.

vations regarding the body surface electrocardiogram waveform features that are suggestive of organization are not in conflict with this concept, but might suggest that a relatively small number of interlacing wavelets of reentry are involved (Clayton et al, in press). Other mechanisms have been proposed and it is likely that an electrocardiographic pattern of ventricular fibrillation may arise by fibrillatory conduction from a rapid, regularly discharging focal generator (Dillon et al, 1993). At present, such a mechanism cannot be inferred reliably from the body surface, but conceivably it might underlie some ventricular fibrillation incidents that arise from degeneration of a rapid, regular ventricular tachycardia.

Critical Components

The critical components of ventricular fibrillation are not easily defined. The arrhythmia arises from a complex interaction of a substrate and a trigger. The interplay and interdependence of substrate and trigger are the basis of the concept of threshold (Gang et al, 1987). The better the arrhythmia substrate is developed, the less powerful must be the trigger to initiate the arrhythmia. When the substrate is poorly developed (i.e., the threshold is high), successful triggering phenomena must be powerful. This relationship of substrate and trigger may be very dynamic as, for instance, in the electrophysiologically volatile first minutes of acute myocardial infarction.

Substrate

Ventricular fibrillation can be supported in the normal heart, a situation in which there is no preexisting abnormal substrate (Cunningham, 1899). In this circumstance, the trigger is so powerful as to create the substrate. A clinical example would be electrocution. Nonetheless, in many patients with a clinical history of ventricular fibrillation, even aggressive pacing protocols may not induce a sustained ventricular arrhythmia. In the globally diseased heart, the ventricular fibrillation threshold is reduced, but perhaps not to the extent that occurs when there are heterogeneous electrical conditions as, for instance, in regional ischemia. Thus, the nature, severity, and territorial extent of underlying cardiac disease are some of the critical substrate components.

Trigger

The trigger is a second critical component. Each of the abnormal electrophysiologic processes that generate a trigger in themselves contain their own critical components that may merit therapeutic attention. Ventricular ectopic beats may be the triggers for ventricular fibrillation; details of their critical components are elaborated in Ch. 12. At one time, it was widely believed that R-on-T ventricular ectopic beats were specific and reliable triggers for the ventricular fibrillation that complicated acute phase myocardial infarction (Lown et al, 1967). Undoubtedly, most incidents of such ventricular fibrillation are associated with the R-on-T phenomenon, but these are neither specific nor sensitive for the arrhythmia (Campbell et al, 1981).

Autonomic Modulation

A final critical component is the autonomic tone that modulates all electrophysiologic process and that, particularly if it operates differentially, will alter the ventricular fibrillation threshold. Autonomic tone may determine whether a rapidly firing ventricular ectopic generator will remain as ventricular tachycardia, will terminate, or will destabilize the rest of the myocardium to produce ventricular fibrillation. One example of the potency of autonomic modulation is seen in the fact that vagal stimulation at the onset of myocardial ischemia can prevent ventricular fibrillation in dogs one month postinfarction (Vanoli et al, 1991).

Prevention and Termination of Ventricular Fibrillation

Prevention of ventricular fibrillation involves modification of either the trigger or the substrate, or better both, to favorably alter the ventricular fibrillation threshold. However, encouraging self-termination of ventricular fibrillation could be an important alternative management strategy. Semantically, this might not seem to be ventricular fibrillation prevention, but it could be argued that, in many instances, fibrillation does not actually begin until after an initial period of rapidly destabilizing but organized electrical activity. This brief time of electrical coherence could be highly susceptible to therapeutic attack. The critical components involved would then be those that supported the initial, possibly single reentrant wavelet and would concern conduction, refractoriness, and the impedance and wavefront energy considerations involved in the transfiber pivots of the wavefront (Janse and Allessie, 1992).

Vulnerable Parameters

It is probably impossible to prevent all the triggers that might initiate ventricular fibrillation. Even a single ventricular ectopic beat produces remarkable heterogeneity of recovery of electrical excitability (Day et al, 1992) and can set the stage for ventricular fibrillation. Total prevention of triggers, while of theoretical interest, is unlikely to be a practical proposition. Creation of a completely ventricular fibrillation-resistant substrate is probably also impossible, particularly given that ventricular fibrillation can be supported in normal myocardium when its persistence is largely a phenomenon of critical mass.

There is unlikely to be a single vulnerable parameter for ventricular fibrillation prevention. The therapeutic approach should be to modify the ventricular fibrillation threshold; this could involve a synergistic attack on several critical components. Moreover, ventricular fibrillation prevention should not be considered as solely a challenge for pharmacologic intervention. In the diseased heart, minimizing electrical inhomogeneity is important and may more appropriately be achieved by modification of the basic disease process than by manipulation of regional or global electrophysiology.

Targets

Potassium Channels

Modulation of repolarizing K currents (including I_K and $I_{K(ATP)}$) could create homogeneous conditions of electrical recovery of excitability (increased ventricular fibrillation threshold). Further, by increasing the wavelength, reentry might be prevented or the number of multiple interlacing circuits might be reduced or their creation prevented.

Sodium Channels

Suppression of fast inward Na^+ current could slow conduction to disrupt reentry and suppress ectopic pacemakers (triggers).

β-Receptors

Blockade of cardiac β-receptors could prevent sympathetically modulated shortening of action potentials (which might encourage more reentrant circuits or destabilize existing circuits) and could suppress ectopic pacemaker activity (triggers).

Evidence from Basic Experiments

A variety of models have been used to investigate the antifibrillatory potency of drugs. All have their limitations. The threshold for induction of ventricular fibrillation or the energy requirements to terminate ventricular fibrillation have been examined in elegant but nonetheless electrophysiologically crude experiments (Babbs et al, 1979; Jung et al, 1992; Singer and Lang, 1992; Usui et al, 1993). These electrical measurements do not reflect the same entity, but Chen et al (1993) have shown a correlation between the two. Table 1 lists the drugs that, in these experiments, have produced a putatively beneficial result (they have increased the energy requirements to produce ventricular fibrillation and/or have decreased the energy needs to stop ventricular fibrillation) and those with a putatively detrimental effect. Many of the beneficial agents are potassium channel blockers or have effects that prolong the duration of the action potential. The detrimental drugs include many that incorporate sodium channel block in their spectrum of activity. As an illustration that such experiments are not entirely robust, amiodarone and flecainide appear in both categories, with these outcomes probably depending on nuances of the test protocol. Moreover, lidocaine, a detrimental drug in this context, is one of the few interventions proven to prevent ventricular fibrillation in clinical practice (Koster and Dunning, 1985). Increased vagal tone increases the threshold for ventricular fibrillation (Kolman et al, 1975), while increased sympathetic activity reduces the threshold (Schwartz et al, 1976).

Evidence from Clinical Practice

Ventricular fibrillation is a serious clinical problem. Its safe and reliable prevention would be a major therapeutic achievement. It is perhaps surprising, then, that there is very little direct clinical evi-

Table 1
Effects of Specific Interventions on Ventricular Fibrillation Threshold and Defibrillation Energy

Drug		
↑ Ventricular Fibrillation Threshold ↓ Defibrillation Energy	↓ Ventricular Fibrillation Threshold ↓ Defibrillation Energy	Reference
Amiodarone		Fain et al, 1987
	Amiodarone	Guldal et al, 1993
		Guarnieri et al, 1987
		Fogoros, 1984
Flecainide		Usui et al, 1993
	Flecainide	Reiffel et al, 1985
Bidisomide (SC-40230)		Hackett et al, 1993
Sotalol		Dorian and Newman, 1993
		Nademanee and Singh, 1990
Ibutilide		Wesley et al, 1993
		Friedrichs et al, 1993
UK-68,798		Black et al, 1991
E-4031		Chi et al, 1991
WAY-123,398		Spinelli et al, 1992
Clofilium		Tacker et al, 1980
		Dorian et al, 1991
Bretylium		Tacker et al, 1980
Dibenzepin		Amitzur et al, 1990
ORG 7797		Janse et al, 1990
	Quinidine	Babbs et al, 1979
	Lidocaine	Babbs et al, 1979
		Dorian et al, 1986
	Diphenylhydantoin	Babbs et al, 1979
	Encainide	Fain et al, 1986
	Propafenone	Peters et al, 1991
	Mexiletine	Marinchak et al, 1988
Vagotonia		Vanoli et al, 1991
	Sympathotonia	Schwartz et al, 1992a

Table 2
Ventricular Fibrillation Prevention in Large Scale Clinical Trials

Proven to Prevent Ventricular Fibrillation	Uncertain Action on Ventricular Fibrillation	Unlikely to Prevent Ventricular Fibrillation
Lidocaine (Koster and Dunning, 1985)	Thrombolysis (Solomon et al, 1994)	Mexiletine (Campbell et al, 1979)
Intravenous atenolol (ISIS-I Investigators, 1986)	Sotalol (Ramsdale et al, 1988)	Tocainide (Campbell et al, 1983)
Intravenous/oral propranolol (Norris et al, 1984)	Amiodarone (Fain et al, 1987)	Magnesium and quinidine (Roffe et al, 1994)
Revascularization (Kelly et al, 1990)*	Angiotensin converting enzyme inhibitors (Cohn et al, 1991)	Procainamide (Koch-Weser et al, 1969)
Left stellate ganglionectomy (Schwartz et al, 1991a)*†		Calcium antagonists (Danish Study Group, 1984)

*: not randomized, not placebo controlled; †: sudden death endpoint

dence of drug actions against ventricular fibrillation (Table 2). Many studies have used the surrogate endpoint of sudden death, but as ventricular fibrillation may merely be the final common pathway for a variety of pathologic cardiac processes, an extrapolation of sudden death reduction to ventricular fibrillation prevention is not valid. The majority of ventricular fibrillation prevention research has been conducted in the earliest phases of acute myocardial infarction when the ventricular fibrillation event rate is high and when patients are under continuous electrocardiographic surveillance.

Perhaps because of its salutary effect in the suppression of ventricular ectopic beats, lidocaine has been extensively investigated. In the first positive study (Valentine et al, 1974), only sudden death was reported, but in three subsequent randomized studies, lidocaine significantly reduced the rate of ventricular fibrillation (Lie et al, 1974; Lie et al, 1978; Koster and Dunning, 1985). That this effect was obtained at the price of an increased incidence of asystole is irrelevant to the current discussion; there is definite clinical evidence that lidocaine can prevent ventricular fibrillation. Smaller studies involving mexiletine (Campbell et al, 1979) and tocainide (Campbell et al, 1983), which are close structural analogues of lidocaine, showed no such effect, but this might reflect aspects of study design (patient numbers, administration schedule, delays, etc.) rather than true drug inefficacy.

β-Blockers are effective in ventricular fibrillation prevention when given intravenously in the earliest phase of acute myocardial infarction (ISIS-I, 1986; Norris et al, 1984). Their subsequent mortality benefits have also been ascribed to an "antiventricular fibrillation" mechanism, but this has never been established.

In individual patients, amiodarone can prevent ventricular fibrillation but, as yet, no large scale randomized study has shown this effect. There is an ever growing list of studies that suggest mortality benefit from which ventricular fibrillation prevention is inferred but unproven (Burkart et al, 1990; Ceremuzynski et al, 1992). Sotalol is widely credited as being effective in preventing ventricular fibrillation (Nademanee and Singh, 1990; Trappe et al, 1990), but this has not been proven except in isolated individual patients who are subject to repetitive ventricular fibrillation.

In situations of their deficiency, potassium and magnesium administration can prevent ventricular fibrillation, but there is no evidence of such a benefit in other contexts. In early studies of prophylactic magnesium use in acute phase myocardial infarction, antiarrhythmic effects were suggested (Rasmussen et al, 1986; Schechter et al, 1990), but this endpoint was an arrhythmia composite that included ventricular arrhythmias other than ventricular fibrillation. In subsequent investigations of magnesium use, neither an antiventricular fibrillation nor indeed an antiarrhythmic effect has been confirmed (Woods et al, 1992).

Angiotensin converting enzyme inhibitors have an important action to reduce mortality in heart failure sufferers (CONSENSUS I, 1987), but until the V-HeFT-1 study (Cohn et al, 1986), there had been no suggestion of an antiarrhythmic effect. In V-HeFT-2 (Cohn et al, 1991), sudden death rates were reduced (although this is not true of all studies), but there is no specific information regarding ventricular fibrillation effects.

Thrombolytic therapy may create transient arrhythmogenesis, but there is growing evidence of the electrophysiologic improvements with successful thrombolysis (reduced late potentials, reduced ventricular tachycardia inducibility, decreased QT dispersion) (Gang et al, 1989; Bourke et al, 1990). Ventricular fibrillation rates following thrombolysis may be lower, suggesting that myocardial salvage by this technique can prevent ventricular fibrillation.

Nonpharmacologic interventions may prevent ventricular fibrillation. There is evidence of the power of revascularization (Kelly et al, 1990; Varnauskas, 1982) and of left cardiac sympathetic denervation (stellate ganglionectomy) (Schwartz et al, 1991a). A more general role for sympathectomy in high-risk survivors of acute myocardial infarction has been investigated. Sudden death rather than ventricular fibrillation was the endpoint. In a subgroup of patients deemed at high risk, left sympathetic denervation reduced the sudden death rate from 21.3% to 3.6%.

In animal experiments, removal of the left ventricular endocardium has increased ventricular fibrillation thresholds, sometimes to levels at which ventricular fibrillation can no longer be produced regardless of the strength of the stimulus (Damiano et al, 1984). There are anecdotal clinical reports of similar human experience, but this intervention has not been systematically investigated.

Drug Termination of Ventricular Fibrillation

It would seem likely that drugs that could terminate the process of ventricular fibrillation might be effective in preventing the arrhythmia. Termination of experimental ventricular fibrillation has been reported for a wide variety of antiarrhythmic drugs including bretylium, ibutilide (Wesley et al, 1993), dibenzepin (Manoach et al, 1979), WAY 123,398 (Spinelli et al, 1992), and UK-68,798 (Black et al, 1991). In clinical ventricular fibrillation, the first recourse is to electrical defibrillation and, not surprisingly, there is no model (nor is there likely to be) for drug use as a first line approach. Shock-resistant ventricular fibrillation, however, is a problem. No antiarrhythmic drug has yet proved effective in this clinical context (i.e., increased defibrillation success). This may more reflect the parlous condition of patients in this situation rather than true drug inefficacy. Nonetheless, clinical resuscitation schedules all suggest the use of adjunctive drugs, the recommendations being derived from experimental studies.

Conclusions

Ventricular fibrillation arises from a breakdown of a variety of safety mechanisms that include the hierarchy of refractory periods of the His-Purkinje system and ventricular myocardium and the cohesive activation of the heart. Disease processes, in complex and dynamic ways, can reduce the threshold for ventricular fibrillation. Stabilizing the myocardium to prevent ventricular fibrillation in such a volatile electrophysiologic milieu is a major challenge. Based on concepts of critical components, a variety of therapeutic strategies present themselves. It is in the spirit of the Sicilian Gambit to identify the vulnerable parameters, i.e., those which might be most sensitive or amenable to attack. So little is known of ventricular fibrillation that this is difficult. Based on the evidence of relatively empirical, basic electrophysiologic experiments, however, an approach based on altering refractoriness would seem well supported. In clinical practice, however, there is still no proof that ventricular fibrillation can be prevented by this method. Positive studies of amiodarone and sotalol have used surrogate endpoints rather than ventricular fibrillation. The new potassium channel blockers may prove too readily capable of provoking torsades de pointes to be used in this context for clinical success.

Surprisingly, the major evidence of clinical benefit comes from studies of lidocaine and β-blockers. Lidocaine would not immediately stand out as a likely preventer of ventricular fibrillation, but its success may relate to its highly specific action on depressed conduction, its very rapid dissociation kinetics (Campbell, 1983), its marked frequency-dependent effects on the sodium channel (Hondeghem and Katzung, 1984), and its relative lack of disturbance to recovery of excitability. The efficacy of β-blockers is an important reminder of the powerful antiarrhythmic effects to be obtained by manipulation of autonomic tone. Even in normal individuals, there is probably a great variation in susceptibility to ventricular fibrillation, which may be explained by vagotonia versus sympathotonia (Schwartz et al, 1992a).

Chapter 15

The Long QT Syndrome

Two hypotheses, relating to "sympathetic imbalance" and to an "intracardiac abnormality," have been invoked to explain the idiopathic long QT syndrome. The primary defect according to the former hypothesis would be lower than normal right cardiac sympathetic neural activity resulting in increased left-sided sympathetic activity. The latter hypothesis invokes an abnormality in either Ca^{2+} or K^+ currents that would sensitize the heart to the actions of catecholamines (Schwartz and Priori, 1990). In either case, the triggering mechanism for the initiation of the arrhythmias in most instances would be a sudden increase in sympathetic activity, largely mediated by the quantitatively dominant left stellate ganglion (Schwartz, 1984; Schwartz, 1985).

With relatively few exceptions, which will be discussed below, most of the syncopal episodes in long QT syndrome occur during conditions associated with stress (Schwartz et al, 1991b). Notable among these conditions are fear, rage, exercise accompanied by an emotional component, swimming, and arousal from sleep by loud noises (thunder, alarm clock, telephone ring). Thus, clinical experience has linked the occurrence of malignant arrhythmias to intense sympathetic activation.

From *Antiarrhythmic Therapy: A Pathophysiologic Approach* edited by Members of the Sicilian Gambit © 1994, Futura Publishing Co., Inc., Armonk, NY.

Probable Mechanisms

Reentry

Reentry has been considered as a potential mechanism by some investigators. The argument, here, is that a predisposition to reentry exists in the setting of dispersion of repolarization and such dispersion exists in the long QT syndrome (Day et al, 1990 and 1991). Favoring the role of QT dispersion and a propensity to reentry is the observation that dispersion decreases toward normal values among those patients in whom antiadrenergic therapy (either β-blockade or left cardiac sympathetic denervation) is effective in preventing arrhythmia recurrences (Priori et al, 1994). This observation gains further credence in light of the fact that QT dispersion remains excessive in those patients who continue to develop arrhythmias and syncope despite β-adrenergic blockade (Priori et al, 1994). The major argument against reentry derives from the observation that the arrhythmias in the overwhelming majority of long QT syndrome patients are not inducible during programmed electrical stimulation in the electrophysiology laboratory (Bhandari et al, 1985).

Triggered Activity

Both early and delayed afterdepolarizations are regarded as likely mechanisms for the ventricular tachyarrhythmias of the long QT syndrome (Jackman et al, 1988; Schwartz et al, in press) and may also contribute to some of the characteristic electrocardiographic abnormalities (Cranefield and Aronson, 1988; Malfatto et al, 1992; Malfatto et al, 1994). Multiple lines of evidence support this concept. In animals and in isolated tissue studies, blockade of repolarizing K^+ currents, using cesium chloride, favors the development of torsades de pointes (Ben-David and Zipes, 1988; Brachmann et al, 1983). When this information is considered in light of the propensity of torsades de pointes to develop after long cardiac cycles, it favors a role for triggered activity as the initiating mechanism. Also, adrenergic activation by stimulation of the left, but not of the right, stellate ganglion enhances cesium-induced early afterdepolarizations and the incidence of ventricular tachycardias (Ben-David et al, 1988).

Several clinical reports indicated that, particularly after administration of epinephrine (Schechter et al, 1984) or isoproterenol (Shimizu et al, 1991), there are abnormalities in ventricular monophasic action potential recordings suggestive of either early or delayed afterdepolarizations. Moreover, the analysis of the changes in the T wave notches that follow long sinus pauses, and of the attendant arrhythmias, is in agreement with the presence of both early and delayed afterdepolarizations in the same patient (Malfatto et al, 1992).

Based on these considerations, it is reasonable to consider that afterdepolarizations may play a critical role in the genesis of the torsades de pointes arrhythmias that cause syncope and cardiac arrest in long QT syndrome patients.

Approach to Therapy

A few general considerations are essential before formally addressing therapeutic strategies. First, lethality is very high in the long QT syndrome. Among untreated patients, more than 20% die within one year of the first syncopal episode (Schwartz, 1985), as shown in Figure 1. These data were obtained from 233 patients for whom detailed clinical information on the time of the first syncope was known and adequate follow-up was available. Second, patients with the long QT syndrome are usually very young. The average age at first syncope in the 233 patients referred to was 14 years, and many patients were below the age of 10. Hence, they depend on their parents for regular administration of therapy. Third, the long QT syndrome cannot now be cured; it requires chronic therapy. The tolerance and lack of side effects of treatment are extremely important, especially in light of the fact that many teenagers are among the patients to be treated. Finally, any new episode of syncope or cardiac arrest may prove fatal. There is no room for error.

Analysis of Critical Components, Vulnerable Parameters, Targets, and Clinical Course

As discussed above, there are two likely mechanisms involved in the genesis of the life-threatening arrhythmias of the long QT syndrome. The first is reentry. The second is triggered activity. These mechanisms incorporate as many as four critical components:

1. adrenergic activation;
2. action potential duration;
3. early or delayed afterdepolarizations;
4. possibly a reentrant circuit.

Adrenergic Activation

Among the critical components listed above, the one that best fits with the definition of vulnerable parameter is adrenergic activa-

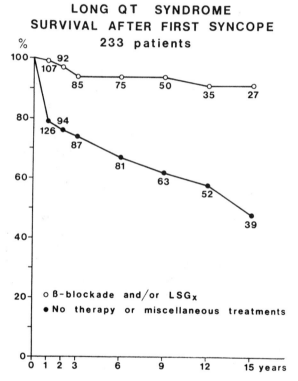

Figure 1. *Effect of therapy on survival, after the first syncopal episode, of 233 patients with idiopathic long QT syndrome. The protective effect of β-blockers and of left stellectomy (LSGₓ) is evident. The mortality rate three years after the initial syncope is 6% in the group treated with antiadrenergic interventions and 26% in the group treated differently or not treated. Fifteen years after the initial syncope, the respective mortality rates are 9% and 53%. Reproduced with permission from Schwartz PJ, Locati E: The idiopathic long QT syndrome. Pathogenetic mechanisms and therapy. Eur Heart J 1985; 6 (suppl D):103–114.*

tion. The most logical targets are the β-adrenergic receptors, the quantitatively dominant (Schwartz, 1984) left-sided cardiac sympathetic nerves and, hypothetically and as yet untested, the α-adrenergic receptors. Interference with the effect of adrenergic activation can be achieved in most instances of the long QT syndrome by blocking the β-adrenergic receptors pharmacologically. Should the results be unsatisfactory, left cardiac sympathetic denervation has been found effective (Schwartz et al, 1991a).

Results with β-adrenergic blockade and with left cardiac sympathetic denervation have been reviewed recently (Schwartz et al, 1991a; Schwartz et al, in press), and they are presented in Figures 1 and 2. Figure 1 shows the dramatic change in survival produced by pharmacologic or surgical antiadrenergic therapy when compared to other therapy or to no treatment. The mortality at 15 years after the first syncope was 9% in the group treated with antiadrenergic therapy (β-blockers and/or left sympathectomy) and was more than 53% in the group not treated or treated by miscellaneous therapies not including β-blockers. These data do not distinguish between the efficacy of β-blockade and that of left cardiac sympathetic denervation. Nonetheless, they conclusively demonstrate that pharmacologic and/or surgical antiadrenergic therapy radically modifies prognosis for symptomatic long QT syndrome patients. More specific information derives from an analysis of left cardiac sympathetic denervation effect in patients who were unresponsive to full-dose β-blockade, as shown by the continuation of cardiac events, i.e., syncope or cardiac arrest (Schwartz et al, 1991b) (Figs. 2 and 3). Left cardiac sympathetic denervation produced impressive decreases in the number of patients with cardiac events (from 99% to 45%), in the number of cardiac events (from 22 ± 32 to 1 ± 3), and in the number of patients with five or more cardiac events (from 71% to 10%) (all $P < .001$). For 62 of these 85 patients, precise information was obtained on the number of cardiac events before and after surgery, and Figure 2 shows that not only the absolute number of episodes but also their yearly incidence, thus adjusting for time, was strikingly reduced after left cardiac sympathetic denervation.

The internal control design of the study did not allow evaluation of whether left cardiac sympathetic denervation actually reduces mortality in the long QT syndrome. On the other hand, since the lethal episodes depend on the same mechanism as the nonfatal ones, it is reasonable to assume that a therapy-induced reduction in the inci-

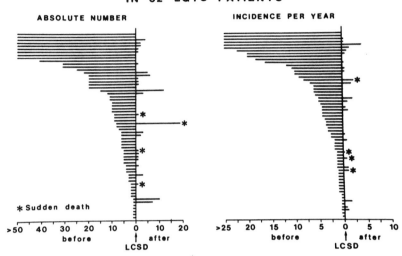

Figure 2. *Incidence of cardiac events before and after left cardiac sympathetic denervation (LCSD) in 62 long QT syndrome (LQTS) patients, in whom the precise number of cardiac events (syncope and/or cardiac arrest) was known. Each horizontal line represents one patient and shows on the left of the vertical line (time of left cardiac sympathetic denervation) the events from the onset of symptoms to surgery, and on the right of the vertical line, the events between left cardiac sympathetic denervation and last follow-up contact. Left panel: Absolute number of cardiac events per each patient before and after left cardiac sympathetic denervation. Right panel: Number of cardiac events per year. This represents the adjustment for the time of exposure to symptoms before (from first syncope to surgery) and after left cardiac sympathetic denervation (from surgery to last follow-up contact). Reproduced with permission from Schwartz PJ, Locati EH, Moss AJ, Crampton RS, Trazzi R, Ruberti U: Left cardiac sympathetic denervation in the therapy of the congenital long QT syndrome. A worldwide report.* Circulation 1991; 84:503–511. Copyright 1991 American Heart Association.

dence of syncope or cardiac arrest also implies a reduction in the risk for fatal events.

Hence, the data available indicate clearly that antiadrenergic interventions have radically modified the long-term prognosis of patients affected by the long QT syndrome and that they constitute the most effective therapy currently available. In this case, the application of the concept of the vulnerable parameter fits with the clinical course.

EFFECT OF LCSD ON QTc AND CARDIAC EVENTS

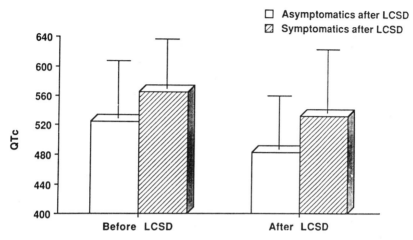

Figure 3. *QT$_c$ of long QT syndrome patients who, after left cardiac sympathetic denervation (LCSD), became completely asymptomatic (n = 45) or still had one or more cardiac events (symptomatic, n = 37). It is evident that 1) before surgery the QT$_c$ was less prolonged among those patients destined to become asymptomatic (P < 0.001); 2) that after left cardiac sympathetic denervation, QT$_c$ shortened to a similar extent in both groups; and 3) because of the different starting point, the QT$_c$ of the patients who became asymptomatic is definitely closer (P < 0.01) to the upper limit of normal values (440 ms). Reproduced with permission from Schwartz PJ, Bonazzi O, Locati EH, Napolitano C, Sala S: Pathogenesis and therapy of the idiopathic long QT syndrome. Ann NY Acad Sci 1992; 644:112–141.*

Action Potential Duration

Action potential duration can be reduced by activating outward repolarizing currents (e.g., I_K), by blocking inward Na$^+$ or Ca^{2+} plateau currents, or by increasing heart rate. At present, there is no experience with K$^+$ channel openers in treating patients with the congenital long QT syndrome. A few patients have received pentisomide, a Na$^+$ channel blocker that shortens the QT interval, but not as sole therapy. Indeed, this has been done in conjunction with antiadrenergic therapy, which has prevented the assessment of the independent value of pentisomide (Pala et al, 1987; Leenhardt et al, 1989).

Contrary to early impressions, left cardiac sympathetic denervation does shorten the QT interval. In the largest series reported so far (Schwartz et al, 1991a), the QT_c was found to shorten by 8%. Given the initial values that were quite prolonged, most patients still had abnormal QT intervals after surgery. The fact that the patients who remained completely free of recurrences during an average of six years of follow-up were those with the less prolonged QT values before and after surgery (Fig. 3) raises the possibility that even a partial acceleration of ventricular repolarization may reduce the probability of episodes of torsades de pointes.

The magnitude of heterogeneity in ventricular repolarization can be quantified, grossly but very feasibly, by measuring QT dispersion from the 12-lead electrocardiogram (Day et al, 1990). Patients with the long QT syndrome have a very marked increase in QT dispersion, the extent of which correlates with long-term outcome of therapy (Priori et al, 1994). Indeed, in 11 patients who continued to have syncope and cardiac arrest despite full-dose β-blockade, left cardiac sympathetic denervation not only abolished the recurrence of these major cardiac events during an average follow-up period of seven years, but also reduced QT dispersion to the values present in the normal control population. This finding further contributes to the evolving concept (Schwartz et al, 1994) that left cardiac sympathetic denervation exerts its protective effect not only by interfering with the trigger but also by modifying the arrhythmogenic substrate in patients with the congenital long QT syndrome. Hence, clinical observation suggests that action potential duration, while not the most easily approachable vulnerable parameter, nonetheless does have a role in therapy.

Early and Delayed Afterdepolarizations

There is growing evidence for an involvement of early afterdepolarizations (Shimizu et al, 1991), particularly in the genesis of the premature ventricular beats that initiates sustained arrhythmias, and of delayed afterdepolarizations (Schechter et al, 1984), particularly in the onset and maintenance of the sustained ventricular tachycardias and of the torsades de pointes. It follows that early and delayed afterdepolarizations are reasonable vulnerable parameters.

Early afterdepolarizations result from an excess of inward over outward currents during the plateau and phase 3 of the action potential, delaying or interrupting repolarization (Cranefield and Aronson, 1988; Damiano and Rosen, 1984). Any intervention that reduces inward plateau currents (e.g., I_{Ca-L}) or increases outward currents (e.g., I_K), thus shortening action potential duration, will tend to diminish or prevent early afterdepolarizations. Early afterdepolarizations tend to arise after long pauses or at low heart rates when action potential duration is maximal (Wit and Rosen, 1992). Hence, not only early afterdepolarizations, but also action potential duration, can be effectively considered as a vulnerable parameter for rhythms dependent on this type of triggered activity.

Delayed afterdepolarizations occur after the termination of the action potential and are induced by β-adrenergic or α-adrenergic stimulation and by increased free intracellular Ca^{2+} levels (Wit and Cranefield, 1976; Boyden et al, 1984; Lazzara and Marchi, 1989). They are also enhanced by rapid heart rates (Wit and Rosen, 1992).

As indicated earlier, action potential duration may be shortened either by blocking inward or by enhancing outward currents. In the first case, Ca^{2+} entry blockers and Mg^{2+} would be the drugs of choice. The alternate possibility, namely, to enhance outward currents, would require an increase in heart rate by β-receptor agonists or vagolytic agents. This is clearly not a therapeutic option in the long QT syndrome because the fine line between reducing the likelihood of the occurrence of early afterdepolarizations and actually increasing the probability of delayed afterdepolarizations would be easily crossed.

The potential role of delayed afterdepolarizations in the arrhythmias of the congenital long QT syndrome has led to the expectation (Jackman et al, 1988; De Ferrari et al, 1994) that drugs such as verapamil could be useful in its management. The data available thus far are largely anecdotal, with mixed results, and do not allow clear conclusions, mainly because Ca^{2+} entry blockers are always used in conjunction with antiadrenergic therapy (Schwartz et al, in press).

There are two reports on the beneficial effect of cardiac pacing in patients with the long QT syndrome (Eldar et al, 1987: Moss et al, 1991). Unfortunately, the fact that pacemaker implant was often associated with concomitant β-blocker therapy or with left cardiac sympathetic denervation makes it difficult to establish the independent therapeutic effect of cardiac pacing. Cardiac pacing is clearly indicated in patients with atrioventricular block and whenever there is evidence of pause-dependent malignant arrhythmias. There are now data on patients who have most of their episodes at night, at rest, or sometimes on arousal from sleep (Schwartz et al, in press). Most of these patients respond well to antiadrenergic therapy; however, pause-dependent arrhythmias are of particular concern in this group and pacemaker implantation has to be considered (Schwartz et al, in press).

Conclusion

The critical components and vulnerable parameters for the long QT syndrome, identified according to the concepts of the Sicilian Gambit fit very well with the successful clinical management of these high-risk patients. Antiadrenergic interventions remain the most effective therapeutic modality. For the approximately 4% to 5% of patients who do not respond to this therapy, several other options remain available, even though none has as yet been convincingly proven as independently effective. Nonetheless, they may be useful in conjunction with antiadrenergic therapy. It is for this selected group of patients at extremely high risk that the implantable defibrillator may be taken into consideration as a fail-safe system and as bridge therapy while less established therapeutic modalities are evaluated.

SECTION IV

Where to Next? Directions in Drug Development

Chapter 16

The Future of Drug Development

The Need for New Antiarrhythmic Drugs

Many types of supraventricular arrhythmias now can be treated by ablating specific structures in the atria or ventricles that are crucial to the operation of the arrhythmogenic mechanism. Nevertheless, it may take quite some time for this mode of treatment to be available and safe worldwide. Also, this type of intervention may not always be acceptable. Further, some supraventricular arrhythmias such as persistent atrial flutter and fibrillation still require drugs that are safer and more effective than available agents. Ventricular arrhythmias present a much more pressing problem. Prevention of sustained ventricular tachycardia cannot be achieved with regularity, and certain prevention of ventricular fibrillation is beyond the capability of all available agents. Further, Na^+ channel and K^+ channel blocking drugs have a significant arrhythmogenic potential.

It thus seems clear that there is a pressing need to develop new antiarrhythmic drugs that are consistently effective and safe.

General Considerations

Although there is a need for new drugs, one should not assume that need can be satisfied by merely adding to the list of available

From *Antiarrhythmic Therapy: A Pathophysiologic Approach* edited by Members of the Sicilian Gambit © 1994, Futura Publishing Co., Inc., Armonk, NY.

local anesthetics and blockers of the delayed rectifier and other repolarizing K^+ channels. For both types of agents, the potential to create new arrhythmias is inseparably linked to their predominant mechanism of action.

Agents that block fast sodium channels decrease the ability of most heart cells to develop an effective action potential. The safety factor for propagation is thus reduced. This is the means by which these agents suppress propagation in depressed areas and probably contributes to their ability to terminate or prevent reentrant excitation. Also, this effect is the cause of any observed QRS prolongation. However, for most agents, the intensity of block of sodium channels is use dependent; i.e., their channel block increases as heart rate increases. The effect of these drugs also is voltage dependent. This means that in partially depolarized areas, the decrease in safety factor for propagation will be greater than in cells with a normal resting potential. These two properties probably contribute to efficacy, but also are responsible for arrhythmogenicity. In many instances, initiation of reentrant excitation depends on unidirectional block and slow propagation in a depressed (partially depolarized) segment. Under these conditions, partial block of sodium channels can convert unidirectional to bidirectional block and either prevent initiation of or terminate reentry. By the same mechanisms, if localized transient ischemia causes partial depolarization and tachycardia, blockade of sodium channels in the involved area can establish the substrate for a new reentrant circuit (Fig. 1). Finally, during the tachycardia, the same effects of these drugs can cause heterogeneous depression of excitability and conduction and convert the tachycardia to fibrillation.

Agents that prolong the action potential and effective refractory period by blocking potassium channels of the delayed rectifier type can terminate a reentrant rhythm presumably by causing changes that eliminate the excitable gap. However, at slow heart rates, all such agents also can cause excessive action potential prolongation that leads to generation of early afterdepolarizations and torsades-like tachyarrhythmias (Dangman and Hoffman, 1981; Roden and Hoffman, 1985). These arrhythmias typically appear after a pause in the dominant rhythm, as on termination of a rapid reentrant rhythm, or during a decrease in heart rate.

The basis for this problem stems from the fact that the drug-induced prolongation of the action potential is minimal at rapid rates and increases progressively as the cycle length increases (Hondeghem

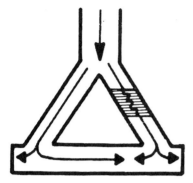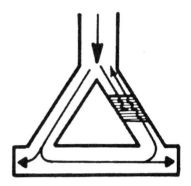

Figure 1. *The diagram shows a schematic representation of a terminal branch of the specialized conducting system where it makes contact with ventricular muscle. The arrows show impulse propagation. On the left, one branch is normal, whereas the other is partially depolarized (cross-hatched zone). In this branch, conduction is slowed and the safety factor for propagation reduced. On the right, a sodium channel blocking drug has further depressed conduction in the abnormal branch so that there is unidirectional block of impulse propagation that permits reentrant excitation.*

and Snyders, 1990). This relationship has been called reverse use-dependence, but this is a misnomer. The relationship obtains for agents that show use-dependent binding to open K^+ channels and also for agents whose binding is not influenced by action potential generation. The excessive prolongation of the action potential at slow heart rates most likely results from the fact that currents other than I_{Kr} and I_{Ks} contribute progressively more to control of action potential duration as rate increases. Thus, to achieve sufficient (antiarrhythmic) prolongation during a tachycardia, the drug-induced block must be so intense that, when the heart slows, repolarization is excessively delayed or incomplete. In the latter case, early afterdepolarizations occur and initiate an arrhythmia.

In addition to these major problems, a number of other often undesirable properties need be mentioned. Most drugs that block the Na^+ channel exert multiple effects by blocking other channels as well (Colatsky et al, 1990). Thus, quinidine causes sufficient block of delayed rectifier currents to cause early afterdepolarizations and torsades de pointes. Also, most available drugs act on atrium, ventricle, and specialized tissues rather than selectively on the site of the arrhythmogenic mechanism. A drug used to treat an atrial arrhythmia thus can impair conduction and initiate a ventricular arrhythmia.

The list of problems could be extended but the main point is clear. For arrhythmias that need to be prevented or terminated, available drugs, for the most part, lack efficacy and have the potential to cause serious arrhythmias. Something better clearly is needed.

General Approach

Identification of needed new agents can be achieved in many ways. The starting point might be derived from clinical experience. Thus, one might, quite correctly, decide that a new drug is needed to prevent ventricular fibrillation. This is an empty statement, however, since it provides no clues as to the nature of the drug.

A more reasonable approach is to employ the Gambit logic sequence (The Sicilian Gambit, 1991). First, the mechanism of initiation is identified as is the mechanism for perpetuation. In relation to these mechanisms, critical components are identified. From among these, the vulnerable parameters (the parameter(s) most susceptible to and suitable for modification by drugs) are selected. This step permits characterization of an intervention that has the desired effect on the vulnerable parameter. Subsequent tests in laboratory models then will demonstrate whether or not the assumptions have been correct.

Obviously, there are many problems with this approach. The arrhythmogenic mechanism may have been identified incorrectly or several abnormalities may provide the mechanism for the arrhythmia. In the worst case, the mechanism is admittedly unknown. This merely demonstrates the need for additional studies, both basic and clinical, that are adequate to identify mechanisms. Alternatively, the mechanisms for initiation may be uncertain but the mechanism for persistence may be quite clear. In this case, the latter becomes the subject of analysis to identify critical components and vulnerable parameters. In other words, even if prevention is impossible, treatment may still be effective.

One additional point deserves comment. New therapeutic interventions will hopefully fall into two categories. One will include agents that normalize electrophysiologic properties so that the arrhythmogenic substrate no longer exists. Obviously, this is the most desirable outcome. However, if this goal is impossible, then the new intervention, which is the second category, should be one that compensates for the causative electrophysiologic abnormality. As an example, one might consider the case in which partial depolarization of a group of fibers causes slow conduction and increases the likelihood of unidirectional block. The preferred approach would be to develop an agent that restored the reduced membrane potential to the normal value. If the partial depolarization has resulted from a change in the inward rectifier conductance, g_{K1}, such that I_{K1} was decreased, the desired agent is one that increases I_{K1} to or towards normal. If this is impossible, then it might be sufficient to augment repolarizing current provided by other K^+ channels such as $I_{K(ACh)}$ or $I_{K(ATP)}$. Tests of such interventions then might show that, even though resting potential could be restored to normal, the intervention had other and undesirable effects such as causing an excessive decrease in action potential duration. If this were so, it would be necessary to select a different target, perhaps blockade of a channel providing an excess inward current.

The main points are clear in any case. What we have is often not good enough. New agents thus are needed. Experience suggests that the approach most likely to provide drugs that are effective, selective, and safe is one that is derived from an understanding of arrhythmogenic mechanisms, the critical components of these mechanisms, and the possible vulnerable parameters that are susceptible to modification of the correct sort. Several examples of this are discussed below.

Drugs Acting on K^+ Channels

Termination of reentrant excitation can be brought about by agents that delay repolarization and thus prolong the effective refractory period and shorten the excitable gap. Sotalol (Spinelli and Hoffman, 1989) and bretylium (Baccaner, 1966) are familiar drugs that act in this way. Unfortunately, these and almost all available agents, including the new and selective blockers of I_{Kr}, often cause insufficient action potential prolongation at rapid rates and cause excessive prolongation when the heart slows. The new selective I_{Kr} blockers provide an excellent example of the bases for their inadequacy.

In developing these agents, the delayed rectifier was selected as the target and an effort made to achieve a high degree of selectively. The selectively was achieved, but the drugs blocked I_{Kr} rather than I_{Ks}. Availability of selective blockers of I_{Kr} allows us to ask if this channel is a suitable target. In general, the current contributed to repolarization by this channel becomes progressively less important as heart rate increases (Jurkiewicz and Sanguinetti, 1993). I_{Ks} thus might have been preferable. One new drug causing strong block of I_{Ks} (NE 10064) is available and appears to cause quite marked prolongation of action potentials of canine ventricular and Purkinje fibers at rapid rates (unpublished observations). However, there are clear and large differences in the importance of I_{Kr}, I_{Ks}, and I_{to1} to repolarization among different types of cardiac fibers and in the same fiber type from different species. Finally, we have no information on the relative roles of these three currents in fibers modified by disease. Selection of the target thus must not be haphazard.

All available drugs that block K^+ channels and prolong repolarization, perhaps excepting amiodarone, exhibit what is called reverse use-dependence. The intensity of effect diminishes as cycle length decreases. It has been suggested that this problem would be overcome by a drug that bound only to open channels (Hondeghem, 1991). Thus, as the frequency of depolarizations increased, more drug would bind to the channel and the intensity of block would increase. This clearly is an oversimplification since the new selective I_{Kr} blockers do bind to open channels but still cause the excessive action potential prolongation at slow rates (Jurkiewicz and Sanguinetti, 1993). This most likely reflects the fact that drugs that bind to open channels typically unbind only when the channel is open.

In light of these and other considerations, it seems reasonable to suggest that a better target is I_{Ks}. However, one also has to consider the effect of binding of a drug to a target. At present, we have drugs that partially block the channel and thus decrease repolarizing currents, but we have seen that this is far from ideal in terms of the therapeutic objective. It well may be that I_{Ks} is a suitable target, but that the drug-induced change should be a modification of kinetics and not solely blockade. The rate-dependent shortening of the action potential has been attributed to the fact that when the I_{Ks} channel closes (deactivates) on repolarization, it does so only slowly (Noble, 1984). As a result, if the cycle length is short, residual (not yet deactivated) current accumulates and speeds repolarization. It thus might be more appropriate to seek an agent that bound selectively to the I_{Ks} channel and, because of the voltage-dependence of binding, strongly modified the rate of deactivation so that, during repolarization, outward current turned off much more rapidly. This action would not modify the repolarization at slow rates, when diastole ordinarily is long enough for deactivation to reach completion, but (if the premise about incomplete deactivation is correct) would reduce the shortening of the action potential during a tachycardia. That such an action is possible is shown by data for endothelin-1 (Argentieri et al, 1993), which blocks the delayed rectifier and significantly speeds deactivation.

Again, as is the case for almost every arrhythmogenic mechanism, we need to know, but usually do not know, how disease has modified the electrophysiologic properties of cardiac fibers and thus influenced both binding of drug to target and effects of that interaction. This lack of information is a problem, but the fact that disease can modify membrane channels may present an advantage in that the targets in the diseased tissues may be more sensitive to desired drug actions than are similar targets in normal cells. Also, disease-induced changes may permit drug effects to be exerted selectively on the abnormal cells. This is considered in more detail below.

Potassium channels other than I_{Kr} and I_{Ks} may well be suitable targets when the objective is to prolong the action potential and effective refractory period. One important example is the inward rectifier (I_{K1}), the channel that sustains the resting potential. This channel does not deliver much repolarizing current because of rectification. However, during the plateau and phase 3, the net membrane current is small and, thus, changes in minor components can have important effects. It has been shown that partial block of I_{K1} quite markedly increases action potential duration (Escande et al, 1992). In spite of the partial block, resting potential of normal cells is not reduced appreciably. This approach to prolonging action potential duration obviously deserves further exploration. For example, at rapid rates, the action potential prolongation may disappear because, with tachycardia, $[K^+]_o$ increases somewhat and an increase in $[K^+]_o$ increases I_{K1}. Also, in abnormal tissues, inward leakage currents may be enhanced and, thus, even a small decrease in I_{K1} might cause excessive depolarization. This might be an undesirable effect, because depolarization can impair conduction.

The transient outward K^+ current, I_{to1}, also deserves further evaluation as a target. This channel causes the phase 1 repolarization of Purkinje fibers and epicardial and midmyocardial ventricular muscle fibers (Tseng and Hoffman, 1989; Sicouri and Antzelevitch, 1991). It also is a major repolarizing current in some atrial fibers. The channel opens and then inactivates on depolarization and recovers rather slowly from inactivation, at least in ventricular muscle. The current thus may not be of much importance during rapid rhythms. Nevertheless, several studies have shown, for nonhuman cardiac tissues, clear effects of channel block on action potential duration as well as configuration. To the extent that I_{to1} is much more important to atrial repolarization than to repolarization in other fiber types (Escande et al, 1987b), agents acting only on this target might provide needed selectivity of action on atrial versus ventricular refractoriness.

Until now, most emphasis has been placed on design of agents to partially block various K^+ channels. The time has come to begin to consider agents that increase, rather than decrease, channel currents. The inward rectifier provides a clear example of the potential usefulness of this approach. In the dog heart, after two-stage ligation of the left anterior descending coronary artery, the infarct typically does not kill the subendocardial Purkinje fibers (Friedman et al, 1973b). These surviving fibers partially depolarize, develop abnormal automaticity, and cause ventricular tachyarrhythmias during the subacute stage of infarction. As a result of the ischemic insult, $[K^+]_i$ is decreased in these fibers and $[Na^+]_i$ is somewhat increased. However, maximum diastolic potential is much more positive than can be accounted for by the decrease in the potassium equilibrium potential (E_K) (Dresdner et al, 1987). If membrane potential is increased to the value of E_K by opening the ATP-regulated channel, $I_{K(ATP)}$, the abnormal automaticity is abolished, the slow response action potential is converted to a fast response, and the action potential configuration is normalized. Several studies have indicated that the depolarization in excess of the change in E_K results from a decrease in I_{K1} (Clarkson and Ten Eick, 1983). An agent that increased I_{K1} would effectively mimic one action of pinacidil (increasing resting potential) without exerting the undesirable effects of $I_{K(ATP)}$ activation. This concept probably can be extended to other cases in which ischemia or inflammation have caused partial depolarization and impairment of impulse propagation. Further, it suggests that channel openers, as well as channel blockers, can be effective antiarrhythmic agents.

In addition to agents that interact directly with target channels to increase or decrease current, it probably will be necessary to give added emphasis to factors that normally regulate channel function. An example can again be drawn from the inward rectifier. Intracellular Mg^{2+} blocks this channel in a concentration-dependent manner. Normally, intracellular ATP binds Mg^{2+} and keeps its concentration low enough to leave the channel unblocked. However, ischemia can reduce [ATP] and thus increase $[Mg^{2+}]_i$ to a level at which channel blockade becomes significant. The Mg^{2+} binding site thus might be an appropriate target for a drug.

Other Channel Types

Currently available drugs have focused attention on fast sodium channels, L-type calcium channels, and delayed rectifier potassium channels. It is time, however, to begin to consider other types of channels as suitable targets. The heart contains at least nine types of K^+ channels, two or more Ca^{2+} channels, probably several types of Na^+ channels, and others. Among these several deserve mention.

It has been known for some time that in the heart there are slowly inactivating Na^+ channels that differ from the fast channel in terms of sensitivity to tetrodotoxin and that deliver inward current contributing to plateau duration (Coraboeuf et al, 1979). In theory, enhancement of current in these channels would prolong the action potential and effective refractory period. Evidence that this actually happens is provided by ibutilide, an agent that interacts with quite a few channels, but in very low concentration augments slowly inactivating or noninactivating Na^+ current and prolongs the atrial and ventricular action potentials (Lee, 1992). An agent interacting only with this class of channel might provide an interesting alternative to K^+ channel blockade.

Cardiac cells also contain or can express several types of Cl^- channels. In guinea pig ventricle, one type of Cl^- channel can be activated by catecholamines and, when activated, causes a loss of resting potential and initiation of abnormal automaticity (Egan et al, 1988). This channel type is not found in normal canine atrial or ventricular cells, but might be expressed under abnormal conditions (Sorota et al, 1991). Another type of Cl^- channel, present in canine atrium and ventricle, is activated with some delay by cell swelling or by agents that modify cell shape (Tseng, 1992). Such a channel might well cause abnormal electrical activity in disease states by contributing to partial depolarization and action potential abbreviation.

One of the two major Ca^{++} channels, I_{Ca-T}, has been shown to contribute inward current during the latter part of phase 4 depolarization of the sinus node where blockade of I_{Ca-T} slows rate. If this channel provides significant current to influence other automatic foci, and if sufficient tissue selectivity could be ensured, an agent blocking I_{Ca-T} might be useful for automatic rhythms.

I_f is the current providing the normal pacemaker current in the sinus node, ectopic atrial pacemakers, and Purkinje fibers (DiFrancesco, 1981a and 1981b; Irisawa et al, 1993). In ventricular muscle, an I_f channel is present but does not activate at normal transmembrane potentials. If disease can shift the voltage-dependence of the I_f channel in the ventricle to the range of transmembrane potentials at which it causes automatic firing, the I_f channel might deserve attention as an antiarrhythmic target.

Effects of Disease on Targets and Mechanisms

Unfortunately, most of what we know about cardiac ion channels and their modification by drugs has been derived from studies on channels in normal cells. It is clear, however, that disease processes modify channel function and regulation, and the affinity of drugs for these modified channels may differ from the affinity for normal cells. The disease-induced change may result from expression of modified channels or from structural alteration of standard channels. In either case, it will be important to extend consideration of available and new antiarrhythmic agents to interactions with targets that have been altered as a result of disease. On one hand, affinity of a drug for the altered channel might be less than for normal channels. As a result, concentrations needed to modify function of the altered channel might exert undesired actions on the normal channels. Conversely, the affinity for the altered channel might be increased enough to provide local selectivity of action. Future studies will have to include tissues, cells, and channels from hearts in which disease processes have modified electrophysiologic properties. Hopefully, single myocytes from human atrium and ventricle will be studied.

Other Types of Interventions

The typical sarcolemmal channel is regulated by the transmembrane potential with depolarization typically causing activation (opening) and inactivation and repolarization causing deactivation (closing) or recovery from inactivation and closing. The voltage sensor in the channel responds to alterations in the transmembrane potential, but also senses fixed charges in the membrane. The density of fixed charges can be altered, as by allowing La^{2+} or other ions to bind to the membrane. A change in the local fixed charge density is necessarily reflected by a change in the apparent voltage-dependence of activation. It is possible to employ agents that bind to the membrane only in the vicinity of one channel type. An example is provided by n-dodecylguanidine, which shows selectivity for the I_{to1} channel and strongly alters its voltage-dependence and kinetics (Tseng-Crank et al, 1993).

A suggestion that agents acting at specific loci to modify surface charge might be useful is provided by findings for canine ventricular muscle fibers surviving infarction in the epicardial border zone (Lue and Boyden, 1992). In these fibers, peak sodium current is markedly reduced at the normal resting potential and only partially restored by strong hyperpolarization. This might result from a change in voltage sensitivity or a change in fixed charge density. In either case, the ability to modify the surface charge might restore sodium channel function towards normal.

Leads from Molecular Biology

Future drug development will be influenced at every step by information derived from molecular biologic studies on channels. It is anticipated that such studies will demonstrate which components of the channel and other target structures are responsible for which functional characteristics. They will localize the site(s) of interaction between drug and target component and thus provide a molecular template to aid drug design. By point mutations, they should tell which sequences of amino acids are crucial to high affinity binding and, thus, tell where and why drug-channel and drug-target interactions are modified by disease. Finally, as a result of disease, channel density may be decreased with consequent change in the contribution of that channel type to the membrane potential. Any or all of these abnormalities can provide leads for development of new types of drugs.

Other Types of Targets

In drug development to date, emphasis has been placed almost exclusively on drugs that interact with sarcolemmal ion channels. This is unfortunate since other targets may well be equally important. A few examples are particularly deserving of consideration.

The heart cell membrane contains protein structures that transport ions across the sarcolemma and, by so doing, control the intracellular environment and generate transmembrane currents. The Na/K ATPase or pump maintains normal values of $[Na^+]_i$ and $[K^+]_i$ and provides a current that contributes to maintenance of resting potential and action potential duration. Disordered pump function permitting a decrease in $[K^+]_i$ and an increase in $[Na^+]_i$ has been demonstrated. Change in these intracellular ion activities has profound effects on electrical properties and function.

Equally important is the Na^+/Ca^{2+} exchanger that maintains $[Ca^{2+}]_i$ at a suitable value. Depending on the value of E_{Ca} and the transmembrane potential, the exchanger can deliver substantial inward and outward currents during electrical activity. Loss of normal regulation of $[Ca^{2+}]_i$ has multiple effects on electrical activity, such as influencing L-type calcium channel inactivation, activating a specific sarcolemmal Cl^- channel, and modifying Ca^{2+} stores in the sarcoplasmic reticulum. Elevation of $[Ca^{2+}]_i$ also decreases the conductance of the gap junctional channels and leads to cellular uncoupling. Other pumps and exchangers also contribute to maintenance of a normal intracellular environment and contribute directly and indirectly to the membrane potential. As studies identify the alterations in these processes caused by disease, it will be essential to design drugs that can compensate for the demonstrated abnormalities.

As has been emphasized throughout this book, there are populations of receptors throughout the heart whose effector coupling processes modulate both normal rhythm and arrhythmias. The greatest attention has been paid to date to β-adrenergic receptors, and there is no question that interventions aimed at β-blockade have improved survival postmyocardial infarction. However, α-adrenergic receptors have been implicated in the genesis of specific arrhythmias, especially in animal experimentation (Sheridan et al, 1980), and the antiarrhythmic potential of block of appropriate receptor subtypes is an area that warrants further exploration. Moreover, the possible antiarrhythmic role of muscarinic agonists that are cardioselective is a subject of interest (Vanoli et al, 1991), and the finding that adenosine, which has a very similar receptor-effector coupling process to that of acetylcholine, is effective both in termination of specific arrhythmias and diagnosis of mechanisms (Lerman, 1993; Lerman et al, 1986) holds out the hope that selective modulation of the muscarinic and purinergic receptor systems will have growing therapeutic application in the future.

It is of interest that whereas, to date, most research into the therapeutic application of receptor modulation has resided at the level of the receptor itself, current technology makes it possible to explore other targets in the effector pathway. Hence, GTP regulatory proteins, second messenger systems, and protein phosphorylation mechanisms all become fair game as therapeutic targets.

Although the potential therapeutic targets discussed in this section go far beyond a rigid consideration of channels, we must remember that the list of candidates goes even beyond this. For example, recent research on the cytoskeleton has implicated both actin and tubulin as having actions that might link into antiarrhythmic therapy. Actin has been shown to modulate transmembrane Na^+ flux (Cantiello et al, 1991). As for tubulin, the effects of a variety of agents to modify its polymerization have been studied. Tubulin binding agents not only can affect contraction (often having a positive inotropic effect) (Lampidis et al, 1992; Chevalier et al, 1994), but selected agents manifest local anesthetic actions on the Purkinje fiber action potential and modulate both automaticity and delayed afterdepolarizations (Chevalier et al, 1994). As these and other structures come under further investigative scrutiny, it is clear that the potential for identifying targets and exploring their therapeutic potential stretches as far as our imaginations.

Summary and Conclusions

The Sicilian Gambit approach to selection of antiarrhythmic drugs for a given arrhythmia indicates that the same considerations can lead to the design of new classes of drugs that may have improved selectivity and effectiveness with a reduced likelihood of unwarranted effects on cardiac electrical activity. One hopes that this approach may be adopted in future attempts to design antiarrhythmic drugs.

References

Adhar G, Platia EV, Griffith LSC, Duran D, Kallman C, Reid PR: Specific cardiac substrate abnormalities predict electrophysiologic study results. J Am Coll Cardiol 1983; 1:606.

Akahane K, Furukawa Y, Ogiwara Y, Haniuda M, Chiba S: β_2 adrenoceptor-mediated effects on sinus rate and atrial and ventricular contractility on isolated, blood-perfused dog heart preparations. J Pharmacol Exp Ther 1989; 248(2):1276–1282.

Akhtar M, Breithardt G, Camm AJ, Coumel P, Janse MJ, Lazzara R, et al: CAST and beyond—Implications of the Cardiac Arrhythmia Suppression Trial. Circulation 1990; 81:1123–1127.

Akhtar M, Damato AN, Batsford WP, Ruskin JN, Ogunkelu JB, Vargas G: Demonstration of re-entry within the His-Purkinje system in man. Circulation 1974; 50:1150–1162.

Akiyama T, Pawitan Y, Greenberg H, Kuo C-S, Reynolds-Haertle RA, the CAST Investigators: Increased risk of death and cardiac arrest from encainide and flecainide in patients after non-Q-wave acute myocardial infarction in the Cardiac Arrhythmia Suppression Trial. Am J Cardiol 1991; 68:1551–1555.

Alboni P, Paparella N, Pirani R, Cappato R, Cucci AM, Rufilli E, et al: Different electrophysiologic modes of action of oral quinidine in man. Eur Heart J 1985; 6:946–953.

Alboni P, Paparella N, Cappato R, Candini GC: Direct and autonomically mediated effects of oral flecainide. Am J Cardiol 1988; 61:759–763.

Alderman EL, Kerber RE, Harrison DC: Evaluation of lidocaine resistance in man using intermittent large-dose infusion techniques. Am J Cardiol 1974; 34:342–347.

Allessie MA, Bonke FIM, Schopman FJG: Circus movement in rabbit atrial muscle as a mechanism of tachycardia. Circ Res 1973; 33:54–62.

Allessie MA, Bonke FIM, Schopman FJG: Circus movement in rabbit atrial muscle as a mechanism of tachycardia. II. The role of nonuniform recovery

From *Antiarrhythmic Therapy: A Pathophysiologic Approach* edited by Members of the Sicilian Gambit © 1994, Futura Publishing Co., Inc., Armonk, NY.

of excitability in the occurrence of unidirectional block, as studied with multiple microelectrodes. Circ Res 1976; 39:168–177.

Allessie MA, Bonke FIM, Schopman FJG: Circus movement in rabbit atrial muscle as a mechanism of tachycardia. III. The "leading circle" concept: A new model of circus movement in cardiac tissue without the involvement of an anatomical obstacle. Circ Res 1977; 41:9–18.

Allessie M, Lammers W, Smeets J, Bonke F, Hollen J: Total mapping of atrial excitation during acetylcholine-induced atrial flutter and fibrillation in the isolated canine heart. In Kulbertus HE, Olsson SB, Schlepper M (eds): Atrial Fibrillation. Molndal, Sweden: A B Hassell, 1982, pp. 44–59.

Allessie MA, Lammers WJEP, Bonke FIM, Hollen J: Intraatrial reentry as a mechanism for atrial flutter induced by acetylcholine in rapid pacing in the dog. Circulation 1984; 70:123–135.

Allessie M, Lammers WJEP, Bonke FI, Hollen J: Experimental evaluation of Moe's multiple wavelet hypothesis of atrial fibrillation. In Zipes DP, Jalife J (eds): Cardiac Electrophysiology and Arrhythmias. New York, NY: Grune & Stratton, 1985, pp. 265–275.

Allessie MA, Rensma W, Brugada J, Smeets JLRM, Penn O, Kirchhof CJHJ: Modes of atrial re-entry. In Touboul P, Waldo AL (eds): Atrial Arrhythmias. Current Concepts and Management. St. Louis, MO: Mosby Year Book, 1990, pp. 112–130.

Amitzur G, El-Sharif N, Gough WB: Electrophysiological effects of a chemical defibrillatory agent, dibenzepin. Cardiovasc Res 1990; 24:781–785.

Anastasiou-Nana MI, Anderson JL, Stewart JR, Crevey BJ, et al: Occurrence of exercise-induced and spontaneous wide complex tachycardia during therapy with flecainide for complex arrhythmias: A probable proarrhythmic effect. Am Heart J 1987; 113:1071–1077.

Anderson JL, Gilbert EM, Alpert BL, Henthorn RW, Waldo AL, Bhandari AK, et al: Prevention of symptomatic recurrences of paroxysmal atrial fibrillation in patients initially tolerating antiarrhythmic therapy: A multicenter, double-blind, cross over study of flecainide and placebo using transtelephonic monitoring. Circulation 1989; 80:1557–1570.

Anderson KP, Walker R, Dustman T, Lux RL, Ershler PR, Kates RE, et al: Rate-related electrophysiologic effects of long-term administration of amiodarone on canine ventricular myocardium in vivo. Circulation 1989; 79: 948–958.

Antmann EM, Andrew D, Beamer AD, Cantillon C, McGowan N, Friedman PL: Therapy of refractory symptomatic atrial fibrillation and atrial flutter: A staged care approach with new antiarrhythmic drugs. J Am Coll Cardiol 1990; 15:698–707.

Antzelevitch C, Jalife J, Moe K: Characteristics of reflection as a mechanism of reentrant arrhythmias and its relationship to parasystole. Circulation 1980; 61:182–191.

Antzelevitch C, Moe GK, Jalife J: Electrotonic modulation of pacemaker activity. Further biological and mathematical observations in the behaviour of modulated parasystole. Circulation 1982; 66:1225–1230.

Antzelevitch CE, Sicouri S, Litovsky SH, Lukas A, Krishnan SC, DiDiego JM, et al: Heterogeneity within the ventricular wall. Electrophysiology and pharmacology of epicardial, endocardial and M-cells. Circ Res 1991; 69: 1427–1449.

Anyukhovsky EP, Rybin VO, Nikashin AV, Budanova OP, Rosen MR: Positive chronotropic responses induced by α_1-adrenergic stimulation of normal and "ischemic" Purkinje fibers have different receptor-effector coupling mechanisms. Circ Res 1992; 71:526–534.

Apkon M, Nerbonne JM: Alpha$_1$-adrenergic agonists selectively suppress voltage dependent K^+ currents in rat ventricular myocytes. Proc Nat Acad Sci 1988; 85:8756–8760.

Argentieri TM, Carroll MS, Colatsky TJ: Effects of endothelin-1 on plateau currents in isolated feline ventricular myocytes. Pharmacologist 1993; 35(3): 179.

Arlock P, Katzung BG: Effects of sodium substitutes on transient inward current and tension in guinea-pig and ferret papillary muscle. J Physiol (Lond) 1985; 360:105–120.

Aronson RS: Afterpotentials and triggered activity in hypertrophied myocardium from rats with renal hypertension. Circ Res 1981; 48:720–727.

Aronson RS, Cranefield PF: The effect of resting potential on the electrical activity of canine cardiac Purkinje fibers exposed to Na-free solution or to ouabain. Pflügers Arch 1974; 347:101–116.

Aronson RS, Gelles JM: The effect of ouabain, dinitrophenol, and lithium on the pacemaker current in sheep cardiac Purkinje fibers. Circ Res 1977; 40: 517–524.

Aronson RS, Gelles JM, Hoffman BF: Effect of ouabain on the current underlying spontaneous diastolic depolarization in cardiac Purkinje fibres. Nature New Biol 1973; 245:118–120.

Aronson RS, Cranefield PF, Wit AL: The effects of caffeine and ryanodine on the electrical activity of the canine coronary sinus. J Physiol (Lond) 1985; 368:593–610.

Atwood JE, Sullivan M, Forbers S: Effect of beta-adrenergic blockade on exercise performance in patients with chronic atrial fibrillation. J Am Coll Cardiol 1987; 10:314–320.

Azuma K, Iwane H, Ibukiyama C, Watabe Y, Shin-Mura H, Iwaoka M, et al: Experimental studies on aconitine-induced atrial fibrillation with microelectrodes. Israeli J Med Sci 1969; 5:470–474.

Babbs CF, Yim GKW, Whistler SJ, Tacker WA, Geddes LA: Elevation of ventricular defibrillation threshold in dogs by antiarrhythmic drugs. Am Heart J 1979; 98:345–350.

Baccaner MG: Bretylium tosylate for the suppression of induced ventricular fibrillation. Am J Cardiol 1966; 17:528–534.

Backx PH, Marban E: Background potassium current active during the plateau of the action potential in guinea pig ventricular myocytes. Circ Res 1993; 72:890–900.

Bagdonas AA, Stuckey JH, Piera J, Amer NS, Hoffman BF: Effects of ischemia and hypoxia on the specialized conducting system of the canine heart. Am Heart J 1961; 61:206–218.

Balser JR, Hondeghem LM, Roden DM: Amiodarone reduces time dependent I_k activation. Circulation 1987a; 75(suppl IV):IV-151.

Balser JR, Hondeghem LM, Roden DM: Quinidine block of I_K accumulates at negative potentials. Circulation 1987b; 76(suppl):IV-149.

Balser JR, Bennett PB, Hondeghem LM, Roden DM: Suppression of time-dependent outward current in guinea pig ventricular myocytes: Actions of quinidine and amiodarone. Circ Res 1991; 69:519–529.

Bardy GH, Olson WH: Clinical characteristics of spontaneous-onset sustained ventricular tachycardia and ventricular fibrillation in survivors of cardiac arrest. In Zipes DP, Jalife J (eds): Cardiac Electrophysiology. From Cell to Bedside. Philadelphia, PA: WB Saunders Co, 1990, pp. 778–790.

Barold SS, Wyndham CRC, Kappenberger LL, Abinader EG, Griffin JC, Falkoff MD: Implanted atrial pacemakers for paroxysmal atrial flutter: Long term efficacy. Ann Intern Med 1987; 107:144–149.

Bassett AL, Fenoglio JJ Jr, Wit AL, Myerburg RJ, Gelband H: Electrophysiologic and ultrastructural characteristics of the canine tricuspid valve. Am J Physiol 1976; 230:1366–1373.

Bean BP: Two kinds of calcium channels in canine atrial cells. Differences in kinetics, selectivity and pharmacology. J Gen Physiol 1985; 86:1–30.

Beckmann J, Hertrampf R, Gundert-Remy U, Mikus G, Gross AS, Eichelbaum M: Is there a genetic factor in flecainide toxicity? Br Med J 1988; 297:1316–1317.

Belardinelli L, Isenberg G: Actions of adenosine and isoproterenol on isolated mammalian ventricular myocytes. Circ Res 1983; 53:287–297.

Belhassen B, Rotmensch HH, Laniado S: Response of recurrent sustained ventricular tachycardia to verapamil. Br Heart J 1981; 46:679–682.

Belhassen B, Pelleg A, Shoshani D, Geva B, Laniado S: Electrophysiologic effects of adenosine-5'-triphosphate on atrioventricular reentrant tachycardia. Circulation 1983; 68:827–833.

Belhassen B, Shapira I, Pelleg A, Copperman I, Kauli N, Laniado S: Idiopathic recurrent sustained ventricular tachycardia responsive to verapamil: An ECG-electrophysiologic entity. Am Heart J 1984; 108:1034–1037.

Ben-David J, Zipes DP: Differential response to right and left ansae subclaviae stimulation of early afterdepolarizations and ventricular tachycardia induced by cesium in dogs. Circulation 1988; 78:1241–1250.

Benditt D: Nodoventricular accessory connections: A misnomer or a structural functional spectrum. J Cardiovasc Electrophysiol 1990; 1:231–237.

Benishin CG, Sorensen RG, Brown WE, Krueger BK, Blaustein MP: Four polypeptide components of green mamba venom selectively block certain potassium channels in rat brain synaptosomes. Mol Pharmacol 1988; 34:152–159.

Berger MD, Waxman HL, Buxton AE, Marchlinski FE, Josephson ME: Spontaneous compared with induced onset of sustained ventricular tachycardia. Circulation 1988; 78:885–892.

Bergfeldt L, Rosenqvist M, Vallin H, Edhag O: Disopyramide induced second and third degree atrioventricular block in patients with bifascicular block: An acute stress test to predict atrioventricular block progression. Br Heart J 1985; 53:328–334.

Bers DM: Excitation-contraction coupling and cardiac contractile force. Boston, MA: Kluwer Academic Publishers, 1993.

Beta-Blocker Heart Attack Research Group: A randomized trial of propranolol in patients with acute myocardial infarction. 1. Mortality results. JAMA 1982; 247:1707–1714.

Beuckelmann D, Näbauer M, Erdmann E: Alterations of K$^+$ currents in isolated human ventricular myocytes from patients with terminal heart failure. Circ Res 1993; 73:379–385.

Bexton RS, Hellestrand KJ, Cory-Pearce R, Spurrell RA, English TA, Camm AJ: The direct electrophysiologic effects of dysopyramide phosphate in the transplanted heart. Circulation 1983a; 67:38–45.

Bexton RS, Milne JR, Cory-Pearce R, English TA, Camm AJ: The effects of beta blockade on exercise response following cardiac transplantation. Br Heart J 1983b; 49:584–588.

Bhandari AK, Shapiro WA, Morady F, Shen EN, Mason J, Scheinman MM: Electrophysiologic testing in patients with the long QT syndrome. Circulation 1985; 71:63–71.

Bigger JT Jr, Goldreyer BN: The mechanism of supraventricular tachycardia. Circulation 1970; 42:673–688.

Bigger JT, Fleiss JL, Steinman RC, Rolnitzky LM, Kleiger RE, Rottman JN: Frequency domain measures of heart period variability and mortality after myocardial infarction. Circulation 1992; 85:164–171.

Binah O, Cohen IS, Rosen MR: The effects of adriamycin on normal and ouabain-toxic canine Purkinje and ventricular muscle fibers. Circ Res 1983; 53:655–662.

Bink-Boelkens MThE, Velvia H, van der Heide JJH, Eygelaar A, Hardijowijono RA: Dysrhythmias after atrial surgery in children. Am Heart J 1983; 106:125–130.

Birgersdotter UM, Wong W, Turgeon J, Roden DM: Stereoselective genetically-determined interaction between chronic flecainide and quinidine in patients with arrhythmias. Br J Clin Pharmacol 1992; 33:275–280.

Black SC, Chi LG, Mu DX, Lucchesi BR: The antifibrillatory actions of UK-68,798, a class III antiarrhythmic agent. J Pharmacol Exp Ther 1991; 258: 416–423.

Blakeman BP, Wilber D: Surgical ablation for idiopathic ventricular tachycardia. Ann Thorac Surg 1990; 49:314–316.

Blum M, Grant DM, McBride W, Heim M, Meyer UA: Human arylamine N-acetyltransferase genes: Isolation, chromosomal localization and functional expression. DNA Cell Biol 1990; 9:193–203.

Boineau JP, Schuessler RB, Mooney CR, Miller CB, Wylds AC, Hudson RD, et al: Natural and evoked atrial flutter due to circus movement in dogs. Am J Cardiol 1980; 45:1167–1181.

Bonke FIM, Bouman LN, van Rijn HE: Change of cardiac rhythm in the rabbit after an atrial premature beat. Circ Res 1969; 24:533–544.

Borggrefe M, Martinez-Rubio A, Karbenn U, Breithardt G: Influence of the site of stimulation on the induction and termination of ventricular tachycardia. Circulation 1988a; 78(suppl):II-631.

Borggrefe M, Podczeck A, Wittmann N, Martinez-Rubio A, Breithardt G:

Vergleich der Auslöse-und Terminierungsbedingungen von ventrikulären Tachykardien durch Stimulation am Ursprungsort und im Bereich der RV-Spitze. Z Kardiol 1988b; 77(suppl I):89. Abstract.

Boudet J, Qing W, Boyer-Chammard A, Del Franco G, et al: Dose-response effects of atropine in human volunteers. Fundam Clin Pharmacol 1991; 5: 635–640.

Bourke JP, Young AA, Richards DAB, Uther JB: Reduction in incidence of inducible ventricular tachycardia after myocardial infarction by treatment with streptokinase during infarct evolution. J Am Coll Cardiol 1990; 16: 1703–1710.

Bowles SK, Reeves RA, Cardozo L, Edwards DJ: Evaluation of the pharmacokinetic and pharmacodynamic interaction between quinidine and nifedipine. J Clin Pharmacol 1993; 33:727–731.

Boyden PA: Activation sequence during atrial flutter in dogs with surgically induced right atrial enlargement. I. Observations during sustained rhythms. Circ Res 1988; 62:596–608.

Boyden PA, Hoffman BF: The effects on atrial electrophysiology and structure of surgically induced right atrial enlargement in dogs. Circ Res 1981; 49: 1319–1331.

Boyden PA, Graziano JN: Activation mapping of reentry around an anatomical barrier in the canine atrium: Observations during the action of class III agent d-sotalol. J Cardiovasc Electrophysiol 1993a; 4:266–279.

Boyden PA, Graziano JN: Multiple modes of termination of re-entrant excitation around an anatomic barrier in the canine atrium during the action of d-sotalol. Eur Heart J 1993b; 14(suppl H):41–49.

Boyden PA, Tilley LP, Pham TD, Liu S, Fenoglio JJ Jr, Wit AL: Effects of left atrial enlargement on atrial transmembrane potentials and structure in dogs with mitral valve fibrosis. Am J Cardiol 1982; 49:1896–1908.

Boyden PA, Tilley LP, Albala A, Liu SK, Fenoglio JJ Jr, Wit AL: Mechanisms for atrial arrhythmias associated with cardiomyopathy: A study of feline hearts with primary myocardial disease. Circulation 1984; 69:1036–1047.

Boyden PA, Frame LH, Hoffman BF: Activation mapping of reentry around an anatomic barrier in the canine atrium. Observations during entrainment and termination. Circulation 1989a; 79:406–416.

Boyden PA, Albala A, Dresdner KP Jr: Electrophysiology and ultrastructure of canine subendocardial Purkinje cells isolated from control and 24-hour infarcted hearts. Circ Res 1989b; 65:955–970.

Brachmann J, Scherlag BJ, Rosenshtraukh LV, Lazzara R: Bradycardia-dependent triggered activity: Relevance to drug induced multiform ventricular tachycardia. Circulation 1983; 68:846–856.

Breithardt G, Borggrefe M, Martinez-Rubio A, Budde T: Pathophysiological mechanisms of ventricular tachyarrhythmias. Eur Heart J 1989; 10(suppl): 9–18.

Breithardt G, Cain ME, El-Sherif N, Flowers NC, Hombach V, Janse M, et al: Standards for analysis of ventricular late potentials using high-resolution or signal-averaged electrocardiography. Circulation 1991; 83:1481–1488.

Brodde OE: β_1- and β_2-adrenoceptors in the human heart: Properties, function, and alterations in chronic heart failure. Pharmacol Rev 1991; 43(2): 203–242.

Broly F, Vandamme N, Caron J, Libersa C, Lhermitte M: Single-dose quinidine treatment inhibits mexiletine oxidation in extensive metabolizers of debrisoquine. Life Sci 1991; 48:123–128.

Brown BB, Acheson GH: Aconitine-induced auricular arrhythmias and their relationship to circus-movement flutter. Circulation 1952; 6:529–537.

Brown HF: Electrophysiology of the sinoatrial node. Physiol Rev 1982; 62: 505–530.

Brown HF, Noble SJ: Membrane currents underlying delayed rectification and pace-maker activity in frog atrial muscle. J Physiol (Lond) 1969; 204:717–736.

Brown HF, DiFrancesco D: Voltage clamp investigations of membrane currents underlying pacemaker activity in rabbit sino-atrial node. J Physiol (Lond) 1980; 308:331–351.

Brown HF, Kimura J, Noble S: The relative contributions of various time-dependent membrane currents to pacemaker activity in the sino atrial node. In Bouman LN, Jongsma HJ (eds): Cardiac Rate and Rhythm: Physiological, Morphological and Developmental Aspects. The Hague, The Netherlands: Martinus-Nijhoff, 1982, pp. 53–68.

Brugada P, Abdollah H, Heddle B, Wellens HJJ: Results of ventricular stimulation protocol using a maximum of 4 premature stimuli in patients without documented or suspected ventricular arrhythmias. Am J Cardiol 1983; 52: 1214.

Buchert E, Woosley RL: Clinical implications of variable antiarrhythmic drug metabolism. Pharmacogenetics 1992; 2:2–11.

Burkart FF, Pfisterer M, Kiowski W, Follath F, Burckhardt D, Jordi H: Effect of antiarrhythmic therapy on mortality in survivors of myocardial infarction with asymptomatic complex ventricular arrhythmias: Basel Antiarrhythmic Study of Infarct Survival (BASIS). J Am Coll Cardiol 1990; 16:1711–1718.

Buxton AE, Waxman HL, Marchlinski FE, Simson MB, Cassidy D, Josephson ME: Right ventricular tachycardia: Clinical and electrophysiological characteristics. Circulation 1983; 68:917–927.

Cabin HS, Clubb KS, Hall C, Perlmutter RA, Feinstein AR: Risk for systemic embolization of atrial fibrillation without mitral stenosis. Am J Cardiol 1990; 61:714–717.

Cahalan MD: Local anesthetic block of sodium channels in normal and pronase treated squid giant axons. Biophys J 1978; 23:285–311.

Calkins H, Maughan WL, Weissman HF, Sugiura S, Sagawa K, Levine JH: Effect of acute volume load on refractoriness and arrhythmia development in isolated chronically infarcted canine hearts. Circulation 1989; 79:687–697.

Callewaert G, Vereecke J, Carmeliet E: Existence of a calcium-dependent potassium channel in the membrane of cow cardiac Purkinje cells. Pflügers Arch 1986; 406:424–426.

Camm AJ: The recognition and management of tachycardias. In Julian DG, Camm AJ, Fox KM, Hall RJC, Poole-Wilson PA (eds): Diseases of the Heart. London: Ballière Tindal, 1989, pp. 509–583.

Camm AJ, Ward DE: Antiarrhythmic drugs. Hospital Update 1981; 11: 1149–1154.

Camm AJ, Garratt CJ: Adenosine and supraventricular tachycardia. N Engl J Med 1991; 325:1621–1629.

Camm AJ, Katritsis D: How to prescribe and manage antiarrhythmic drug therapy. Eur Heart J 1992; 13(suppl F):44–52.

Camm J, Ward D, Spurrell R: Response of atrial flutter to overdrive atrial pacing and intravenous disopyramide phosphate singly and in combination. Br Heart J 1980; 44:240.

Camm AJ, Katritsis D, Nunain SO: Effects of flecainide on atrial electrophysiology in the Wolff-Parkinson-White syndrome. Am J Cardiol 1992; 70: 33A–37A.

Campbell DL, Rasmusson RL, Qu Y, Strauss HC: The calcium-independent transient outward potassium current in isolated ferret right ventricular myocytes. I. Basic characterization and kinetic analysis. J Gen Physiol 1993a; 101:571–601.

Campbell DL, Qu Y, Rasmusson RL, Strauss HC: The calcium-independent transient outward potassium current in isolated ferret right ventricular myocytes. II. Closed state reverse use-dependent block by 4-aminopyridine. J Gen Physiol 1993b; 101:603–626.

Campbell DL, Rasmusson RL, Comer MB, Strauss HC: The cardiac calcium independent transient outward potassium current: Kinetics, molecular properties, and role in ventricular repolarization. In Zipes DP, Jalife J (eds): Cardiac Electrophysiology: From Cell to Bedside. Philadelphia, PA: WB Saunders Co, 1994.

Campbell RWF, Achuff SC, Pottage A, Murray A, Prescott LF, Julian DG: Mexiletine in the prophylaxis of ventricular arrhythmias during acute myocardial infarction. J Cardiovasc Pharmacol 1979; 1:43–52.

Campbell RWF, Murray A, Julian DG: Ventricular arrhythmias in first 12 hours of acute myocardial infarction. Natural history study. Br Heart J 1981; 46:351–357.

Campbell RWF, Hutton I, Elton R, Goodfellow RM, Taylor E: Prophylaxis of primary ventricular fibrillation with tocainide in acute myocardial infarction. Br Heart J 1983; 49:557–563.

Campbell TJ: Kinetics of onset of rate-dependent effects of class I antiarrhythmic drugs are important in determining their effects on refractoriness in guinea-pig ventricle, and provide a theoretical basis for their subclassification. Cardiovasc Res 1983; 17:344–352.

Cannell MB, Lederer WJ: The arrhythmogenic current I_{TI} in the absence of electrogenic sodium-calcium exchange in sheep cardiac Purkinje fibres. J Physiol (Lond) 1986; 374:201–219.

Cantiello HF, Stow JL, Prat AG, Ausiello OA: Actin filaments regulate epithelial Na^+ channel activity. Am J Physiol 1991; 261:C882–C888.

Cappato R, Alboni P, Codecia L, Guardiglia G, Toselli T, Antonioli GE: Direct and autonomically mediated effects of oral quinidine on RR/QT relation after an abrupt increase in heart rate. J Am Coll Cardiol 1993; 22:99–105.

Capucci A, Rubino I, Boriani G, Della Casa S, Sanguinetti M, Magnani B: A placebo controlled study comparing oral propafenone to quinidine plus digoxin in conversion of recent onset atrial fibrillation. Eur Heart J 1990; 12:338. Abstract.

Capucci A, Tiziano L, Boriani G, Trisolino G, Binetti N, Cavazza M, et al: Effectiveness of loading oral flecainide for converting recent-onset atrial fibrillation to sinus rhythm in patients without organic heart disease or with only systemic hypertension. Am J Cardiol 1992; 70:69–72.

Caraco Y, Sheller JR, Wood AJJ: Polymorphic drug metabolism and codeine pharmacodynamics. Clin Res 1993; 41:204A.

The Cardiac Arrhythmia Suppression Trial (CAST) Investigators: Effect of encainide and flecainide on mortality in a randomized trial of arrhythmia suppression after myocardial infarction. N Engl J Med 1989; 321:406–412.

The Cardiac Arrhythmia Suppression Trial-II (CAST) Investigators: Effect of the antiarrhythmic agent moricizine on survival after myocardial infarction. N Engl J Med 1992; 327:227–233.

Cardinal R, Vermeulen M, Shenasa M, Roberge F, Pagé P, Helie F, et al: Anisotropic conduction and functional dissociation of ischemic tissue during reentrant ventricular tachycardia in canine myocardial infarction. Circulation 1988; 77:112–117.

Carlson MD, Schoenfeld MH, Garan H, Choong CY, et al: Programmed ventricular stimulation in patients with left ventricular dysfunction and ventricular tachycardia: Effect of acute hemodynamic improvement due to nitroprusside. J Am Coll Cardiol 1989; 14:1744–1752.

Carmeliet E: Existence of pacemaker current i_f in human atrial appendage fibres. J Physiol (Lond) 1984; 357:125P. Abstract.

Carmeliet E: Electrophysiologic and voltage clamp analysis of the effects of sotalol on isolated cardiac muscle and Purkinje fibers. J Pharmacol Exp Ther 1985; 232:817–825.

Carmeliet E: Voltage- and time-dependent block of the delayed K^+ current in cardiac myocytes by dofetilide. J Pharmacol Exp Ther 1993; 262:809–817.

Carmeliet E, Storms L, Vereecke J: The ATP-dependent K channel and metabolic inhibition. In Zipes DP, Jalife J (eds): Cardiac Electrophysiology: From Cell to Bedside. Philadelphia, PA: WB Saunders Co, 1990, pp. 103–108.

Carroll MS, Colatsky TJ: Effects of endothelin-1 on plateau currents in isolated feline ventricular myocytes. Pharmacologist 1993; 35(3):179.

Carrupt PE, Tayar NE, Karlen A, Testa B: Molecular electrostatic potentials for characterizing drug-biosystem interactions. In Langone JJ (ed): Methods in Enzymology. Vol. 203. London: Academic Press, 1991, pp. 638–677.

Catterall WA: Cellular and molecular biology of voltage-gated sodium channels. Physiol Rev 1992; 72:S15–S48.

Catterall WA, Gainer M: Interaction of brevitoxin A with a new receptor site on the sodium channel. Toxicon 1985; 23:497–504.

Cerbai E, Klockner U, Isenberg G: Ca-antagonistic effects of adenosine in guinea pig atrial cells. Am J Physiol 1988; 255:H872–H878.

Ceremuzynski L, Kleczar E, Krzeminska-Pakula M, Kuch J, Nartowicz E, Smielak-Korombel J, et al: Effect of amiodarone on mortality after myocardial infarction: A double-blind, placebo-controlled, pilot study. J Am Coll Cardiol 1992; 20:1056–1062.

Chen PS, Feld GK, Kriett JM, Mower MM, Tarazi RY, Fleck RP, et al: Relations between upper limit of vulnerability and defibrillation threshold in humans. Circulation 1993; 88:186–192.

Chevalier P, Kuznetsov V, Robinson RB, Rosen MR: The tubulin binding agent, CI-980, has positive inotropic and local anesthetic actions. J Cardiovasc Pharmacol 1994; 23:944–951.

Chi LG, Mu DX, Lucchesi BR: Electrophysiology and antiarrhythmic actions of E-4031 in the experimental animal model of sudden coronary death. J Cardiovasc Pharmacol 1991; 17:285–295.

Chicchi GG, Giminez-Gallego G, Ber E, Garcia ML, Winquist R, Cascieri MA: Purification and characterization of a unique, potent inhibitor of Apamin binding from Leirus quinquestriatus hebraeus venom. J Biol Chem 1988; 263: 10192–10197.

Clarkson CW, Ten Eick RE: On the mechanism of lysophosphatidylcholine-induced depolarization of cat ventricular myocardium. Circ Res 1983; 52: 543–556.

Clayton RH, Murray A, Higham PD, Campbell RWF: Self-terminating ventricular tachyarrhythmias—a diagnostic dilemma. Lancet 1993; 341:93–95.

Clayton RH, Murray A, Campbell RWF: Changes in the surface electrocardiogram during the onset of spontaneous ventricular fibrillation in man. Eur Heart J. In press.

Clerc L: Directional differences of impulse spread in trabecular muscle from mammalian heart. J Physiol (Lond) 1976; 255:335–346.

Clusin WT, Bristow MR, Baim DS, Schroeder JS, Jaillon P, Brett P, et al: The effects of diltiazem and reduced serum ionized calcium on ischemic ventricular fibrillation in the dog. Circ Res 1982; 50:518–526.

Coelho A, Palileo EV, Ashley WW, Swiryn S, Petropoulos T, Welch W, et al: Tachyarrhythmias in young athletes. J Am Coll Cardiol 1986; 7:237–243.

Coggins DL, Sweeney J, Chien W, Epstein L, Lee R, Cohen T, et al: Radiofrequency ablation of non-coronary ventricular tachycardia. Circulation 1992; 86(suppl I):I-520.

Cohn JN, Archibald DG, Ziesche S, Franciosa JA, Harston WE, Tristani FE, et al: Effect of vasodilator therapy on mortality in chronic congestive heart failure. Results of a Veterans Administration Co-operative Study. N Engl J Med 1986; 314:1547–1552.

Cohn JN, Johnson G, Ziesche RN, Cobb F, Francis G, Tristani F, et al: A comparison of enalapril with hydralazine-isosorbide dinitrate in the treatment of chronic congestive heart failure. N Engl J Med 1991; 325:303–310.

Colatsky TJ: Mechanisms of action of lidocaine and quinidine on action potential duration in rabbit cardiac Purkinje fibers. An effect on steady state sodium currents. Circ Res 1982; 50:17–27.

Colatsky TJ: Modulation of cardiac repolarization currents by antiarrhythmic drugs. In Rosen MR, Janse MJ, Wit AL (eds): Cardiac Electrophysiology. A Textbook. Mount Kisco, NY: Futura Publishing Company, 1990, pp. 1043–1062.

Colatsky TJ, Follmer CH, Starmer CF: Channel specificity in antiarrhythmic drug action. Mechanism of potassium channel block and its role in suppressing and aggravating cardiac arrhythmias. Circulation 1990; 82: 2235–2242.

Collin T, Wang J-J, Nargeot J, Schwartz A: Molecular cloning of three isoforms of the L-type voltage-dependent calcium channel β subunit from normal human heart. Circ Res 1993; 72:1337–1344.

Colquhoun D, Neher E, Reuter H, Stevens CF: Inward current channels activated by intracellular Ca in cultured cardiac cells. Nature 1981; 294:752–754.

Comer MB, Campbell DL, Rasmusson RL, Lamson DR, Morales MJ, Zhang Y, et al: Cloning and characterization of an I_{to}-like potassium channel from ferret ventricle. Am J Physiol (Heart and Circ Physiol) In press.

Connors SP, Terrar DA: The effect of forskolin on activation and de-activation of time-dependent potassium current in ventricular cells isolated from guinea-pig heart. J Physiol (Lond) 1990; 429:109P. Abstract.

The Consensus Trial Study Group: Effects of enalapril on mortality in severe congestive heart failure: Results of the Co-operative North Scandinavian Enalapril Survival Study (CONSENSUS). N Engl J Med 1987; 316: 1429–1435.

Cooper MJ, Krall R, Moddrelle D, Kates RE, Anderson KP: Proarrhythmic effects of flecainide acetate in the normal canine heart. Circulation 1989; 80(suppl II):326. Abstract.

Coplen SE, Antman EM, Berlin JA, Hewitt P, Chalmers TC: Efficacy and safety of quinidine therapy for maintenance of sinus rhythm after cardioversion. A meta-analysis of randomized control trials. Circulation 1990; 82:1106–1116.

Coraboeuf E: Voltage clamp studies of the slow inward current. In Zipes DP, Bailey JC, Elharrar V (eds): The Slow Inward Current and Cardiac Arrhythmias. The Hague, The Netherlands: Martinus Nijhoff, 1980, pp. 25–95.

Coraboeuf E, Carmeliet E: Existence of two transient outward currents in sheep cardiac Purkinje fibers. Pflügers Arch 1982; 392:352–359.

Coraboeuf E, Deroubaix E, Coulomb A: Effect of tetrodotoxin on action potentials of the conducting system in the dog heart. Am J Physiol (Heart Circ Physiol) 1979; 5(4):H561–H567.

Coronel R, Wilms-Schopman FJG, Opthof T, Cinca J, Fiolet JWT, Janse MJ: Reperfusion arrhythmias in isolated perfused pig hearts. Inhomogeneities in extracellular potassium, ST and TQ potentials, and transmembrane action potentials. Circ Res 1992; 71:1131–1142.

Cosio FG: Endocardial mapping of atrial flutter. In Touboul P, Waldo AL (eds): Atrial Arrhythmias. St. Louis, MO: Mosby Year Book, 1990, pp. 229–240.

Cosio FG, Lopez-Gil M, Giocolea A, Arribas F, Barroso JL: Radiofrequency ablation of the inferior vena cava-tricuspid valve isthmus in common atrial flutter. Am J Cardiol 1993; 71:705–709.

Coulombe A, Coraboeuf E, Deroubaix E: Computer simulation of acidosis-induced abnormal repolarization and repetitive activity in dog Purkinje fibers. J Physiol (Paris) 1980; 76:107–112.

Coumel P: Neural aspects of paroxysmal atrial fibrillation. In Falk RH, Podrid PJ (eds): Atrial Fibrillation Mechanisms and Management. New York, NY: Raven Press Ltd, 1992, pp. 109–125.

Coumel P, Cabrol C, Fabiato A, et al: Tachycardie permanent par rhythm reciproque. Arch Mal Coeur 1967; 60:1830–1864.

Coumel P, Attuel P, Lavallée JP, Flammang D, Leclerc JF, Slama R: Syndrome d'arythmie auriculaire d'origine vagale. Arch Mal Coeur 1978; 71:645–656.

Coumel P, Rosengarten MD, Leclerc J-F, Attuel P: Role of sympathetic nervous system in non-ischemic ventricular arrhythmias. Br Heart J 1982; 47: 137–147.

Coumel P, Leclerc JF, Zimmermann M, Funck-Brentano JL: Antiarrhythmic therapy: Non-invasive guided strategy versus empirical or invasive strategies. In Brugada P, Wellens HJJ (eds): Cardiac Arrhythmias: Where to Go from Here? Mount Kisco, NY: Futura Publishing Company, 1987, pp. 403–419.

Cox MM, Berman I, Myerburg RJ, Smets MJD, Kozlovskis PL: Morphometric mapping of regional myocyte diameters after healing of myocardial infarction in cats. J Mol Cell Cardiol 1991; 23:127–135.

Cox JL, Canaven TE, Schuessler RB, Cain ME, Lindsay BD, Stone C, et al: The surgical treatment of atrial fibrillation. II. Intraoperative electrophysiologic mapping and description of the electrophysiologic basis of atrial flutter and atrial fibrillation. J Thorac Cardiovasc Surg 1991; 101:406–426.

Cramer G: Early and late results of conversion of atrial fibrillation with quinidine: A clinical and hemodynamic study. Acta Med Scand Suppl 1968; 490: 5–102.

Cramer M, Siegal M, Bigger JT Jr, Hoffman BF: Characteristics of extracellular potentials recorded from the sinoatrial pacemaker of the rabbit. Circ Res 1977; 41:292–300.

Cranefield PF: The Conduction of the Cardiac Impulse: The Slow Response and Cardiac Arrhythmias. Mount Kisco, NY: Futura Publishing Co, 1975.

Cranefield PF: Action potentials, afterpotentials and arrhythmias. Circ Res 1977; 41:415–423.

Cranefield PF, Aronson RS: Initiation of sustained rhythmic activity by single propagated action potentials in canine cardiac Purkinje fibers exposed to sodium-free solution or to ouabain. Circ Res 1974; 34:477–481.

Cranefield PF, Aronson RS: Cardiac Arrhythmias: The Role of Triggered Activity and Other Mechanisms. Mount Kisco, NY: Futura Publishing, 1988.

Cranefield PF, Klein HO, Hoffman BF: Conduction of the cardiac impulse. I. Delay, block and one-way block in depressed Purkinje fibers. Circ Res 1971; 28:199–219.

Cranefield PF, Wit AL, Hoffman BF: Genesis of cardiac arrhythmias. Circulation 1973; 47:190–204.

Crest M, Jacquet G, Gola M, Zerrouk H, Benslimane A, Rochat H, et al: Kaliotoxin, a novel peptidyl inhibitor of neuronal BK-type Ca^{2+} activated K^+ channels characterized from Androctonus mauretanicus venom. J Biol Chem 1992; 267:1640–1647.

Cunningham RH: Death by electricity. Electrical World Engineer 1899; xxxiv: 1–8.

Cupples LA, Gagnon DR, Kannel WB: Long- and short-term risk of sudden coronary death. Circulation 1992; 85(suppl I):I-11–I-18.

Damiano BP, Rosen MR: Effects of pacing on triggered activity induced by early afterdepolarizations. Circulation 1984; 69:1013–1025.

Damiano RJ, Smith PK, Tripp HF, Lowe JE, Ideker RE, Cox JL: The effect of superficial endocardial ablation on ventricular fibrillation threshold. Circulation 1984; 70:(suppl II):224. Abstract.

Dangman KH, Hoffman BF: In vivo and in vitro antiarrhythmic and arrhythmogenic effects of N-acetyl procainamide. J Pharmacol Exp Ther 1981; 217: 851–862.

Dangman KH, Hoffman BF: Studies on overdrive stimulation of canine cardiac Purkinje fibers: Maximal diastolic potential as a determinant of the response. J Am Coll Cardiol 1983; 2:1183–1190.

Dangman KH, Hoffman BF: The effects of single premature stimuli on automatic and triggered rhythms in isolated canine Purkinje fibers. Circulation 1985; 71:813–822.

Dangman KH, Dresdner KP, Zaim S: Automatic and triggered impulse initiation in canine subepicardial ventricular muscle cells from border zone of 24-hour transmural infarcts. Circulation 1988; 78:1020–1030.

Danish Study Group on Verapamil in Myocardial Infarction: Verapamil in acute myocardial infarction. Eur Heart J 1984; 5:516–528.

Data JL, Wilkinson GR, Nies AS: Interaction of quinidine with anticonvulsant drugs. N Engl J Med 1976; 294:699–702.

Davidenko JM, Cohen L, Goodrow R, Antzelevitch C: Quinidine-induced action potential prolongation, early afterdepolarizations, and triggered activity in canine Purkinje fibers. Effects of stimulation rate, potassium, and magnesium. Circulation 1989; 79:674–686.

Davies M, Giffin K, Liang CD, Russell MA, Butler A, Salkoff L, et al: Verapamil inhibits the human cardiac delayed rectifier (Kv1.5) channel. Biophys J 1992; 61:A376.

Davis LD: Effect of changes in cycle length on diastolic depolarization produced by ouabain in canine Purkinje fibers. Circ Res 1973; 32:206–214.

Day CP, McComb JM, Campbell RWF: QT dispersion: An indication of arrhythmia risk in patients with long QT intervals. Br Heart J 1990; 63: 342–344.

Day CP, McComb JM, Campbell RWF: Reduction in QT dispersion by sotalol following myocardial infarction. Eur Heart J 1991; 12:423–427.

Day CP, McComb JM, Campbell RWF: QT dispersion in sinus beats and ventricular extrasystoles in normal hearts. Br Heart J 1992; 67:39–41.

Debbas NMG, Nathan AW, Chochrane T, Levy AM, Camm AJ: Characterization of atrial repolarization from the surface ECG. Effect of antiarrhythmic drugs and atrial pacing. PACE 1984; 7:458–463.

DeBin JA, Maggio JE, Strichartz GR: Purification and characterization of chlorotoxin, a chloride channel ligand from the venom of the scorpion. Am J Physiol 1993; (Cell Physiol 33) 264:C361–C369.

DeBoer S: Herzwühlen, Flimmern, Flattern, gehäufte Extrasystolie, paroxysmale Tachykardie. Pflügers Arch Ges Physiol 1921; 193:183.

Deck KA: Aenderungen des Ruhepotentials und der Kabeleigenschaften von Purkinje-Faden bei der Dehnung. Pflügers Arch 1964; 280:131–140.

De Ferrari GM, Nador F, Beria G, Sala S, Lotto A, Schwartz PJ: Effect of calcium channel blocker on the wall motion abnormality of the idiopathic long QT syndrome. Circulation 1994; 89:2126–2132.

Deitmer JW, Ellis D: The intracellular sodium activity of cardiac Purkinje fibres during inhibition and re-activation of the Na-K pump. J Physiol (Lond) 1978; 284:241–259.

DeLacey WA, Nath S, Haines DE, Barber MJ, DiMarco JP: Adenosine and verapamil-sensitive ventricular tachycardia originating from the left ventricle: Radiofrequency catheter ablation. PACE 1992; 15:2240–2244.

De la Fuente D, Sasyniuk BI, Moe GK: Conduction through a narrow isthmus in isolated canine atrial tissue. A model of the WPW syndrome. Circulation 1971; 44:803–809.

del Balzo U, Rosen MR, Malfatto G, Kaplan LM, Steinberg SF: Specific α_1-adrenergic receptor subtypes modulate catecholamine induced increases and decreases in ventricular automaticity. Circ Res 1990; 67:1535–1551.

DeMello WC: Effect of intracellular injection of calcium and strontium on cell communication in heart. J Physiol (Lond) 1975; 250:231–245.

Désilets M, Baumgarten CM: Isoproterenol directly stimulates the Na^+-K^+ pump in isolated cardiac myocytes. Am J Physiol 1986; 251:H218–H225.

de Weille JR: Modulation of ATP sensitive potassium channels. Cardiovasc Res 1992; 26:1017–1020.

de Weille JR, Schweitz H, Maes P, Tartar A, Lazdunski M: Calciseptine, a peptide isolated from black mamba venom, is a specific blocker of the L-type calcium channel. Proc Natl Acad Sci USA 1991; 88:2437–2440.

Dietrich H, Borchard U, Hafner D, Hirth C: Antiarrhythmic and electrophysiological actions of flecainide, bepridil and amiodarone on isolated heart preparations during controlled hypoxia. Arch Int Pharmacodyn Ther 1985; 274:267–282.

DiFrancesco D: A new interpretation of the pace-maker current in calf Purkinje fibres. J Physiol (Lond) 1981a; 314:359–376.

DiFrancesco D: A study of the ionic nature of the pace-maker current in calf Purkinje fibres. J Physiol (Lond) 1981b; 314:377–393.

DiFrancesco D: The cardiac hyperpolarizing-activated current, I_f. Origins and developments. Prog Biophys Mol Biol 1985; 46:163–183.

DiFrancesco D: Characterization of single pacemaker channels in cardiac sino-atrial node cells. Nature 1986; 324:470–473.

DiFrancesco D: The hyperpolarization-activated current, I_f, and cardiac pace-making. In Rosen MR, Janse MJ, Wit AL (eds): Cardiac Electrophysiology: A Textbook. Mount Kisco, NY: Futura Publishing Co, 1990, pp. 117–132.

DiFrancesco D: The contribution of the pacemaker current (I_f) to generation of spontaneous activity in rabbit sino-atrial node myocytes. J Physiol (Lond) 1991; 434:23–40.

DiFrancesco D, Ojeda C: Properties of the current I_f in the sino-atrial node of the rabbit compared with those of the current I_{K2} in Purkinje fibres. J Physiol (Lond) 1980; 308:353–367.

DiFrancesco D, Noble D: A model of cardiac electrical activity incorporating ionic pumps and concentration changes. Philos Trans R Soc Lond (Biol) 1985; 307:353–398.

DiFrancesco D, Tortora P: Direct activation of cardiac pacemaker channels by intracellular cyclic AMP. Nature 1991; 351:145–147.

DiFrancesco D, Zaza A: The cardiac pacemaker current I_f. J Cardiovasc Electrophysiol 1992; 3:334–344.

DiFrancesco D, Ferroni A, Mazzanti M, Tromba C: Properties of the hyperpolarizing-activated current (I_f) in cells isolated from the rabbit sino-atrial node. J Physiol (Lond) 1986; 377:61–88.

DiFrancesco D, Ducouret P, Robinson RB: Muscarinic modulation of cardiac rate at low acetylcholine concentrations. Science 1989; 243:669–671.

Dillon S, Allessie MA, Ursell PC, Wit AL: Influence of anisotropic tissue structure on reentrant circuits in the subepicardial border zone of subacute canine infarcts. Circ Res 1988; 63:182–206.

Dillon SM, Coromilas J, Waldecker B, Wit AL: Effects of overdrive stimulation on functional reentrant circuits causing ventricular tachycardia in the canine heart: Mechanisms for resumption or alteration of tachycardia. J Cardiovasc Electrophysiol 1993; 4:393–411.

DiMarco JP, Sellers D, Lerman BB, Greenberg ML, Berne RM, Belardinelli L: Diagnostic and therapeutic use of adenosine in patients with supraventricular tachyarrhythmias. J Am Coll Cardiol 1985; 6:417–425.

Dodge FA, Cranefield PF: Nonuniform conduction in cardiac Purkinje fibers. In Carvalho AP, Hoffman BF, Lieberman M (eds): Normal and Abnormal Conduction in the Heart. Mount Kisco, NY: Futura Publishing Co, 1982, pp. 379–395.

Doerr T, Denger R, Trautwein W: Calcium currents in single SA nodal cells of the rabbit heart studied with action potential clamp. Pflügers Arch 1989; 413:599–603.

Dorian P, Newman D: Effect of sotalol on ventricular fibrillation and defibrillation in humans. Am J Cardiol 1993; 72(4):72A–79A.

Dorian P, Fain ES, Davy JM, Winkle RA, et al: Lidocaine causes a reversible, concentration-dependent increase in defibrillation energy requirements. J Am Coll Cardiol 1986; 8:327–332.

Dorian P, Wang M, David I, Poindel C: Oral clofilium produces sustained lowering of defibrillation energy requirements in a canine model. Circulation 1991; 83:614–621.

Downar E, Janse MJ, Durrer D: The effect of acute coronary artery occlusion on subepicardial transmembrane potentials in the intact porcine heart. Circulation 1977; 56:217–224.

Drayer DE, Lowenthal DT, Woosley RL, Nies AS, et al: Cumulation of N-acetylprocainamide, an active metabolite of procainamide, in patients with impaired renal function. Clin Pharmacol Ther 1977; 22:63–69.

Drayer DE, Reidenberg MM: Clinical consequences of polymorphic acetylation of basic drugs. Clin Pharmacol Ther 1977; 22:251–258.

Dresdner KP, Kline RP, Wit AL: Intracellular K^+ activity, intracellular Na^+ activity and maximum diastolic potential of canine subendocardial Purkinje cells from one-day-old infarcts. Circ Res 1987; 60:122–132.

Duchatelle-Gourdon I, Hartzell CH, Lagrutta AA: Modulation of the delayed rectifier potassium current in frog cardiomyocytes by beta-adrenergic agonists and magnesium. J Physiol (Lond) 1989; 415:251–274.

Duff HJ, Offord J, West J, Catterall WA: Class I and IV antiarrhythmic drugs and cytosolic calcium regulate mRNA encoding the sodium channel alpha subunit in rat cardiac muscle. Mol Pharmacol 1992; 42:570–574.

Durrer D, Schoo L, Schuilenburg RM, Wellens HJJ: The role of premature beats in the initiation and the termination of supraventricular tachycardia in the Wolff-Parkinson-White syndrome. Circulation 1967; 36:644–662.

Earm YE, Shimoni Y, Spindler AJ: A pace-maker-like current in the sheep atrium and its modulation by catecholamines. J Physiol (Lond) 1983; 342: 569–590.

Echt DS, Lee JT, Murray KT, Vorperian V, Borganelli SM, Crawford DM, et al: A randomized, double-blind, placebo-controlled dose-ranging study of intravenous UK-68,798 (dofetilide) in patients with inducible sustained ventricular tachyarrhythmias. Circulation 1991b; 84:II-714.

Echt DS, Liebson PR, Mitchell LB, Peters RW, Obias-Manno D, Barker AH, et al: Mortality and morbidity in patients receiving encainide, flecainide, or placebo. N Engl J Med 1991a; 324:781–788.

Egan TM, Noble SJ, Powell T, Twist VW, Yamaoka K: On the mechanism of isoprenaline- and forskolin-induced depolarization of single guinea-pig ventricular myocytes. J Physiol (Lond) 1988; 400:299–320.

Ehara T, Noma A, Ono K: Calcium-activated non-selective cation channel in ventricular cells isolated from adult guinea-pig hearts. J Physiol (Lond) 1988; 403:117–133.

Eichelbaum M, Gross AS: The genetic polymorphism of debrisoquine/sparteine metabolism—clinical aspects. Pharmacol Ther 1990; 46:377–394.

Eisner DA, Lederer WJ: Inotropic and arrhythmogenic effects of potassium-depleted solutions on mammalian cardiac muscle. J Physiol (Lond) 1979; 294:255–277.

Eisner DA, Lederer WJ: Na-Ca exchange: Stoichiometry and electrogenicity. Am J Physiol 1985; 248:C189–C202.

Eisner DA, Smith TW: The Na-K pump and its effectors in cardiac muscle. In Fozzard HA, Haber E, Jennings RB, Katz AM, Morgan HE (eds): The Heart and Cardiovascular System. Scientific Foundations. New York, NY: Raven Press, 1992, pp. 863–901.

Eldar M, Griffin JY, Abbott JA, Benditt D, Bhandari A, Herre JM, et al: Permanent cardiac pacing in patients with the long QT syndrome. J Am Coll Cardiol 1987; 10:600–607.

Elharrar V, Bailey JC, Lathrop DA, Zipes DP: Effects of aprindine HC1 on slow channel action potentials and transient depolarizations in canine Purkinje fibers. J Pharmacol Exp Ther 1978;205:410–417.

El-Sherif N, Lazzara R: Reentrant ventricular arrhythmias in the late myocardial infarction period. 7. Effects of verapamil and D-600 and role of the "slow channel." Circulation 1979; 60:605–615.

El-Sherif N, Scherlag BJ, Lazzara R, Hope RR: Reentrant ventricular arrhythmias in the late myocardial infarction period. 1. Conduction characteristics in the infarction zone. Circulation 1977a; 55:686–702.

El-Sherif N, Hope RR, Scherlag BJ, Lazzara R: Reentrant ventricular arrhythmias in the late myocardial infarction period. 2. Patterns of initiation and termination of reentry. Circulation 1977b; 55:702–719.

El-Sherif N, Smith RA, Evans K: Canine ventricular arrhythmias in the late myocardial infarction period. 8. Epicardial mapping of reentrant circuits. Circ Res 1981; 49:255–265.

El-Sherif N, Gough WB, Zeiler RH, Mehra R: Triggered ventricular rhythms in one-day-old myocardial infarction in the dog. Circ Res 1983; 52:566–579.

El-Sherif N, Gough WB, Zeiler RH, Hariman R: Reentrant ventricular arrhythmias in the late myocardial infarction period. 12. Spontaneous versus induced reentry and intramural versus epicardial circuits. J Am Coll Cardiol 1985; 6:124–132.

Engelmann TW: Über den Ursprung der Herzbewegung und die physiologischen Eigenschaften der großen Herznerven des Frosches. Pflügers Arch 1896; 65:109.

Engle G, Hoyer D, Berthold R, Wagner H: ($\pm$)-[125-iodo]cyanopindolol, a new ligand for β-adrenoceptors: Identification and quantification of subclasses of β-adrenoceptors in guinea-pig. Naunyn-Schmiedeberg's Arch Pharmacol 1981; 317:277–285.

Escande D, Coraboeuf E, Planche C: Abnormal pacemaking is modulated by sarcoplasmic reticulum in partially-depolarized myocardium from dilated right atria in humans. J Mol Cell Cardiol 1987a; 19:231–241.

Escande D, Coulombe A, Faiure JF, Deroubaix E, Coraboeuf E: Two types of transient outward current in adult human atrial cells. Am J Physiol 1987b; 252:H142–148.

Escande D, Mestre M, Cavero I, Brugada J, Kirchhof C: RP 58866 and its active enantiomer RP 62719 (Terikalant) blockers of the inward rectifier K^+ current acting as pure class III antiarrhythmic agents. J Cardio Pharm 1992; 20:S106–S113.

Fabiato A: Calcium-induced release of calcium from the cardiac sarcoplasmic reticulum. Am J Physiol 1983; 245:C1–C14.

Fabiato A, Fabiato F: Contractions induced by a calcium-triggered release of calcium from the sarcoplasmic reticulum of single skinned cardiac cells. J Physiol (Lond) 1975; 249:469–495.

Fain ES, Dorian P, Davy JM, Kates RE, Winkle RA: Effects of encainide and its metabolites on energy requirements for defibrillation. Circulation 1986; 73:1334–1341.

Fain ES, Lees JT, Winkle RA: Effects of acute intravenous and chronic oral amiodarone on defibrillation energy requirements. Am Heart J 1987; 114: 8–17.

Falk RH: Proarrhythmic responses to atrial antiarrhythmic therapy. In Falk RH, Podrid PJ (eds): Atrial Fibrillation. Mechanisms and Management. New York, NY: Raven Press, 1992, pp. 283–306.

Falk RH, Leavitt JI: Digoxin for atrial fibrillation: A drug whose time has gone? Ann Intern Med 1991; 14:573–575.

Falk RH, Knowlton AA, Bernard SA, Gotlieb NE, Battinelli NJ: Digoxin for converting recent-onset atrial fibrillation to sinus rhythm. A randomized double-blinded trial. Ann Intern Med 1987; 106:503–506.

Faniel R, Schoenfeld PH: Efficiency of i.v. amiodarone in converting rapid atrial fibrillation and flutter to sinus rhythm in intensive care patients. Eur Heart J 1983; 4:180–185.

Fedida DY, Shimoni S, Giles WR: A novel effect of norepinephrine on cardiac cells is mediated by α_1 adrenoceptors. Am J Physiol 1989; 256:H1500–1504.

Feld GK: Atrial fibrillation: Is there a safe and highly effective pharmacological treatment? Circulation 1990; 82:2248–2250.

Feld GK, Shahandeh-Rad F: Mechanism of double potentials recorded during sustained atrial flutter in the canine right atrial crush-injury model. Circulation 1992; 86:628–641.

Feld GK, Fleck P, Cheng P-S, Boyce K, Bahnson TD, Stein JB, et al: Radiofrequency catheter ablation for the treatment of human Type I atrial flutter. Identification of a critical zone in the reentrant circuit by endocardial mapping techniques. Circulation 1992; 86:1233–1240.

Ferrier GR: Effects of transmembrane potential on oscillatory afterpotentials induced by acetylstrophanthidin in canine ventricular tissues. J Pharm Exp Ther 1980; 215:332–341.

Ferrier GR, Moe GK: Effect of calcium on acetylstrophanthidin-induced transient depolarizations in canine Purkinje tissue. Circ Res 1973; 33:508–515.

Ferrier GR, Rosenthal JE: Automaticity and entrance block induced by focal depolarization of mammalian ventricular tissues. Circ Res 1980; 47:238–248.

Ferrier GR, Saunders JH, Mendez C: A cellular mechanism for the generation of ventricular arrhythmias by acetylstrophanthidin. Circ Res 1973; 32: 600–609.

Fields JZ, Roeske WR, Morkin E, Yamamura HI: Cardiac muscarinic cholinergic receptors: Biochemical identification and characterization. J Biol Chem 1978; 253:3251–3258.

Flaker GC, Blackshear JL, McBride R, Kronmal RA, et al: Antiarrhythmic drug therapy and cardiac mortality in atrial fibrillation. The Stroke Prevention in Atrial Fibrillation Investigators. J Am Coll Cardiol 1992; 20:527–532.

Flinn CJ, Wolff GS, Dick M II, Campbell RM, Borkat G, Cast A, et al: Cardiac rhythm after the Mustard operation for complete transposition of the great arteries. N Engl J Med 1984; 310:1625–1638.

Fogoros RN: Amiodarone-induced refractoriness to cardioversion. Ann Intern Med 1984; 100:699–700.

Folander K, Smith JS, Antanavage J, Bennett C, Stein RB, Swanson R: Cloning and expression of the delayed-rectifier I_{SK} channel from neonatal rat heart and diethylstilbesterol-primed rat uterus. Proc Natl Acad Sci USA 1990; 87: 2975–2979.

Follmer CH, Colatsky TJ: Block of delayed rectifier potassium current, I_K, by flecainide and E-4031 in cat ventricular myocytes. Circulation 1990; 82: 289–293.

Follmer CH, Cullinan CA, Colatsky TJ: Amiodarone: Delayed rectifier block selectivity in cat ventricular myocytes. Circulation 1990; 82:III–11. Abstract.

Fozzard HA: Conduction of the action potential. In Berne RM (ed): The Cardiovascular System. Bethesda, MD: The American Physiological Society, 1979, pp. 335–356.

Fozzard HA, Hanck DA: Sodium channels. In Fozzard HA, Haber E, Jennings

RB, Katz AM, Morgan HE (eds): The Heart and Cardiovascular System. Scientific Foundations. New York, NY: Raven Press, 1992, pp. 1091–1119.

Frame LH, Simson MB: Oscillations of conduction, action potential duration, and refractoriness. A mechanism for spontaneous termination of reentrant tachycardias. Circulation 1988; 78:1277–1287.

Frame LH, Page RL, Hoffman BF: Atrial reentry around an anatomic barrier with a partially refractory excitable gap. A canine model of atrial flutter. Circ Res 1986; 58:495–511.

Frame LH, Page RL, Boyden PA, Fenoglio JJ Jr, Hoffman BF: Circus movement in the canine atrium around the tricuspid ring during experimental atrial flutter and during reentry in vivo. Circulation 1987; 76:1155–1175.

Franz MR: Method and theory of monophasic action potential. Prog Cardiovasc Dis 1991; 33:347–368.

Frech GC, VanDongen MJ, Schuster G, Brown AM, Joho RH: A novel potassium channel with delayed rectifier properties isolated from rat brain by expression cloning. Nature 1989; 340:642–645.

Friedman L, Schron E, Yusuf S: Risk-benefit assessment of antiarrhythmic drugs. An epidemiological perspective. Drug Safety 1991; 6:323–331.

Friedman PL, Manwaring JH, Roseman RH, Donion G: Clinical and pathological differentiation in coronary artery disease. JAMA 1973a; 225:1319–1328.

Friedman PL, Stewart JR, Fenoglio JJ Jr, Wit AL: Survival of subendocardial Purkinje fibers after extensive myocardial infarction in dogs. In vitro and in vivo correlations. Circ Res 1973b; 33:597–611.

Friedrichs GS, Chi L, Black SC, Manley PJ, et al: Antifibrillatory effects of ibutilide in the rabbit isolated heart: Mediation via ATP-dependent potassium channels. J Pharmacol Exp Ther 1993; 266:1348–1354.

Funck-Brentano C, Kroemer HK, Lee JT, Roden DM: Propafenone. N Engl J Med 1990; 322:518–525.

Furukawa T, Kimura S, Castellanos A, Bassett AL, Myerburg RJ: In vivo induction of "focal" triggered ventricular arrhythmias and responses to overdrive pacing in the canine heart. Circulation 1990; 82:549–559.

Furukawa T, Kimura S, Furukawa N, Bassett AL, Myerburg RJ: Role of cardiac ATP-regulated potassium channels in differential responses of endocardial and epicardial cells to ischemia. Circ Res 1991a; 68:1693–1702.

Furukawa T, Moroe K, Mayrovitz HN, Sampsell R, Furukawa N, Myerburg RJ: Arrhythmogenic effects of graded coronary blood flow reduction superimposed upon prior myocardial infarction in dogs. Circulation 1991b; 84: 368–377.

Furukawa T, Kimura S, Furukawa N, Bassett AL, Myerburg RJ: Potassium rectifier currents differ in myocytes of endocardial and epicardial origin. Circ Res 1992; 70:91–103.

Furukawa T, Bassett AL, Kimura S, Furukawa N, Myerburg RJ: The ionic mechanism of reperfusion-induced early afterdepolarizations in feline left ventricular hypertrophy. J Clin Invest 1993; 91:1521–1531.

Furukawa T, Myerburg RJ, Furukawa N, Kimura S, Bassett AL: Metabolic inhibition of $I_{Ca,L}$ and I_K differs in feline left ventricular hypertrophy. Am J Physiol. In press.

Gadsby DC: The Na/K pump of cardiac cells. Annu Rev Biophys Bioeng 1984; 13:373–378.

Gadsby DC, Cranefield PF: Electrogenic sodium extrusion in cardiac Purkinje fibers. J Gen Physiol 1979; 73:819–837.

Gaita F, Leclercq JF, Haissaguerre M, Libero L, Guistetto C, Richiardi E, et al: Clinical features and long-term follow-up of idiopathic fascicular tachycardias. Eur Heart J 1992; 13(suppl):135.

Gallagher JJ, Pritchett ELC, Sealy WC, Kasell J, Wallace AG: The preexcitation syndromes. Prog Cardiovasc Dis 1978; 20:285–327.

Gallagher JJ, Smith WM, Kasell JH, Benson DW Jr, et al: Role of Mahaim fibers in cardiac arrhythmias in man. Circulation 1981; 64:176–189.

Galvez A, Gimenez-Gallego G, Reuben JP, Roy-Contancin L, Feigenbaum P, Kaczorowski GJ, et al: Purification and characterization of a unique, potent, peptidyl probe for the high conductance calcium-activated potassium channel from venom of the scorpion *Buthus tamulus*. J Biol Chem 1990; 265: 11083–11090.

Gang ES, Peter T, Karagueuzian HS, Mandel WJ, Meesmann M: Decline in ventricular fibrillation threshold after successive premature extrastimuli: A possible explanation for the induction of ventricular fibrillation during programmed stimulation with multiple extrastimuli. Cardiovasc Res 1987; 21:790–795.

Gang ES, Lew AS, Hong M, Wang FZ, Siebert CA, Peter T: Decreased incidence of ventricular late potentials after successful thrombolytic therapy for acute myocardial infarction. New Engl J Med 1989; 321:712–716.

Gardner PI, Ursell PC, Fenoglio JJ, Wit AL: Electrophysiologic and anatomic basis for fractionated electrograms recorded from healed myocardial infarcts. Circulation 1985; 72:596–611.

Garson A Jr, Gillette PC, Moak JP, Perry JC, Ott DA, Cooley DA: Supraventricular tachycardia due to multiple atrial ectopic foci: A relatively common problem. J Cardiovasc Electrophysiol 1990; 132–138.

German LD, Packer DL, Bardy GH, Gallagher JJ: Ventricular tachycardia induced by atrial stimulation in patients without symptomatic cardiac disease. Am J Cardiol 1983; 52:1202–1207.

Gettes LS: Electrolyte abnormalities underlying lethal ventricular arrhythmias. Circulation 1992; 85(suppl I):I-70–I-76.

Gettes LS, Reuter H: Slow recovery from inactivation of inward currents in mammalian myocardial fibres. J Physiol (Lond) 1974; 240:703–724.

Giles WR, Imaizumi Y: Comparison of potassium currents in rabbit atrial and ventricular cells. J Physiol (Lond) 1988; 405:123–145.

Gilliam FR III, Starmer CF, Grant AO: Blockade of rabbit atrial sodium channels by lidocaine. Characterization of continuous and frequency-dependent blocking. Circ Res 1989; 65:723–739.

Gilman AG: G proteins: Transducers of receptor-generated signals. Ann Rev Biochem 1987; 56:615–649.

Gilmour RF Jr, Zipes DP: Abnormal automaticity and related phenomena. In Fozzard HA, Haber E, Jennings RB, Katz AM, Morgan HE (eds): The Heart and Cardiovascular System. Scientific Foundations. New York, NY: Raven Press, Ltd, 1986, pp. 1239–1257.

Gintant GA, Cohen IS: Advances in cardiac cellular electrophysiology: Implications for automaticity and therapeutics. Ann Rev Pharmacol Toxicol 1988; 28:61–81.

Ginzton LE, Conant R, Rodrigues DM, Laks MM: Functional significance of hypertrophy of the non-infarcted myocardium after myocardial infarction in humans. Circulation 1989; 80:816–822.

Glicksman FL, Huikuri HV, Dwyer EM, Anthony RM, Castellanos A, Myerburg RJ: Differential prognostic significance of 2–5 or ≥6 repetitive ventricular ectopic beats. Circulation 1988; 78(suppl II):II-70.

Glitsch HG: Characteristics of active Na transport in intact cardiac cells. Am J Physiol 1979; 236:H189–H199.

Goethals M, Raes A, van Bogaert P: Use-dependent block of the pacemaker current, I_f, in rabbit sinoatrial node cells by zatebradine (UL-FS 49). Circulation 1993; 88(5):2389–2401.

Goicolea A, Cosio FG, Lopez-Gil M, Kallmeyer C: Conversion of recurrent atrial flutter with implanted pacemakers programmable to high rate AOO mode. Eur J C P E 1992; 2:19–21.

Goldreyer BN, Bigger JT Jr: Site of reentry in paroxysmal supraventricular tachycardia in man. Circulation 1971; 43:15–26.

Goldreyer BN, Damato AN: The essential role of atrioventricular conduction delay in the initiation of paroxysmal supraventricular tachycardia. Circulation 1971; 43:679–687.

Gorgels APM, Vos MA, Smeets JLRM, Kriek E, Brugada P, Wellens HJJ: Delayed afterdepolarizations and atrial and ventricular arrhythmias. In Rosen MR, Janse MJ, Wit AL (eds): Cardiac Electrophysiology: A Textbook. Mount Kisco, NY: Futura Publishing Co, 1990; pp. 3–7; 341–354.

Gorgels APM, Vos MA, Leunissen JDM, Dijkman B, Smeets JLRM, Wellens HJJ: Flunarizine as a specific drug to identify triggered activity based on delayed afterdepolarizations. In Josephson ME, Wellens HJJ (eds): Tachycardias: Mechanisms and Management. Mount Kisco, NY: Futura Publishing Co, 1993; pp. 87–97.

Gosselink ATM, Crijns HJGM, Van Gelder K, Hillige H, Wiesfeld ACP, Liek I: Low-dose amiodarone for maintenance of sinus rhythm after cardioversion of atrial fibrillation or flutter. JAMA 1992; 267:3289–3293.

Goto M, Sakamoto Y, Imanaga I: Aconitine-induced fibrillation of the different muscle tissues of the heart and the action of acetylcholine. In Sano T, Matsuda K, Mizuhira B (eds): Electrophysiology and Ultrastructure of the Heart. New York, NY: Grune & Stratton, 1967, pp. 199–209.

Gough WB, Zeiler RH, El-Sherif N: Basis for reduced transmembrane potentials associated with triggered activity in ischemic subendocardial Purkinje fibers. Circulation 1982; 66:II-156.

Gough WB, Zeiler RH, El-Sherif N: Effects of diltiazem on triggered activity in canine 1-day-old infarction. Cardiovasc Res 1984; 18:339–343.

Gough WB, Hu D, El-Sherif N: Effects of clofilium in ischemic subendocardial Purkinje fibers 1 day postinfarction. J Am Coll Cardiol 1988; 11:431–437.

Goy JJ, Kaufmann L, Kappenberger L, Sigwart U: Restoration of sinus rhythm with flecainide in patients with atrial fibrillation. Am J Cardiol 1988; 62: 38D–40D.

Grant AO, Starmer CF, Strauss HC: Antiarrhythmic drug action: Blockade of the inward sodium current. Circ Res 1984; 55:427–439.

Greenberg GM, Dustman TJ, Fuller MS, Lux RL, Anderson KP: Initiation of spontaneous sustained monomorphic ventricular tachycardia. Circulation 1990; 82(suppl):III-580.

Grubb BP: The use of oral labetalol in the treatment of arrhythmias associated with the long QT syndrome. Chest 1991; 100:1724–1726.

Guarnieri T, Levine JH, Veltri EP, Griffith LSC, Watkins L Jr, Juanteguy J, et al: Success of chronic defibrillation and the role of antiarrhythmic drugs with the automatic implantable cardioverter defibrillator. Am J Cardiol 1987; 60:1061–1064.

Guldal M, Karaoguz R, Akalin H, Bayar M, Akyol T: Is there an effect of amiodarone on the defibrillation threshold? Jpn Heart J 1993; 34:221–226.

Gursoy S, Schlüter M, Kuck K-H: Radiofrequency current catheter ablation for control of supraventricular arrhythmias. J Cardiovasc Electrophysiol 1993; 4:194–205.

Hackett AM, Gardiner P, Garthwaite SM: The effect of bidisomide (SC-40230), a new Class Ia/Ib antiarrhythmic agent, on defibrillation energy requirements in dogs with healed myocardial infarctions. PACE 1993; 16:317–326.

Hagiwara N, Irisawa H, Kameyama M: Contribution of two types of calcium currents to the pacemaker potentials of rabbit sino-atrial node cells. J Physiol (Lond) 1988; 395:223–253.

Hagiwara N, Irisawa H, Kasanuki H, Hosoda S: Background current in sino-atrial node cells of rabbit heart. J Physiol (Lond) 1992; 448:53–72.

Haissaguerre M, Warin JF, Le Metayer P, Maraud L, et al: Catheter ablation of Mahaim fibers with preservation of atrioventricular nodal conduction. Circulation 1990; 82:418–427.

Halpern SW, Ellrodt G, Singh BN, Mandel WJ: Efficacy of intravenous procainamide infusion in converting atrial fibrillation to sinus rhythm. Relation to left atrial size. Br Heart J 1980; 44:589–595.

Hamer AW, Karagueuzian HS, Sugi K, Zaher CA, Mandel WJ, Peter T: Factors related to the induction of ventricular fibrillation in the normal canine heart by programmed electrical stimulation. J Am Coll Cardiol 1984; 3:751–759.

Hamra M, Rosen MR: Alpha-adrenergic receptor stimulation during simulated ischemia and reperfusion in canine cardiac Purkinje fibers. Circulation 1988; 78:1495–1502.

Hariman RJ, Gough WB: Delayed afterdepolarization-induced triggered activity as a mechanism of ventricular arrhythmias in vivo. In Rosen MR, Janse MJ, Wit AL (eds): Cardiac Electrophysiology: A Textbook. Mount Kisco, NY: Futura Publishing Co, 1990; pp. 323–331.

Harrison DA: Antiarrhythmic drug classification: New science and practical applications. Am J Cardiol 1985; 56:185–187.

Harrison DA, Winkle RA, Sami M, Mason J: Encainide: A new and potent antiarrhythmic agent. In Harrison DC (ed): Cardiac Arrhythmias: A Decade of Progress. Boston, MA: GK Hall, 1981, pp. 315–330.

Hartmann HA, Kirsch GE, Drewe JA, Taglialatela RH, Joho RH, Brown AM:

Exchange of conduction pathways between two related K$^+$ channels. Science 1991; 251:942–944.

Hartzell HC: Regulation of cardiac ion channels by catecholamines, acetylcholine and second messenger systems. Prog Biophys Mol Biol 1988; 52: 165–247.

Hartzell HC, Duchatelle-Gourdon I: Structure and neural modulation of cardiac calcium channels. J Cardiovasc Electrophysiol 1993; 3:567–578.

Harvey RD, Hume JR: Autonomic regulation of the delayed rectifier K$^+$ current in mammalian heart involves G proteins. Am J Physiol 1989a; 257: H818–H823.

Harvey RD, Hume JR: Isoproterenol activates a chloride current, not the transient outward current, in rabbit ventricular myocytes. Am J Physiol 1989b; 257:C1177–C1181.

Harvey RD, Clark CD, Hume JR: Chloride current in mammalian cardiac myocytes. J Gen Physiol 1990; 95:1077–1102.

Hashimoto K, Moe GK: Transient depolarizations induced by acetylstrophanthidin in specialized tissue of dog atrium and ventricle. Circ Res 1973; 32: 618–624.

Hauswirth O, Noble D, Tsien RW: The mechanism of oscillatory activity at low membrane potentials in cardiac Purkinje fibres. J Physiol (Lond) 1969; 200:255–265.

Hellestrand KJ: Intravenous flecainide acetate for supraventricular tachycardias. Am J Cardiol 1988; 62:16D–22D.

Henning B, Wit AL: The time course of action potential repolarization affects delayed afterdepolarization amplitude in atrial fibers of the canine coronary sinus. Circ Res 1984; 55:110–115.

Henthorn RW, Okumura K, Olshansky B, Plumb VJ, Hess PG, Waldo AL: A fourth criterion for transient entrainment: The electrogram equivalent of progressive fusion. Circulation 1988; 77:1003–1012.

Hescheler J, Trautwein W: Modulation of calcium current of ventricular cells. In Piper HM, Isenberg G (eds): Isolated Adult Cardiomyocytes. Boca Raton, FL: CRC Press Inc, 1989, pp. 128–154.

Hess P, Weingart R: Intracellular free calcium modified by pH$_i$ in sheep cardiac Purkinje fibres. J Physiol (Lond) 1980; 307:60P–61P.

Hewett K, Gessman L, Rosen MR: Effects of procaine amide, quinidine and ethmozin on delayed afterdepolarizations. Eur J Pharmacol 1983; 96:21–28.

Hille B: Ionic Currents of Excitable Membranes. Sunderland, MA: Sinauer Associates, 1992.

Hirano Y, Fozzard HA, January CT: Characteristics of L- and T-type Ca^{2+} currents in canine cardiac Purkinje cells. Am J Physiol 1989; 256: H1478–H1492.

Hiraoka M: Membrane current changes induced by acetylstrophanthidin in cardiac Purkinje fibers. Jpn Heart J 1977; 18:851–859.

Hiromasa S, Coto H, Li ZY, Maldonado C, Kupersmith J: Dextrorotatory isomer of sotalol: Electrophysiologic effects and interaction with verapamil. Am Heart J 1988; 116:1552–1557.

Ho K, Nichols CG, Lederer WJ, Lytton J, Vassilev PM, Kanazirska MV, et al:

Cloning and expression of an inwardly rectifying ATP-regulated potassium channel. Nature 1993; 362:35–37.

Ho SY, McComb JM, Scott CD, Anderson RH: Morphology of the cardiac conduction system in patients with electrophysiologically proven dual atrioventricular nodal pathways. J Cardiovasc Electrophysiol 1993; 4:504–512.

Hoffman BF, Cranefield PF: Electrophysiology of the Heart. New York, NY: McGraw-Hill, 1960.

Hoffman BF, Rosen MR: Cellular mechanisms for cardiac arrhythmias. Circ Res 1981; 49:1–15.

Hoffman BF, Dangman KH: Are arrhythmias caused by automatic impulse generation? In Paes de Carvalho A, Hoffman BF, Lieberman M (eds): Normal and Abnormal Conduction in the Heart. Mount Kisco, NY: Futura Publishing Co, 1982, pp. 429–448.

Hogan PM, Davis LD: Evidence for specialized fibers in the canine right atrium. Circ Res 1968; 23:387–396.

Hogan PM, Wittenberg SM, Klocke FJ: Relationship of stimulation frequency to automaticity in the canine Purkinje fiber during ouabain administration. Circ Res 1973; 32:377–384.

Hondeghem LM: Antiarrhythmic agents: Modulated receptor applications. Circulation 1987; 75:514–520.

Hondeghem LM: Ideal antiarrhythmic agents: Chemical defibrillators. J Cardiovasc Electrophysiol 1991; 2(suppl):S169–S177.

Hondeghem LM, Katzung BG: Time- and voltage-dependent interactions of antiarrhythmic drugs with cardiac sodium channels. Biochim Biophys Acta 1977; 472:377–398.

Hondeghem LM, Katzung BG: Antiarrhythmic agents. The modulated receptor mechanism of action of sodium and calcium channel blocking agents. Ann Rev Pharmacol Toxicol 1984; 24:387–423.

Hondeghem LM, Snyders DJ: Class III antiarrhythmic agents have a lot of potential but a long way to go. Reduced effectiveness and dangers of reverse use dependence. Circulation 1990; 81:686–690.

Honerjager P: New aspects of the molecular effects of anti-arrhythmia agents. Herz 1990; 15:70–78.

Honig PK, Woosley RL, Zamani K, Conner DP, Cantilena LR Jr: Changes in the pharmacokinetics and electrocardiographic pharmacodynamics of terfenadine with concomitant administration of erythromycin. Clin Pharmacol Ther 1992; 52:231–238.

Honig PK, Wortham DC, Zamani K, Conner DP, Mullin JC, Cantilena LR: Terfenadine-ketoconazole interaction: Pharmacokinetic and electrocardiographic consequences. JAMA 1993; 269:1513–1518.

Hope RR, Scherlag BJ, El-Sherif N, Lazzara R: Hierarchy of ventricular pacemakers. Circ Res 1976; 39:883–888.

Horacek TH, Neumann M, von Mutius S, Budden M, Meesmann W: Nonhomogenous electrophysiological changes and bimodal distribution of early ventricular arrhythmias during acute coronary artery occlusion. Basic Res Cardiol 1984; 79:649–667.

Horowitz LN, Spear JF, Moore EN: Subendocardial origin of ventricular arrhythmias in 24-hour-old experimental myocardial infarction. Circulation 1976; 53:56–63.

Huikuri HV, Linnaluoto MK, Seppanen T, Kessler KM, Takkunen JT, Myerburg RJ: Heart rate variability and its circadian rhythm in survivors of cardiac arrest. Am J Cardiol 1992; 70:610–615.

Huikari HV, Valkama JO, Airaksinen KEJ, Seppanen T, Kessler KM, Takkunen JT, et al: Frequency domain measures of heart rate variability before the onset of non-sustained and sustained ventricular tachycardia in patients with coronary artery disease. Circulation 1993; 87:1220–1228.

Idle JR, Mahgoub A, Lancaster R, Smith RL: Hypotensive response to debrisoquine and hydroxylation phenotype. Life Sci 1978; 22:979–984.

Ilvento JP, Provet J, Danilo P Jr, Rosen MR: Fast and slow idioventricular rhythms in the canine heart. A study of their mechanism using antiarrhythmic drugs and electrophysiologic testing. Am J Cardiol 1982; 49:1909–1916.

Imanishi S, Surawicz B: Automatic activity in depolarized guinea pig ventricular myocardium. Circ Res 1976; 39:751–759.

Inoue H, Matsuo H, Takayanagi K, Murao S: Clinical and experimental studies of the effects of extrastimulation and rapid pacing on atrial flutter: Evidence of macroreentry with an excitable gap. Am J Cardiol 1981; 48:623–631.

Irisawa H, Giles WR: Sinus and atrioventricular node cells: Cellular electrophysiology. In Zipes DP, Jalife J (eds): Cardiac Electrophysiology: From Cell to Bedside. Philadelphia, PA: WB Saunders Co, 1990, pp. 95–102.

Irisawa H, Brown HF, Giles W: Cardiac pacemaking in the sinoatrial node. Physiol Rev 1993; 73:197–227.

Isenberg G, Belardinelli L: Ionic basis for the antagonism between adenosine and isoproterenol in isolated mammalian ventricular myocytes. Circ Res 1984; 55:309–325.

Ishii F, Yamagishi T, Taira N: Cloning and functional expression of a cardiac inward rectifier K^+ channel. FEBS Lett 1994; 338:107–111.

ISIS-1: First International Study of Infarct Survival Collaborative Group. Randomised trial of intravenous atenolol among 16,027 cases of suspected acute myocardial infarction. Lancet 1986; 2:57–66.

Isom LL, De Jongh KS, Patton DE, Reber BF, Offord J, Charbonneau H, et al: Primary structure and functional expression of the beta-1 subunit of the rat brain sodium channel. Science 1992; 256:839–842.

Jackman WM, Friday KJ, Anderson JL, Aliot EM, Clark M, Lazarra R: The long QT syndrome: A critical review, new clinical observations, and a unifying hypothesis. Prog Cardiovasc Dis 1988; 32:115–172.

Jackman WM, Beckman KJ, McClelland JH, Wang X, et al: Treatment of supraventricular tachycardia due to atrioventricular nodal reentrant tachycardia by radiofrequency catheter ablation of slow-pathway conduction. N Engl J Med 1992; 327:313–318.

Jalife J, Moe GK: Excitation, conduction and reflection of impulses in isolated bovine and canine cardiac Purkinje fibers. Circ Res 1981; 49:233–247.

Jalife J, Davidenko JM, Michaels DC: A new perspective on the mechanisms of arrhythmias and sudden cardiac death: Spiral waves of excitation in heart muscle. J Cardiovasc Electrophysiol 1991; 2:(suppl 3):S133–S152.

James TN, Isobe JH, Urthaler F: Correlative electrophysiologic and anatomical studies concerning the site of origin of escape rhythm during complete atrioventricular block in the dog. Circ Res 1979; 45:108–119.

Jan LY, Jan YN: Structural elements involved in specific K$^+$ channel functions. Ann Rev Physiol 1992; 54:537–555.

Janse MJ: *The Effect of Changes in Heart Rate on the Refractory Period of the Heart.* Mondeel-Offsetdrukkerij, Amsterdam: University of Amsterdam, 1971. Thesis.

Janse MJ: Electrophysiological effects of myocardial ischaemia. Relationship with early ventricular arrhythmias. Eur Heart J 1986; 7(suppl A):35–43.

Janse MJ: Arrhythmias during acute ischemia in experimental models. In Brugada P, Wellens HJJ (eds): Cardiac Arrhythmias. Where to Go from Here? Mount Kisco, NY: Futura Publishing Co, 1987, pp. 105–128.

Janse MJ: Putting the Sicilian Gambit to the test. Eur Heart J 1992; 13(suppl F):30–37.

Janse MJ, van Capelle FJL: Electrotonic current flow across a region of block as a cause for ventricular premature beats during acute regional myocardial ischemia. A study in intact hearts and computer models. Circ Res 1982; 50:527–537.

Janse MJ, Allessie MA: Experimental observations in atrial fibrillation. In Falk RH, Podrid PJ (eds): Atrial Fibrillation: Mechanisms and Management. New York, NY: Raven Press Ltd, 1992, pp. 41–57.

Janse MJ, van der Steen ABM, van Dam RTh, Durrer D: Refractory period of the dog's ventricular myocardium following sudden changes in frequency. Circ Res 1969; 24:251–262.

Janse MJ, Van Capelle FJL, Morsink H, Kleber AG, Wilms-Schopman FJG, Cardinal R, et al: Flow of "injury" current and patterns of excitation during early ventricular arrhythmias in acute regional myocardial ischemia in isolated porcine and canine hearts. Evidence for two different arrhythmogenic mechanisms. Circ Res 1980; 47:151–165.

Janse MJ, Schwartz PJ, Wilms-Schopman F, Peters RJG, Durrer D: Effects of unilateral stellate ganglion stimulation and ablation on electrophysiologic changes induced by acute myocardial ischemia in dogs. Circulation 1985; 72:585–595.

Janse MJ, Kleber AG, Capucci A, Coronel R, Wilms-Schopman F: Electrophysiological basis for arrhythmias in acute ischemia. Role of the subendocardium. J Mol Cell Cardiol 1986; 18:339–355.

Janse MJ, Wilms-Schopman F, Opthof T: Mechanism of antifibrillatory action of Org 7797 in regionally ischemic pig heart. J Cardiovasc Pharmacol 1990; 15:633–643.

Janse MJ, Anderson RH, McGuire MA, Ho SY: "AV nodal" re-entry: Part I: "AV nodal" reentry revisited. J Cardiovasc Electrophysiol 1993; 4:561–572.

January CP, Fozzard HA: Delayed afterdepolarizations in heart muscles: Mechanisms and relevance. Pharmacol Rev 1988; 30:219–227.

January CT, Riddle JM: Early afterdepolarizations: Mechanism of induction and block. A role for L-type Ca^{2+} current. Circ Res 1989; 64:977–990.

Jazayeri MR, VanWyhe G, Avitall B, McKinnie J, Tchou P, Akhtar M: Isoproterenol reversal of antiarrhythmic effects in patients with inducible sustained ventricular tachyarrhythmias. J Am Coll Cardiol 1989; 14:705–711.

Jazayeri MR, Sra JS, Deshpande SS, Blanck Z, Dhala AA, Krum DP, et al: Electrophysiologic spectrum of atrioventricular nodal behavior in patients with atrioventricular nodal reentrant tachycardia undergoing selective fast or slow pathway ablation. J Cardiovasc Electrophysiol 1993; 4:99–111.

Jenkins KJ, Walsh EP, Colan SD, Bergau DM, et al: Multipolar endocardial mapping of the right atrium during cardiac catheterization: Description of a new technique. J Am Coll Cardiol 1993; 22:1105–1110.

Johnson NJ, Rosen MR: The distinction between triggered activity and other cardiac arrhythmias. In Brugada P, Wellens HJJ (eds): Cardiac Arrhythmias: Where to Go from Here. Mount Kisco, NY: Futura Publishing Co, 1987, pp. 129–145.

Johnson NJ, Danilo P, Wit AL, Rosen MR: Characteristics of initiation and termination of catecholamine-induced triggered activity in atrial fibers of the coronary sinus. Circulation 1986; 74:1168–1179.

Joho RH: Toward a molecular understanding of voltage-gated potassium channels. J Cardiovasc Electrophysiol 1993; 3:589–601.

Jones SB, Euler DE, Hardie E, Randall WC, Brynjolfsson G: Comparison of SA nodal and subsidiary atrial pacemaker function and location in the dog. Am J Physiol 1978; 234:H471–H476.

Jones CR, Molenaar P, Summers RJ: New views of human cardiac beta-adrenoceptors. J Mol Cell Cardiol 1989; 21:519–535.

Jonkman FAM, Boddeke HWGM, van Zwieten PA: Protective activity of calcium entry blockers against ouabain intoxication in anesthetized pigs. J Cardiovasc Pharmacol 1986; 8:1009–1013.

Josephson ME: Tachycardia Mechanism and Management. Mt. Kisco, NY: Futura Publishing Co, 1992.

Josephson ME, Gottlieb CD: Ventricular tachycardias associated with coronary artery disease. In Zipes DP, Jalife J (eds): Cardiac Electrophysiology. From Cell to Bedside. Philadelphia, PA: WB Saunders Co, 1990, pp. 571–580.

Juberg EN, Minneman KP, Abel PW: β_1- and β_2-adrenoceptor binding and functional response in right and left atria of rat heart. Naunyn-Schmiedeberg's Arch Pharmacol 1985; 330:193–202.

Jung W, Manz M, Luderitz B: Effects of antiarrhythmic drugs on defibrillation threshold in patients with the implantable cardioverter defibrillator. PACE 1992; 15:545–548.

Jurkiewicz NK, Sanguinetti MC: Rate-dependent prolongation of cardiac action potentials by a methanesulfonanilide Class III antiarrhythmic agent. Specific block of rapidly activating delayed rectifier K^+ current by dofetilide. Circ Res 1993; 72:75–83.

Juul-Moller S, Edvardsson N, Rehnqvist-Ahlberg N: Sotalol versus quinidine for the maintenance of sinus rhythm after direct current conversion of atrial fibrillation. Circulation 1990; 82:1932–1939.

Kamb A, Tseng-Crank J, Tanouye MA: Multiple products of the *Drosophila*

Shaker gene may contribute to potassium channel diversity. Neuron 1988; 1:421–430.

Kammerling JJ, Green FJ, Watanabe AM, Inoue H, Barber MJ, Henry DP, et al: Denervation supersensitivity of refractoriness in non-infarcted areas apical to transmural myocardial infarction. Circulation 1987; 76:383–393.

Kannel WB, Abbott RD, Savage DD, McNamara PM: Epidemiologic features of atrial fibrillation. The Framingham Study. N Engl J Med 1982; 306: 1018–1022.

Kaplinsky E, Ogawa S, Balke W, Dreifus LS: Role of endocardial activation in malignant ventricular arrhythmias associated with acute ischemia. J Electrocardiol 1979a; 12:299–306.

Kaplinsky E, Ogawa S, Balke CW, Dreifus LS: Two periods of early ventricular arrhythmias in the canine acute infarction model. Circulation 1979b; 60: 397–403.

Karagueuzian H, Katzung BG: Relative inotropic and arrhythmogenic effects of five cardiac steroids in ventricular myocardium: Oscillatory afterpotentials and the role of endogenous catecholamines. J Pharm Exp Ther 1981; 218:348–356.

Karagueuzian HS, Katzung BG: Voltage-clamp studies of transient inward current and mechanical oscillations induced by ouabatin in ferret papillary muscle. J Physiol (Lond) 1982; 327:255–271.

Kass RS, Scheuer T: Slow inactivation of calcium channels in the cardiac Purkinje fiber. J Mol Cell Cardiol 1982; 14:615–618.

Kass RS, Tsien RW, Weingart R: Ionic basis of transient inward current induced by strophantidin in cardiac Purkinje fibres. J Physiol (Lond) 1978a; 281:209–226.

Kass RS, Lederer WJ, Tsien RW, Weingart R: Role of calcium ions in transient inward currents and aftercontractions induced by strophanthidin in cardiac Purkinje fibres. J Physiol (Lond) 1978b; 281:187–208.

Katritsis D, Camm AJ: New class III antiarrhythmic agents. Eur Heart J. In Press.

Katz LN, Pick A: Clinical Electrocardiography, Part I: The Arrhythmias. Philadelphia, PA: Lea and Febiger, 1956.

Katzung BG, Morgenstern JA: Effects of extracellular potassium on ventricular automaticity and evidence for a pacemaker current in mammalian ventricular myocardium. Circ Res 1977; 40:105–111.

Katzung BG, Hondeghem LM, Grant AO: Cardiac ventricular automaticity induced by current of injury. Pflügers Arch 1975; 360:193–197.

Katzung BG, Hondeghem LM, Clarkson CW, Matsubara T: Mechanisms for selective actions and interactions of antiarrhythmic drugs. In Zipes DP, Jalife J (eds): Cardiac Electrophysiology and Arrhythmias. Orlando, FL: Grune & Stratton, 1985, pp. 199–205.

Kay GN, Bubien RS, Epstein AE, Plumb VJ: Effect of catheter ablation of the atrioventricular junction on quality of life and exercise tolerance in paroxysmal atrial fibrillation. Am J Cardiol 1988; 62:741–744.

Kay GN, Epstein AE, Daily SM, Plumb VJ: Role of radiofrequency ablation in the management of supraventricular arrhythmias: Experience in 760 consecutive patients. J Cardiovasc Electrophysiol 1993; 4:371–389.

Kelly P, Ruskin JN, Vlahakes GJ, Buckley MJ, Freeman CS, Garan H: Surgical coronary revascularization in survivors of pre-hospital cardiac arrest: Its effect on inducible ventricular arrhythmias and long-term survival. J Am Coll Cardiol 1990; 15:267–273.

Kent AFS: The right lateral auriculoventricular junction of the heart. J Physiol (Lond) 1914; 48:22–24.

Kessler KM, Kissane B, Cassidy J, Pefkaros KC, Kozlovskis P, Hamburg C, et al: Dynamic variability of binding of antiarrhythmic drugs during the evolution of acute myocardial infarction. Circulation 1984; 70:472–478.

Kimura E, Kato K, Murao S, Ajisaka H, Koyama S, Omiya Z: Experimental studies on the mechanism of auricular flutter. Tohoku J Exp Med 1954; 60: 197–207.

Kimura S, Cameron JS, Kozlovskis PL, Bassett AL, Myerburg RJ: Delayed afterdepolarizations and triggered activity induced in feline Purkinje fibers by alpha-adrenergic stimulation in the presence of elevated calcium levels. Circulation 1984; 70:1074–1082.

Kimura S, Bassett AL, Kohya T, Kozlovskis PL, Myerburg RJ: Simultaneous recording of action potentials from endocardium and epicardium during ischemia in the isolated cat ventricles. Circulation 1986a; 74:401–409.

Kimura S, Bassett AL, Saoudi NC, Cameron JC, Kozlovskis PL, Myerburg RJ: Cellular electrophysiological changes and "arrhythmias" during experimental ischemia and reperfusion in isolated cat ventricular myocardium. J Am Coll Cardiol 1986b; 7:833–842.

Kimura S, Bassett AL, Xi H, Myerburg RJ: Early afterdepolarizations and triggered activity induced by cocaine: A possible mechanism of cocaine arrhythmogenesis. Circulation 1992; 85:2227–2235.

Kimura T, Imanishi S, Arita M, Hadama T, Shirabe J: Two differential mechanisms of automaticity in diseased human atrial fibers. Jpn J Physiol 1988; 38:851–867.

Kinoshita O, Kamakura S, Ohe T, Yutani C, Matsuhisa M, Aihara N, et al: Spectral analysis of signal-averaged electrocardiograms in patients with idiopathic ventricular tachycardia of left ventricular origin. Circulation 1992; 85:2054–2059.

Kirchberger MA, Tada M, Katz AM: Adenosine $3'$-$5'$-monophosphate dependent protein kinase-catalyzed phosphorylation reaction and its relationship to calcium transport in cardiac sarcoplasmic reticulum. J Biol Chem 1974; 249:6166–6173.

Kirsch GE, Codina J, Birnbaumer L, Brown AM: Coupling of ATP-sensitive K^+ channels to A_1 receptors by G proteins in rat ventricular myocytes. Am J Physiol 1990; 259:H820–H826.

Kirsch GE, Drewe JE: Gating-dependent mechanism of 4-aminopyridine block in two related potassium channels. J Gen Physiol 1993; 102:797–816.

Kiyosue T, Arita M: Late sodium current and its contribution to action potential configuration in guinea pig ventricular myocytes. Circ Res 1989; 64: 389–397.

Kleber AG, Janse MJ, van Capelle FJL, Durrer D: Mechanism and time course of ST and TQ segment changes during acute regional myocardial ischaemia in the pig heart determined by extracellular and intracellular recordings. Circ Res 1978; 42:603–613.

Kleiger RE, Miller JP, Bigger JT, Moss AJ, the Multicenter Post-Infarction Research Group: Decreased heart rate variability and its association with increased mortality after acute myocardial infarction. Am J Cardiol 1987; 59:256–262.

Klein GJ, Bashore TM, Sellers TD, Pritchett ELC, Smith WM, Gallagher JJ: Ventricular fibrillation in the Wolff-Parkinson-White syndrome. N Engl J Med 1979; 301:1080–1085.

Klein GJ, Millman PJ, Yee R: Recurrent ventricular tachycardia responsive to verapamil. PACE 1984; 7:938–940.

Klein HO, Cranefield PF, Hoffman BF: Effect of extrasystoles on idioventricular rhythm. Circ Res 1972; 30:651–665.

Klein HO, Lebson R, Cranefield PF, Hoffman BF: Effect of extrasystoles on idioventricular rhythm. Clinical and electrophysiologic correlation. Circulation 1973; 47:758–764.

Klein LS, Hackett FK, Zipes DP, Miles WM: Radiofrequency catheter ablation of "Mahaim fibers" at the tricuspid annulus. Circulation 1993; 87:738–747.

Kline RP, Hanna MS, Dresdner KP, Wit AL: Time course of changes in intracellular K^+, Na^+, and pH of subendocardial Purkinje cells during the first 24 hours after coronary occlusion. Circ Res 1992; 70:566–575.

Koch-Weser J, Klein SW, Foo-Canto LL, Kastor JA, DeSanctis RW: Antiarrhythmic prophylaxis with procainamide in acute myocardial infarction. N Engl J Med 1969; 281:1253–1260.

Kocovic D, Shea J, Friedman PL: Evidence for parasympathetic denervation of the sinus node after radiofrequency modification of the A-V node in patients with A-V nodal reentry. J Am Coll Cardiol 1992; 19:271. Abstract.

Kokubun S, Nishimura M, Noma A, Irisawa H: The spontaneous action potential of rabbit atrioventricular node cells. Jpn J Physiol 1980; 30:529–540.

Kokubun S, Nishimura M, Noma A, Irisawa H: Membrane currents in the rabbit atrioventricular node cell. Pflügers Arch 1982; 393:15–22.

Kolhardt M, Fichtner U, Frobe U, Herzing JW: On the mechanism of drug-induced blockade of Na^+ currents: Interaction of antiarrhythmic drugs with DPI-modified single cardiac Na^+ channels. Circ Res 1989; 64:867–881.

Kolman BS, Verrier RL, Lown B: The effect of vagus nerve stimulation upon vulnerability of the canine ventricle. Circulation 1975; 52:578–585.

Kopeyan C, Martinez G, Rochat H: Primary structure of toxin IV of Leirus quinquestriatus: Characterization of a new group of scorpion toxins. FEBS Lett 1985; 181:211–216.

Koster RW, Dunning AJ: Intramuscular lidocaine for prevention of lethal arrhythmias in the prehospitalization phase of acute myocardial infarction. N Engl J Med 1985; 313:1105–1110.

Kostis JB, Byington R, Friedman LM, Goldstein S, Furberg C, for the BHAT Study Group: Prognostic significance of ventricular ectopic activity in survivors of acute myocardial infarction. J Am Coll Cardiol 1987; 10:231–242.

Kou WH, Nelson SD, Lynch JJ, Montgomery DG, DiCarlo L, Lucchesi BR. Effect of flecainide acetate on prevention of electrical induction of VT and occurrence of ischemic ventricular fibrillation during the early postmyocardial infarction period: Evaluation in a conscious canine model of sudden death. J Am Coll Cardiol 1987; 9:359–365.

Kramer JB, Saffitz JE, Witkowski FX, Corr PB: Intramural reentry as a mechanism of ventricular tachycardia during evolving myocardial infarction. Circ Res 1985; 56:736–748.

Kubo Y, Baldwin TJ, Jan YN, Jan LY: Primary structure and functional expression of a mouse inward rectifier potassium channel. Nature 1993a; 362:127–133.

Kubo Y, Reuveny E, Slesinger P, Jan YN, Jan LY: Primary structure and functional expression of a rat G-protein-coupled muscarinic potassium channel. Nature 1993b; 364:802–806.

Kuck KH, Kunze KP, Schluter M: Transcatheter modulation by radiofrequency current of atrioventricular nodal conduction in patients with atrial fibrillation and flutter. In Luderitz B, Saksena S (eds): Interventional Electrophysiology. Mount Kisco, NY: Futura Publishing Co, 1991, pp. 271–278.

Kulakowski P, Bashir Y, Heald S, et al: Effects of procainamide on the signal-averaged electrocardiogram in relation to the results of programmed ventricular stimulation in patients with sustained monomorphic ventricular tachycardia. J Am Coll Cardiol 1993; 21:1428–1439.

Kulbertus HE: Antiarrhythmic treatment of atrial arrhythmias. J Cardiovasc Pharm 1991; 17(suppl 6):S32–S35.

Kurachi Y, Nakajima T, Sugimoto T: On the mechanism of activation of muscarinic K^+ channels by adenosine in isolated atrial cells: Involvement of GTP-binding proteins. Pflügers Arch 1986; 407:264–274.

Lab MJ: Contraction-excitation feedback in myocardium: Physiologic basis and clinical relevance. Circ Res 1982; 50:757–766.

Lacombe P, Cointe R, Metge M, Bru P, Gérard R, Lévy S: Intravenous flecainide in the management of acute supraventricular tachyarrhythmias. J Electrophysiol 1988; 2:19–22.

Lammers WJEP, Wit AL, Allessie MA: Effects of anisotropy on functional reentrant circuits: Preliminary results of computer simulation studies. In Sideman S, Beyar R (eds): Activation, Metabolism, and Perfusion of the Heart. Dordrecht, The Netherlands: Martinus Nijhoff, 1987, pp. 133–150.

Lampidis TJ, Kolonias D, Savaraj N, Rubin RW: Cardiostimulatory and antiarrhythmic activity of tubulin-binding agents. Proc Natl Acad Sci USA 1992; 89:1256–1260.

LaRovere MT, Specchia G, Mortara A, Schwartz PJ: Baroreflex sensitivity, clinical correlates and cardiovascular mortality among patients with a first myocardial infarction. A prospective study. Circulation 1988; 78:816–824.

Lawrie GM, Pacifico A, Kaushik R: Transannular cryoablation of ventricular tachycardia. Surgical technique and results. J Thorac Cardiovasc Surg 1989; 98:1030–1036.

Lazzara R, Marchi S: Electrophysiologic mechanisms for the generation of arrhythmias with adrenergic stimulation. In Brachmann J, Schomig A (eds): Adrenergic System and Ventricular Arrhythmias in Myocardial Infarction. Berlin: Springer-Verlag, 1989, pp. 231–238.

Lederer WJ, Tsien RW: Transient inward current underlying arrhythmogenic effects of cardiotonic steroids in Purkinje fibres. J Physiol (Lond) 1976; 263:73–100.

Lederman SN, Wenger TL, Bolster DE, Strauss HC: Effects of flecainide on occlusion and reperfusion arrhythmias in dogs. J Cardiovasc Pharmacol 1989; 13:541–546.

Lee CO, Dagostino M: Effect of strophanthidin on intracellular Na ion activity and twitch tension of constantly driven canine cardiac Purkinje fibers. Biophys J 1982; 40:185–198.

Lee H-C, Matsuda JJ, Reynertson SI, Martins JB, Shibata EF: Reversal of lidocaine effects on sodium currents by isoproterenol in rabbit hearts and heart cells. J Clin Invest 1993; 91:693–701.

Lee JH, Rosen MR: Modulation of delayed afterdepolarizations by α_1-adrenergic receptor subtypes. Cardiovasc Res 1993; 27:839–844.

Lee JH, Rosen MR: Alpha$_1$ adrenergic receptor modulation of repolarization in canine Purkinje fibers. J Cardiovasc Electrophysiol 1994; 5:232–248.

Lee JH, Rosen MR: Use-dependent actions and effects on transmembrane action potentials of flecainide, encainide, and ethmozine in canine purkinje fibers. J Cardiovasc Pharmacol 1991; 18(2):285–292.

Lee JT, Kroemer HT, Silberstein D, Funck-Brentano C, Lineberry MD, Wood AJJ, et al: The role of genetically determined polymorphic drug metabolism in the beta-blockade produced by propafenone. N Engl J Med 1990; 322: 1764–1768.

Lee KS: Ibutilide: A new compound with potent Class III antiarrhythmic activity. Activates a slow inward Na^+ current in guinea pig ventricular cells. J Pharm Exper Ther 1992; 262:99–108.

Leenhardt A, Coumel P, Haouala H, Zimmermann M, Munoz A, Maisonblanche P, et al: QT interval shortening by penticainide in patients with the long QT syndrome. Eur Heart J 1989; 10(abstr suppl):300.

Leitch L, Klein GJ, Yee R, Murdock C: New concepts on nodoventricular pathways. J Cardiovasc Electrophysiol 1990; 1:220–230.

Lemery R, Brugada P, Della Bella P, Dugernier T, van den Dool A, Wellens HJJ: Nonischemic ventricular tachycardia. Clinical course and long-term follow-up in patients without clinically overt heart disease. Circulation 1989; 79:990–999.

Lerman BB: Response of nonreentrant catecholamine-mediated ventricular tachycardia to endogenous adenosine and acetylcholine. Evidence for myocardial receptor-mediated effects. Circulation 1993; 87:382–390.

Lerman BB, Belardinelli L, West GA, Berne RM, DiMarco JP: Adenosine-sensitive ventricular tachycardia: Evidence suggesting cyclic AMP-mediated triggered activity. Circulation 1986; 74:270–280.

Levitan ES, Hemmick LM, Birnberg NC, Kaczmarek LK: Dexamethasone increases potassium channel messenger RNA and activity in clonal pituitary cells. Mol Endocrinol 1991; 5:1903–1908.

Lévy S, Lauribe Ph, Dolla E, Kou W, Kadish A, Calkins H, et al: A randomized comparison of external and internal cardioversion of chronic atrial fibrillation. Circulation 1992; 86:1415–1420.

Lewis DL, Soler F, Joho RH: Verapamil and quinidine block two human brain K^+ channels. Biophys J 1992; 61:A381.

Lewis T, Feil HS, Stroud WD: Observations upon flutter and fibrillation. Part II. The nature of auricular flutter. Heart 1920; 7:191–245.

Lie KE, Wellens HJJ, Von Capell FJ, Durrer D: Lidocaine in the prevention of primary ventricular fibrillation. N Engl J Med 1974; 291:1324–1326.

Lie KE, Liem KL, Louridtz WL, Janse MJ, Willebrands AF, Durrer D: Efficacy of lignocaine in preventing ventricular fibrillation within 1 hour after a 300 mg intramuscular injection. A double blind randomised study of 300 hospitalised patients with acute myocardial infarction. Am J Cardiol 1978; 42:486–488.

Lin FC, Finley CD, Rahimtoola SH, Wu D: Idiopathic paroxysmal ventricular tachycardia with a QRS pattern of right bundle branch block and left axis deviation: A unique clinical entity with specific properties. Am J Cardiol 1983; 52:95–100.

Lindemann JP, Jones RL, Hathaway BG, Henry BG, Watanabe A: Beta-adrenergic stimulation of phospholamban phosphorylation and Ca^{2+} ATPase activity in guinea pig ventricles. J Biol Chem 1983; 258:464–471.

Lindemann JP, Watanabe AM: Mechanisms of adrenergic and cholinergic regulation of myocardial contractility. In Sperelakis N (ed): Physiology and Pathophysiology of the Heart. Second Edition. Boston, MA: Kluwer Academic Publishers, 1989, pp. 423–452.

Lipp P, Pott L: Transient inward current in guinea-pig atrial myocytes reflects a change of sodium-calcium exchange current. J Physiol (Lond) 1988; 397: 601–630.

Lipsius SL, Gibbons WR: Membrane currents, contractions, and aftercontractions in cardiac Purkinje fibers. Am J Physiol 1982; 243:H77–H86.

Litovsky SH, Antzelevitch CE: Transient outward current prominent in canine epicardium but not endocardium. Circ Res 1988; 62:116–126.

Livingstone DJ: Pattern recognition methods in rational drug design. In Langone JJ (ed): Methods in Enzymology. Vol. 203. London, UK: Academic Press, 1991, pp. 613–638.

Lloyd EA, Gersh BJ, Forman R: The efficacy of quinidine and disopyramide in the maintenance of sinus rhythm after electroconversion from atrial fibrillation: A double blind study comparing quinidine, disopyramide and placebo. S Afr Med J 1984; 65:367–369.

Locati E, Schwartz PJ: Prognostic value of QT interval and prolongation in post myocardial infarction patients. Eur Heart J 1987; 8:121–126.

Lombardi F, Finocchiaro ML, Dalla Vecchia L, Rech R, et al: Effects of mexiletine, propafenone and flecainide on signal-averaged electrocardiogram. Eur Heart J 1992; 13:517–525.

Lown B, Fakhro AM, Hood WB Jr, Thorn GW: The coronary care unit: New perspectives and directions. JAMA 1967; 199:188–198.

Lubinski A, Vogt B, Hindricks G, Haverkamp W, Shenasa M, Borggrefe M, et al: Inhomogeneity of conduction after flecainide and sotalol in infarcted canine myocardium. PACE 1992; 15:556. Abstract.

Lue W-M, Boyden PA: Abnormal electrical properties of myocytes from chronically infarcted canine heart. Circ Res 1992; 85:1175–1188.

Lumma WC Jr, Wohl RA, Davey DD, Argentieri TM, DeVita RJ, Gomez RP, et al: Rational design of 4-[(methylsulfonyl)amino] benzamides as class III antiarrhythmic agents. J Med Chem 1987; 30:755–758.

Lundstrom T, Ryden L: Ventricular rate control and exercise performance in chronic atrial fibrillation: Effects of diltiazem and verapamil. J Am Coll Cardiol 1990; 16:86–90.

Luo C-H, Rudy Y: A dynamic model of the cardiac ventricular action potential: I. Simulations of ionic currents and concentration changes. Circ Res 1994. In press.

Lyons CJ, Burgess MJ: Demonstration of reentry within the canine specialized conduction system. Am Heart J 1979; 98:595–603.

MacKinnon R, Yellen G: Mutations affecting TEA blockade and ion permeation in voltage-activated K^+ channels. Science 1990; 250:276–279.

Mahgoub A, Idle JR, Dring LG, Lancaster R, Smith RL: Polymorphic hydroxylation of Debrisoquine in man. Lancet 1977; ii:584–586.

Mahmarian JJ, Verani MS, Hohmann T, Hill R, et al: The hemodynamic effects of sotalol and quinidine: Analysis by use of rest and exercise gated radionuclide angiography. Circulation 1987; 76:324–331.

Makita N, Bennett PB, George AL: Recombinant human Na^+ channel 1 subunit functionally associates with skeletal muscle but not cardiac α subunit. Circulation 1993; 88:I-185.

Malfatto G, Rosen TS, Rosen MR: The response to overdrive pacing of triggered atrial and ventricular arrhythmias in the canine heart. Circulation 1988; 77:1139–1148.

Malfatto G, Rosen MR, Foresti A, Schwartz PJ: Idiopathic long QT syndrome exacerbated by β-adrenergic blockade and responsive to left cardiac sympathetic denervation: Implications regarding electrophysiologic substrate and adrenergic modulation. J Cardiovasc Electrophysiol 1992; 3:295–305.

Malfatto G, Beria G, Sala S, Bonazzi O, Schwartz PJ: Quantitative analysis of T wave abnormalities and of their prognostic implications in the idiopathic long QT syndrome. J Am Coll Cardiol 1994; 23:296–301.

Manning AS, Hearse DJ: Reperfusion-induced arrhythmias: Mechanisms and prevention. J Mol Cell Cardiol 1984; 16:497–518.

Manoach M, Kauli N, Netz H, Beker B, Assael M: Dibenzepin as an antifibrillatory agent for spontaneously terminating electrically induced ventricular fibrillation. Isr J Med Sci 1979; 15:443–447.

Manolis AS, Estes NAM: Reversal of electrophysiologic effects of flecainide on the accessory pathway by isoproterenol in the Wolff-Parkinson-White syndrome. Am J Cardiol 1989; 64:194–198.

Marinchak RA, Friehling TD, Kline RA, Stohler J, Koweuy PR: Effect of antiarrhythmic drugs on defibrillation threshold: Case report of an adverse effect of mexiletine and review of the literature. PACE 1988; 11:7–12.

Martin YC: Computer-assisted rational drug design. In Langone JJ (ed): Methods in Enzymology. Vol. 203. London, UK: Academic Press, 1991, pp. 587–613.

Mary-Rabine L, Hordof AJ, Danilo P Jr, Malm JR, Rosen MR: Mechanisms for impulse initiation in isolated human atrial fibers. Circ Res 1980; 47:267–277.

Masini I, Porciatti F, Borea PA, Barbieri M, Cerbai E, Mugelli A: Cardiac β-adrenoceptors in the normal and failing heart: Electrophysiological aspects. Pharmacol Res 1991; 24(suppl 1):21–27.

Mason JW: Amiodarone. N Engl J Med 1987; 316:455–466.

Mason JW: A comparison of seven antiarrhythmic drugs in patients with ventricular tachyarrhythmias. Electrophysiologic Study versus Electrocardiographic Monitoring (ESVEM) Investigators. N Engl J Med 1993; 329: 452–458.

Matsubara H, Suzuki J, Inada M: Shaker-related potassium channel, Kv1.4 mRNA regulation in cultured rat heart myocytes and differential expression of Kv1.4 and Kv1.5 genes in myocardial development and hypertrophy. J Clin Invest 1993; 92:1659–1666.

Matsuda JJ, Lee H, Shibata EF: Enhancement of rabbit cardiac sodium channels by beta-adrenergic stimulation. Circ Res 1992; 70:199–207.

Mattioni TA, Zheutlin TA, Sarmiento JJ, Parker M, Lesch M, Kehoe RF: Amiodarone in patients with previous drug-mediated torsade de pointes. Ann Intern Med 1989; 111(7):574–580.

McDonald TV, Courtney KR, Clusin WT: Use-dependent block of single sodium channels by lidocaine in guinea pig ventricular myocytes. Biophys J 1989; 55:1261–1277.

McGuire MA, Janse MJ, Ross DL: "AV nodal' reentry: Part II: AV nodal, AV junctional or atrionodal reentry? J Cardiovasc Electrophysiol 1993; 4: 573–586.

McKibbin JK, Pocock WA, Barlow JB, Millar RNS, Obel IWP: Sotalol, hypokalaemia, syncope, and torsade de pointes. Br Heart J 1984; 51:157–162.

Mendez C, Mueller WJ, Merideth J, Moe GK: Interaction of transmembrane potentials in canine Purkinje fibers and at Purkinje fiber-muscle junctions. Circ Res 1969; 24:361–372.

Middlekauff HR, Stevenson WG, Stevenson LW: Pronostic significance of atrial fibrillation in advanced heart failure. Circulation 1991; 84:40–48.

Mikus G, Gross AS, Beckmann J, Hertrampf R, Gundert-Remy U, Eichelbaum M: The influence of the sparteine/debrisoquin phenotype on the disposition of flecainide. Clin Pharmacol Ther 1989; 45:562–567.

Miller C, Moczydlowski E, Latorre R, Phillips M: Charybdotoxin, a protein inhibitor of single Ca^{2+}-activated K^+ channels from mammalian skeletal muscle. Nature 1985; 313:316–318.

Milne JR, Hellestrand KJ, Bexton RS, Burnett PJ, Debbas NMG, Camm AJ: Class I antiarrhythmic drugs—a subdivision based on surface electrocardiographic effect. Characteristic electrocardiographic differences when assessed by atrial and ventricular pacing. Eur Heart J 1984; 5:99–107.

Mines GR: On circulating excitation in heart muscles and their possible relations to tachycardia and fibrillation. Trans Roy Soc Can (Ser III, sec IV) 1914; 8:43–52.

Mirro MJ, Manalan AS, Bailey JC, Watanabe AM: Anticholinergic effects of disopyramide and quinidine on guinea-pig myocardium: Mediation by direct muscarinic receptor blockade. Circ Res 1980; 47:855–865.

Mitchell LB, Jutzy KR, Lewis SJ, Schroeder JS, Mason JW: Intracardiac electrophysiologic study of intravenous diltiazem and combined diltiazem-digoxin in patients. Am Heart J 1982; 103:57–65.

Mitrani R, Klein LS, Hackett K, Zipes DP, Miles WM: Radiofrequency ablation for atrioventricular nodal reentrant tachycardia: Comparison between fast (anterior) versus slow (posterior) pathway ablation. J Am Coll Cardiol 1992; 2:432–441.

Miyajima S, Koyama S, Satoh M, Aizawa Y, Shibata A, Kimura M: A case of idiopathic ventricular tachycardia of RBBB and LAD morphology that is related to catecholamine. Respir Circ 1987; 35:993–997.

Moak JP, Rosen MR: Induction and termination of triggered activity by pacing in isolated canine Purkinje fibers. Circulation 1984; 69:149–162.

Moe GH, Jalife J, Mueller WJ: Reciprocation between pacemaker sites: Re-entrant parasystole? In Kulbertus HE (ed): Re-entrant Arrhythmias. Mechanisms and Treatment. Lancaster, PA: MTP Press, 1977, pp. 271–293.

Moe GK, Abildskov JA: Atrial fibrillation as a self sustaining arrhythmia independent of focal discharge. Am Heart J 1959; 58:59–70.

Moe GK, Rheinboldt WC, Abildskov JA: A computer model of atrial fibrillation. Am Heart J 1964; 67:200–220.

Molenaar P, Smolich JJ, Russel FD, McMartin LR, Summers RJ: Differential regulation of β_1 and β_2 adrenoceptors in guinea pig atrioventricular conducting system after chronic ($-$)-isoproterenol infusion. J Pharmacol Exp Ther 1990; 255:393–400.

Mont L, Seixas T, Brugada P, Brugada J, Simonis F, Kriek E, et al: The electrocardiographic, clinical and electrophysiologic spectrum of idiopathic monomorphic ventricular tachycardia. Am Heart J 1992; 124:746–753.

Morad M, Rolett EL: Relaxing effects of catecholamines on mammalian heart. J Physiol (Lond) 1972; 224:537–558.

Morganroth J: Drug-induced early and late proarrhythmia. Cardiol Clin 1992; 10:397–401.

Morganroth J, Horowitz LN: Flecainide: Its proarrhythmic effect and expected changes on the surface electrocardiogram. Am J Cardiol 1984; 53(suppl): 89B–94B.

Mörike KE, Roden DM: Quinidine-enhanced beta-blockade during treatment with propafenone in extensive metabolizer human subjects. Clin Pharmacol Ther 1994; 55:28–34.

Moss AJ, Bigger JT Jr, Odoroff CL: Postinfarct risk stratification. Prog Cardiovasc Dis 1987; 29:389–412.

Moss AJ, Liu JE, Gottlieb S, Locati EH, Schwartz PJ, Robinson JL: Efficacy of permanent pacing in the management of high risk patients with long QT syndrome. Circulation 1991; 84:1524–1529.

Motomura S, Hashimoto K: β_2-adrenoceptor-mediated positive dromotropic effects on atrioventricular node of dogs. Am J Physiol 1992; 262:H123–H129.

Mullins LJ: The generation of electric currents in cardiac fibers by Na/Ca exchange. Am J Physiol 1979; 236:C103–C110.

Mullins LJ: Ion Transport in the Heart. New York, NY: Raven Press, 1981.

Multiple Risk Factor Intervention Trial Research Group: Multiple-risk factor intervention trial: Risk factor changes and mortality results. JAMA 1982; 248:1465–1477.

Muroi M, Kimura I, Kimura M: Blocking effects of hypaconitine and aconitine on nerve action potentials in phrenic nerve-diaphragm muscles of mice. Neuropharmacology 1990; 29:567–572.

Myerburg RJ, Kessler KM, Luceri RM, Zaman L, Trohman RG, Estes D, et al: Classification of ventricular arrhythmias based on parallel hierarchies of frequency and form. Am J Cardiol 1984; 54:1355–1358.

Myerburg RJ, Kessler KM, Castellanos A: Pathophysiology of sudden cardiac death. PACE 1991; 14(part II):935–943.

Myerburg RJ, Kessler KM, Castellanos A: Sudden cardiac death: Structure, function, and time-dependence of risk. Circulation 1992a; 85(suppl I):I-2–-I-10.

Myerburg RJ, Kessler KM, Kimura S, Castellanos A: Sudden cardiac death: Future approaches based on identification and control of transient risk factors. J Cardiovasc Electrophysiol 1992b; 3:626–640.

Myerburg RJ, Kessler KM, Castellanos A: Sudden cardiac death: Epidemiology, transient risk, and intervention assessment. Ann Intern Med 1993; 119:1187–1197.

Myerburg RJ, Kessler KM, Castellanos A: Recognition, clinical assessment, and management of arrhythmias and conduction disturbances. In Schlant RC, Alexander RW (eds): Hurst's: The Heart. Eighth edition. New York, NY: McGraw-Hill, 1994, pp. 705–758.

Nademanee K, Singh BN: Effects of sotalol on ventricular tachycardia and fibrillation produced by programmed electrical stimulation: Comparison with other agents. Am J Cardiol 1990; 65:53A–57A.

Nademanee K, Stevenson WG, Weiss JN, Frame VB, Antimisiaris MG, Suithichaiyakul T, et al: Frequency-dependent effects of quinidine on the ventricular action potential and QRS duration in humans. Circulation 1990; 81: 790–796.

Nakai J, Imagawa Y, Hakamata Y, Shigekawa M, Takeshima H, Numa S: Primary structure and functional expression from cDNA of the cardiac ryanodine receptor/calcium release channel. FEBS Lett 1990; 271:169–177.

Narahashi T: Toxins that modulate the sodium channel gating mechanism. In Kao CY, Levinson SR (eds): Tetrodotoxin Saxitoxin and the Molecular Biology of the Sodium Channel. Ann NY Acad Sci 1986; 479:133–151.

The NHLBI Working Group on Atrial Fibrillation (Antman E, DiMarco J, Domanski MJ, Knatterud GL, Scheinman MM, Singer D, et al: Atrial fibrillation: Current understandings and research imperative. J Am Coll Cardiol 1993; 22:1830–1834.

Niwano S, Ortiz J, Abe H, Gonzalez X, Waldo AL: Evaluation of resetting in a functionally determined reentrant circuit. PACE 1993; 16:II-864.

Niwano S, Ortiz J, Abe H, Gonzalez HX, Rudy Y, Waldo AL: Characterization of excitable gap in a functionally determined reentry circuit. Studies in the sterile pericarditis model of atrial flutter. Circulation. In Press.

Noble D: The surprising heart: A review of recent progress in cardiac electrophysiology. J Physiol (Lond) 1984; 353:1–50.

Noble D, Tsien RW: The kinetics and rectifier properties of the slow potassium current in cardiac Purkinje fibres. J Physiol (Lond) 1968; 195:185–214.

Nordin C, Gilat E, Aronson RS: Delayed afterdepolarizations and triggered activity in ventricular muscle from rats with streptozotocin-induced diabetes. Circ Res 1985; 57:28–34.

Norris RM, Barnaby PF, Brown MA, Geary GG, et al: Prevention of ventricular fibrillation during acute myocardial infarction by intravenous propranolol. Lancet 1984; ii:883–886.

Nozaki A, Shimizu A, Henthorn RW, Waldo AL: Unexpected effects of ouabain on atrial flutter induced in conscious dogs with sterile pericarditis. PACE 1989; 12:I-670.

O'Doherty M, Taylor DI, Quinn E, Vincent R, Camberlain DA: Five hundred patients with myocardial infarction monitored within one hour of symptoms. Br Med J 1983; 286:1405.

Offord J, Catterall WA: Electrical activity, cAMP, and cytosolic calcium regulate mRNA encoding sodium channel α subunits in rat muscle cells. Neuron 1989; 2:1447–1452.

Ohe T: Idiopathic verapamil-sensitive sustained left ventricular tachycardia. Clin Cardiol 1993; 16:139–141.

Ohe T, Shimomura K, Aihara N, Kamakura S, Matsuhisa M, Sato I, et al: Idiopathic sustained left ventricular tachycardia: Clinical and electrophysiologic characteristics. Circulation 1988; 77:560–568.

Okumura K, Waldo AL: Effects of N-acetylprocainamide on experimental atrial flutter and atrial electrophysiologic properties in conscious dogs with sterile pericarditis: Comparison with the effect of quinidine. J Am Coll Cardiol 1987; 9:1332–1338.

Okumura K, Henthorn RW, Epstein AE, Plumb VJ, Waldo AL: Further observations on transient entrainment: Importance of pacing site and properties of the components of the reentry circuit. Circulation 1985; 72:1293.

Okumura K, Olshansky B, Henthorn RW, Epstein RE, Plumb VJ, Waldo AL: Demonstration of the presence of slow conduction during sustained ventricular tachycardia in man. Circulation 1987; 75:369–378.

Okumura K, Matsuyama K, Miyagi H, Tsuchiya T, Yasue H: Entrainment of idiopathic ventricular tachycardia of left ventricular origin with evidence for reentry with an area of slow conduction and effect of verapamil. Am J Cardiol 1988; 62:727–732.

Olshansky B, Martin JB: Usefulness of isoproterenol facilitation of ventricular tachycardia induction during extrastimulus testing in predicting effective chronic therapy with beta-adrenergic blockade. Am J Cardiol 1987; 59: 573–577.

Olshansky B, Okumura K, Hess PG, Henthorn RW, Waldo AL: Use of procainamide with rapid atrial pacing for successful conversion of atrial flutter to sinus rhythm. J Am Coll Cardiol 1988; 11:359–364.

Ono K, Fozzard HA, Hanck DA: Mechanism of cAMP-dependent modulation of cardiac sodium channel current kinetics. Circ Res 1993; 72:807–815.

Ortiz J, Igarashi M, Gonzalez X, Johnson NJ, Waldo AL: A new, reliable atrial fibrillation model with a clinical counterpart. J Am Coll Cardiol 1993; 21: 183A. Abstract.

Ortiz J, Niwano S, Abe H, Gonzalez HX, Rudy Y, Johnson NJ, et al: Mapping the conversion of atrial flutter to atrial fibrillation and atrial fibrillation to atrial flutter—Insights into mechanism. Circ Res 1994; 74:882–894.

Ortiz J, Nozaki A, Shimizu A, Khrestian C, Rudy Y, Waldo AL: Mechanism of interruption of atrial flutter by moricizine: Electrophysiologic and multiplexing studies in the canine sterile pericarditis model of atrial flutter. Circulation 1994. In Press.

Packer M: Sudden unexpected death in patients with congestive heart failure: A second frontier. Circulation 1985; 72:681–685.

Page E, Manjunath CK: Communicating junctions between cardiac cells. In Fozzard HA, Haber E, Jennings RB, Katz AM, Morgan HE (eds): Heart and the Cardiovascular System. New York, NY: Raven Press, 1986, pp. 573–600.

Pagé P, Plumb VJ, Okumura K, Waldo AL: A new model of atrial flutter. J Am Coll Cardiol 1986; 8:872–879.

Pala M, Locati E, Priori SG, Munoz A, Schwartz PJ: QT interval shortening by penticainide in patients with ventricular arrhythmias with and without the long QT syndrome. Circulation 1987; 76(suppl IV):414.

Palileo EV, Ashley WW, Swiryn S, Bauernfeind RA, Strasberg B, Petropoulos T, et al: Exercise provocable right ventricular outflow tract tachycardia. Am Heart J 1982; 104:185–193.

Paparella N, Pirani R, Cappato R, Candini GC, Alboni P: Method for differentiating in humans the direct effects of anti-arrhythmic drugs from those mediated by the autonomic nervous system. Effects of quinidine and propafenone. G Ital Cardiol 1986; 16:762–769.

Pappano AJ, Carmeliet E: Epinephrine and the pacemaking mechanism at plateau potentials in sheep cardiac Purkinje fibers. Pflügers Arch 1979; 382: 17–26.

Pappano AJ, Mubagwa K: Actions of muscarinic agents and adenosine on the heart. In Fozzard HA, Haber E, Jennings RB, Katz AM, Morgan HE (eds): The Heart and Cardiovascular System. Scientific Foundations. New York, NY: Raven Press Ltd, 1992, pp. 1765–1776.

Paspa P, Vassalle M: Mechanism of caffeine-induced arrhythmias in canine cardiac Purkinje fibers. Am J Cardiol 1984; 53:313–319.

Patterson E, Gibson JK, Lucchesi BR: Electrophysiologic actions of lidocaine in a canine model of chronic myocardial ischemic damage—arrhythmogenic actions of lidocaine. J Cardiovasc Pharmacol 1982; 4:925–934.

Peck CC, Temple R, Collins JM: Understanding consequences of current therapy. JAMA 1993; 269:1550–1552.

Pederson TR, the Norwegian Multicenter Study Group: Six-year follow-up of the Norwegian multicenter study on timolol after acute myocardial infarction. N Engl J Med 1985; 313:1055–1058.

Pelzer D, Pelzer S, MacDonald TF: Properties and regulation of calcium channels in muscle cells. Rev Physiol Biochem Pharmacol 1990; 114:107–207.

Penkoske PA, Sobel BE, Corr PB: Disparate electrophysiological alterations accompanying dysrhythmias due to coronary occlusion and reperfusion in the cat. Circulation 1978; 58:1023–1035.

Penny WJ: The deleterious effects of myocardial catecholamines on cellular electrophysiology and arrhythmias during ischemia and reperfusion. Eur Heart J 1984; 5:960–973.

Peralta EG, Ashkenazi A, Winslow JW, Smith DH, Ramachandran J, Capon DJ: Distinct primary structures, ligand-binding properties and tissue-specific expression of four human muscarinic acetylcholine receptors. EMBO J 1987; 6:3923–3929.

Peters W, Gang ES, Solingen S, et al: Acute effects of intravenous propafenone on the internal ventricular defibrillation energy requirements in the anesthetized dog. J Am Coll Cardiol 1991; 17:129A. Abstract.

Pfisterer M, Kiowski W, Burckhardt D, Follath F, Burkart F: Beneficial effect of amiodarone on cardiac mortality in patients with asymptomatic complex ventricular arrhythmias after acute myocardial infarction and preserved but not impaired left ventricular function. Am J Cardiol 1992; 69:1399–1402.

Pfisterer ME, Kiowski W, Brunner H, Burckhardt D, Burkart F: Long-term benefit of 1-year amiodarone treatment for persistent complex ventricular arrhythmias after myocardial infarction. Circulation 1993; 87:309–311.

Pinto JMB, Graziano JN, Boyden PA: Endocardial mapping of reentry around an anatomical barrier in the canine right atrium: Observations during the action of the class IC agent, flecainide. J Cardiovasc Electrophysiol 1993; 4: 672–685.

Po S, Roberds S, Snyders DJ, Tamkun MM, Bennett PB: Heteromultimeric assembly of human potassium channels. Circ Res 1993; 72:1326–1336.

Pogwizd SM, Corr PB: Reentrant and nonreentrant mechanisms contribute to arrhythmogenesis during early myocardial ischemia: Results using 3-dimensional mapping. Circ Res 1987; 61:352–371.

Pogwizd SM, Onufer JR, Kramer JB, Sobel BE, Corr PB: Induction of delayed afterdepolarizations and triggered activity in canine Purkinje fibers by lysophosphoglycerides. Circ Res 1986; 59:416–426.

Pongs P: Molecular biology of voltage-dependent potassium channels. Physiol Rev 1992; 72:S69–S88.

Pragnell M, Snay KJ, Trimmer JS, Maclusky NJ, Naftolin F, Kaczmarek LK, et al: Estrogen induction of a small, putative K^+ channel mRNA in rat uterus. Neuron 1991; 4:807–812.

Pratt CM, Roberts R: Chronic beta blockade therapy in patients after myocardial infarction. Am J Cardiol 1983; 52:661–664.

Price-Evans DAP, Manley KA, McKusick VA: Genetic control of isoniazid metabolism in man. Br Med J 1960; 2:485–491.

Priori SG, Mantica M, Napolitano C, et al: Early afterdepolarizations induced in vivo by reperfusion of ischemic myocardium. Circulation 1990; 81: 1911–1920.

Priori SG, Napolitano C, Diehl L, Schwartz PJ: Dispersion of the QT interval. A marker of therapeutic efficacy in the idiopathic long QT syndrome. Circulation 1994; 89:1681–1689.

Pritchett ELC, McCarthy EA, Wilkinson WE: Propafenone treatment of symptomatic paroxysmal supraventricular arrhythmias: A randomized, placebo-controlled, crossover trial in patients tolerating oral therapy. Ann Intern Med 1991; 114:539–544.

Puech P: L'Activite electrique auriculaire normale et pathologique. Paris: Masson & Cie, 1956, p. 214.

Puech P, Latour H, Grolleau R: Le flutter et ses limites. Arch Mal Coeur 1970; 63:116–144.

Qu Y, Campbell DL, Strauss HC: Modulation of L-type Ca^{2+} current by extra-cellular ATP in ferret isolated right ventricular myocytes. J Physiol (Lond) 1993; 471:295–317.

Quan W, Rudy Y: Unidirectional block and reentry of cardiac excitation: A model study. Circ Res 1990; 66:367–382.

Racker DK: Transmission and reentrant activity in the sinoventricular conduction system and in the circumferential lamina of the tricuspid valve. J Cardiovasc Electrophysiol 1993; 4:513–525.

Ragsdale DS, Catterall WA, Scheuer T: Verapamil blocks type IIA brain Na channels expressed in Chinese hamster ovary cells. Biophys J 1992; 61: A112.

Ramsdale DR, Llewellyn MJ, Pidgeon J, Faragher EB, Charles RG: Effects of intravenous sotalol on the QT interval and incidence of ventricular arrhythmias early in acute myocardial infarction. Am J Noninv Cardiol 1988; 2: 52–58.

Rasmussen HS, McNair P, Norregard P, Backer V, Lindeneg O, Balslev S: Intravenous magnesium in acute myocardial infarction. Lancet 1986; i: 234–236.

Rasmusson RL, Clark JW, Giles WR, Robinson K, Clark RB, Shibata EF, et al: A mathematical model of electrical activity in the bullfrog atrial cell. Am J Physiol 1990; 259:H370–H389.

Rasmusson RL, Campbell DL, Qu Y, Strauss HC: Conformation-dependent drug binding to cardiac potassium channels. In Spooner PM, Brown AM, Catterall WA, Kaczorowski GJ, Strauss HC (eds): Ion Channels in the Cardiovascular System: Function and Dysfunction. Armonk, NY: Futura Publishing Co, 1994, pp. 387–414.

Rawles J: Atrial fibrillation. London: Springer-Verlag, 1992, pp. 181–197.

Reddy CP, Gettes LS: Use of isoproterenol as an aid to electric induction of chronic recurrent ventricular tachycardia. Am J Cardiol 1979; 44:705–713.

Redfors A: Digoxin dosage and ventricular rate at rest and exercise in patients with atrial fibrillation. Acta Med Scand 1971; 190:321–333.

Reiffel JA, Coromilas JM, Zimmerman JM, Spotnitz HM: Drug-device interactions: Clinical considerations. PACE 1985; 8:369–373.

Reimold SC, Cantillon CO, Friedman PL, Antman EM: Propafenone versus sotalol for suppression of recurrent symptomatic atrial fibrillation. Am J Cardiol 1993; 71:558–563.

Reuter H: Ion channels in cardiac cell membranes. Annu Rev Physiol 1984; 46:473–484.

Reuter H, Seitz N: The dependence of calcium efflux from cardiac muscle on temperature and external ion composition. J Physiol (Lond) 1968; 195: 451–470.

Roberds S, Knoth K, Po S, Blair TA, Bennett P, Hartshorne R, et al: Molecular biology of the voltage-gated potassium channels of the cardiovascular system. J Cardiovasc Electrophysiol 1993; 4:68–80.

Roberts DE, Hersh LT, Scher AM: Influence of cardiac fiber orientation on wavefront voltage, conduction velocity and tissue resistivity in the dog. Circ Res 1979; 44:701–712.

Roberts R, Husain A, Ambos HD, Oliver GC, Cox JR Jr, Sobel BE: Relation between infarct size and ventricular arrhythmia. Br Heart J 1975; 37: 1169–1175.

Robertson DW, Steinberg MI: Potassium channel modulators: Scientific applications and therapeutic promise. J Med Chem 1990; 33:1529–1541.

Roden DM: Current status of class III antiarrhythmic therapy. Am J Cardiol 1993; 72(suppl):44B–49B.

Roden DM, Hoffman BF: Action potential prolongation and induction of abnormal automaticity by low quinidine concentrations in canine Purkinje fibers. Relationship to potassium and cycle length. Circ Res 1985; 56: 857–867.

Roden DM, Woosley RL, Primm RK: Incidence and clinical features of the quinidine-associated long QT syndrome: Implications for patient care. Am Heart J 1986; 111:1088–1093.

Roden DM, Bennett PB, Snyders DJ, Balser JR, Hondeghem LM: Quinidine delays I_K activation in guinea pig ventricular myocytes. Circ Res 1988; 62: 1055–1058.

Roffe C, Fletcher S, Woods KL: Investigation of the effects of intravenous magnesium sulphate on cardiac rhythm in acute myocardial infarction. Br Heart J 1994; 71:141–145.

Rosen KM, Lau SH, Damato AN: Simulation of atrial flutter by rapid coronary sinus pacing. Am Heart J 1969; 78:635–642.

Rosen KM, Mehta A, Miller RA: Demonstration of dual atrioventricular nodal pathways in man. Am J Cardiol 1972; 33:291–294.

Rosen MR: Is the response to programmed electrical stimulation diagnostic of mechanisms for arrhythmias? Circulation 1986; 73(suppl II):18–27.

Rosen MR: Mechanisms of arrhythmias: Contributions of cellular electrophysiology. In Josephson ME, Wellens HJJ (eds): Tachycardias: Mechanisms and Management. Mount Kisco, NY: Futura Publishing Co, 1993, pp. 1–11.

Rosen MR, Danilo P Jr: Effects of tetrodotoxin, lidocaine, verapamil, and AHR-2666 on ouabain-induced delayed afterdepolarizations in canine Purkinje fibers. Circ Res 1980; 46:117–124.

Rosen MR, Reder RF: Does triggered activity have a role in the genesis of cardiac arrhythmias? Ann Int Med 1981; 94:794–801.

Rosen MR, Gelband H, Hoffman BF: Correlation between effects of ouabain on the canine electrocardiogram and transmembrane potentials of isolated Purkinje fibers. Circulation 1973a; 47:65–72.

Rosen MR, Gelband H, Merker C, Hoffman BF: Mechanisms of digitalis toxicity. Effects of ouabain on phase four of canine Purkinje fiber transmembrane potentials. Circulation 1973b; 47:681–689.

Rosen MR, Hordof AJ, Ilvento JP, Danilo PJ: Effects of adrenergic amines on electrophysiological properties and automaticity in neonatal and adult canine Purkinje fibers: Evidence for alpha and beta adrenergic actions. Circ Res 1977; 40:390–400.

Rosen MR, Fisch C, Hoffman BF, Danilo P Jr, Lovelace DE, Knoebel SB:

Can accelerated atrioventricular junctional escape rhythms be explained by delayed afterdepolarizations? Am J Cardiol 1980; 45:1272–1284.

Rosen MR, Danilo P Jr, Weiss RM: Action of adenosine on normal and abnormal impulse initiation in canine ventricle. Am J Physiol 1983; 244: H715–H721.

Rosen MR, Steinberg SF, Chow YK, Bilezikian JP, Danilo P Jr: The role of a pertussis toxin-sensitive protein in the modulation of canine Purkinje fiber automaticity. Circ Res 1988; 62:315–323.

Rosenblueth A, Garcia Ramos J: Studies on flutter and fibrillation. II. The influence of artificial obstacles on experimental auricular flutter. Am Heart J 1947; 33:677–684.

Rosenthal JE, Ferrier GR: Contribution of variable entrance and exit block in protected foci to arrhythmogenesis in isolated ventricular tissues. Circulation 1983; 67:1–8.

Rozanski GJ: Electrophysiological properties of automatic fibers in rabbit atrioventricular valves. Am J Physiol 1987; 253:H720–H727.

Rozanski GJ, Lipsius SL: Electrophysiology of functional subsidiary pacemakers in canine right atrium. Am J Physiol 1985; 249:H594–H603.

Rozanski GJ, Lipsius SL, Randall WC: Functional characteristics of sinoatrial and subsidiary pacemaker activity in the canine right atrium. Circulation 1983; 67:1378–1387.

Rozanski GJ, Jalife J, Moe GK: Reflected reentry in nonhomogeneous ventricular muscle as a mechanism of cardiac arrhythmias. Circulation 1984; 69: 163–173.

Rudy Y, Quan W: A model study of the effects of the discrete cellular structure on electrical propagation in cardiac tissue. Circ Res 1987; 61:815–823.

Ruskin JN: The cardiac arrhythmia suppression trial (CAST). N Engl J Med 1989; 321:386–388.

Russell DC, Oliver MF: Ventricular refractoriness during acute myocardial ischemia and its relationship to ventricular fibrillation. Cardiovasc Res 1978; 12:221–227.

Saito T, Otoguro M, Matsubara T: Electrophysiological studies on the mechanism of electrically induced sustained rhythmic activity in the rabbit right atrium. Circ Res 1978; 42:199–206.

Sakai T, Ogawa S, Miyazaki T, Hosokawa M, Sakurai K, Yoshino H, et al: Electrophysiological effects of acute ischemia on electrically stable myocardial infarction. Cardiovasc Res 1989; 23:169–176.

Sakmann B, Noma A, Trautwein W: Acetylcholine activation of single muscarinic K channels in isolated pacemaker cells of the mammalian heart. Nature 1983; 303:250–253.

Sakurai M, Yoshida I, Nishino T, Sato A, Yotsukura A, Yasuda H: The mechanism of verapamil-sensitive ventricular tachycardia: Is it reentry or triggered activity? Eur Heart J 1990; 11(suppl):156.

Salata JJ, Wasserstrom JA: Effects of quinidine on action potentials and ionic currents in isolated canine ventricular myocytes. Circ Res 1988; 62:324–337.

Sanguinetti MC, Jurkiewicz NK: Two components of cardiac delayed rectifier K^+ current. Differential sensitivity to block by Class III antiarrhythmic agents. J Gen Physiol 1990; 96:195–215.

Sanguinetti MC, Jurkiewicz NK, Scott A, Siegl PKS: Isoproterenol antagonizes prolongation of refractory period by the Class III antiarrhythmic agent E-4031 in guinea pig myocytes. Mechanism of action. Circ Res 1991; 68:77–84.

Saoudi N, Atallah G, Kirkorian G, Touboul P: Catheter ablation of the atrial myocardium in human type I atrial flutter. Circulation 1990; 81:762–771.

Sasyniuk BI, Mendez C: A mechanism for reentry in canine ventricular tissue. Circ Res 1971; 28:3–15.

Satin J, Kyle J, Chen M, Rogart R, Fozzard H: The cloned cardiac Na channel alpha-subunit expressed in xenopus oocytes shows gating and blocking properties of native channels. J Membrane Biol 1992; 130:11–22.

Scalabrini A, Okumura K, Olshansky B, Waldo AL: Effects of class IC drugs on induced atrial flutter in a dog model with sterile pericarditis. Circulation 1986; 74:II-251.

Schalij MJ: *Anisotropic Conduction and Ventricular Tachycardia.* Maastrict, The Netherlands: University of Limburg, 1988. Thesis.

Schamroth L: The genesis and evolution of ectopic ventricular rhythm. Br Heart J 1966; 28:244.

Schamroth L: The physiological basis of ectopic ventricular rhythm: A unifying concept. In Sandoe E, Julian DG, Bell JW (eds): Management of Ventricular Tachycardia: Role of Mexiletine. Amsterdam/Oxford: Excerpta Medica, 1987, pp. 83–1281.

Schamroth L, Marriott HJL: Intermittent ventricular parasystole with observations on its relationship to extrasystolic bigeminy. Am J Cardiol 1961; 7: 799.

Schechter E, Freeman CC, Lazzara R: Afterdepolarizations as a mechanism for the long QT syndrome. Electrophysiologic studies of a case. J Am Coll Cardiol 1984; 3:1556–1561.

Schechter M, Hod H, Marks N: Beneficial effect of magnesium sulfate in acute myocardial infarction. Am J Cardiol 1990; 66:271–274.

Scheinman MM: Catheter techniques for ablation of supraventricular tachycardia. N Engl J Med 1989; 320:460–461.

Scherf D: Studies on auricular tachycardia caused by aconitine administration. Proc Exp Biol Med 1947; 64:233–239.

Scherf D, Terranova R: Mechanism of auricular flutter and fibrillation. Am J Physiol 1949; 159:137–142.

Scherf D, Romano FJ, Terranova R: Experimental studies on auricular flutter and auricular fibrillation. Am Heart J 1958; 36:241–251.

Scherlag BJ, El-Sherif N, Hope RR, Lazzara R: Characterization and localization of ventricular arrhythmias resulting from myocardial ischemia and infarction. Circ Res 1974; 35:372–383.

Schmid PG, Nelson LD, Mark AL, Heistad DD, Abboud FM: Inhibition of adrenergic vasoconstriction by quinidine. J Pharmacol Exp Ther 1974; 188: 124–134.

Schmitt FO, Erlanger J: Directional differences in the conduction of the impulse through heart muscle and their possible relation to extrasystolic and fibrillatory contractions. Am J Physiol 1928; 87:326–347.

Schoels W, Yang H, Gough WB, El-Sherif N: Circus movement atrial flutter in the canine sterile pericarditis model. Differential effects of procainamide on the components of the reentrant pathway. Circ Res 1991; 68:1117–1126.

Schömig A, Dart AM, Dietz R, Mayer E, Kübler W: Release of endogenous catecholamines in the ischemic myocardium of the rat. Part A: Locally mediated release. Circ Res 1984; 55:689–701.

Schubert B, Vandongen AMJ, Kirsch GE, Brown AM: Inhibition of cardiac Na$^+$ currents by isoproterenol. Am J Physiol 1990; 258:H977–H981.

Schuessler RB, Grayson TM, Bromberg BI, Cox JL, Boineau JP: Cholinergically mediated tachyarrhythmias induced by a single extrastimulus in the isolated canine right atrium. Circ Res 1992; 71:1254–1276.

Schwartz PJ: Sympathetic imbalance and cardiac arrhythmias. In Randall WC (ed): Nervous Control of Cardiovascular Function. New York, NY: Oxford University Press, 1984, pp. 225–252.

Schwartz PJ: Idiopathic long QT syndrome: Progress and questions. Am Heart J 1985; 109:399–411.

Schwartz PJ, Locati E: The idiopathic long QT syndrome. Pathogenetic mechanisms and therapy. Eur Heart J 1985; 6(suppl D):103–114.

Schwartz PJ, Priori SG: Sympathetic nervous system and cardiac arrhythmias. In Zipes DP, Jalife J (eds): Cardiac Electrophysiology. From Cell to Bedside. Philadelphia, PA: WB Saunders, 1990, pp. 330–343.

Schwartz PJ, Zaza A: The Sicilian Gambit revisited. Theory and Practice. Eur Heart J 1992; 13(suppl F):23–29.

Schwartz PJ, Snebold NG, Brown AM: Effects of unilateral cardiac sympathetic denervation on the ventricular fibrillation threshold. Am J Cardiol 1976; 37:1034–1041.

Schwartz PJ, Locati E, Moss AJ, Crampton RS, Trazzi R, Ruberti U: Left cardiac sympathetic denervation in the therapy of the congenital long QT syndrome. A worldwide report. Circulation 1991a; 84:503–511.

Schwartz PJ, Zaza A, Locati E, Moss AJ: Stress and sudden death. The case of the long QT syndrome. Circulation 1991b; 83(suppl II):II71–II80.

Schwartz PJ, La Rovere MT, Vanoli E: Autonomic nervous system and sudden cardiac death. Experimental basis and clinical observations for post-myocardial infarction risk stratification. Circulation 1992a; 85(suppl I):I77–I91.

Schwartz PJ, Bonazzi O, Locati EH, Napolitano C, Sala S: Pathogenesis and therapy of the idiopathic long QT syndrome. Ann NY Acad Sci 1992b; 644:112–141.

Schwartz PJ, Motolese M, Pollavini G, Lotto A, Ruberti U, Trazzi R, et al: Prevention of sudden cardiac death after a first myocardial infarction by pharmacologic or surgical antiadrenergic interventions. J Cardiovasc Electrophysiol 1992c; 3:2–15.

Schwartz PJ, Moss AJ, Vincent GM, Crampton RS: Diagnostic criteria for the long QT syndrome: An update. Circulation 1993; 88:782–784.

Schwartz PJ, Locati EH, Napolitano C, Priori SG: The long QT syndrome. In Zipes DP, Jalife J (eds): Cardiac Electrophysiology. From Cell to Bedside. Second Edition. Philadelphia, PA: WB Saunders Co. In press.

Sethi KK, Manoharan S, Mohan JC, Gupta MP: Verapamil in idiopathic ventricular tachycardia of right bundle branch block morphology: Observations during electrophysiologic and exercise testing. PACE 1986; 9:8–16.

Shah A, Cohen IS, Rosen M: Stimulation of cardiac alpha receptors increases Na/K pump current and decreases g_k via a pertussis toxin sensitive pathway. Biophys J 1988; 54:219–225.

Sheridan DJ, Penkoske PA, Sobel BE, Corr PB: Alpha adrenergic contributions to dysrhythmia during myocardial ischemia and reperfusion in cats. J Clin Invest 1980; 65:161–171.

Sherman SJ, Catterall WA: Electrical activity and cytosolic calcium regulate levels of tetrodotoxin-sensitive sodium channels in cultured rat muscle cells. Proc Natl Acad Sci USA 1984; 81:262–266.

Sheu S-S, Lederer WJ: Lidocaine's negative inotropic and antiarrhythmic actions. Dependence on shortening of action potential duration and reduction of intracellular sodium activity. Circ Res 1985; 57:578–590.

Sheu S-S, Blaustein MP: Sodium/calcium exchange and control of cell calcium and contractility in cardiac and vascular smooth muscles. In Fozzard HA, Haber E, Jennings RB, Katz AM, Morgan HE (eds): The Heart and Cardiovascular System. Scientific Foundations. New York, NY: Raven Press, 1992, pp. 903–943.

Shih HT, Miles WM, Klein LS, Hubbard JH, Zipes DP: Multiple accessory pathways in the permanent form of junctional reciprocating tachycardia. Am J Cardiol. In press.

Shimizu A, Igarashi M, Rudy Y, Waldo AL: Insights into atrial flutter from experimental models. PACE 1991a; 14:627. Abstract.

Shimizu A, Nozaki A, Rudy Y, Waldo AL: Multiplexing studies of effects of rapid atrial pacing on the area of slow conduction during atrial flutter in canine pericarditis model. Circulation 1991b; 83:983–994.

Shimizu A, Nozaki A, Rudy Y, Waldo AL: Onset of induced atrial flutter in the canine pericarditis model. J Am Coll Cardiol 1991c; 17:1223–1234.

Shimizu W, Ohe T, Kurita T, Takaki H, Aihara N, Kamamura S, et al: Early afterdepolarizations induced by isoproterenol in patients with congenital long QT syndrome. Circulation 1991; 84:1915–1923.

The Sicilian Gambit: A new approach to the classification of antiarrhythmic drugs based on their actions on arrhythmogenic mechanisms. Task force of the working group on arrhythmias of the European Society of Cardiology. Circulation 1991; 84:1831–1851. (Simultaneously published in Eur Heart J 1991; 12:1112–1131.)

Sicouri S, Antzelevitch C: A subpopulation of cells with unique electrophysiological properties in the deep subepicardium of the canine ventricle. Circ Res 1991; 68:1729–1741.

Siddoway LA, Thompson KA, McAllister CB, Wang T, Wilkinson GR, Roden DM, et al: Polymorphism of propafenone metabolism and disposition in man: Clinical and pharmacokinetic consequences. Circulation 1987; 75: 785–791.

Simurda J, Simurdova M, Christé G: Use-dependent effects of 4-aminopyridine on transient outward current in dog ventricular muscle. Pflügers Arch 1989; 415:244–246.

Singer I, Lang D: Defibrillation threshold: Clinical utility and therapeutic implications. PACE 1992; 15:932–949.

Slama R, Leclercq JF, Coumel P: Paroxysmal ventricular tachycardia in patients with apparently normal hearts. In Zipes DP, Jalife F (eds): Cardiac Electrophysiology and Arhythmias. Orlando, FL: Grune and Stratton, 1985, pp. 545–552.

Smeets JLRM, Rodriguez LM, Metzger J, Weide A, Constantinou L, Wellens HJJ: How to select the site for successful catheter ablation of idiopathic ventricular tachycardia using radiofrequency energy. J Am Coll Cardiol 1993; 21:265A.

Snyders DJ, Bennett PB, Hondeghem LM: Mechanisms of drug-channel interaction. In Fozzard HA, Haber E, Jennings RB, Katz AM, Morgan HE (eds): The Heart and Cardiovascular System. New York, NY: Raven Press, 1992a, pp. 2164–2193.

Snyders DJ, Knoth KM, Roberds SL, Tamkun MM: Time-, voltage-, and state-dependent block by quinidine of a cloned human cardiac potassium channel. Mol Pharmacol 1992b; 41:322–330.

Solomon SD, Ridker PM, Antman EM: Ventricular arrhythmias in trials of thrombolytic therapy for acute myocardial infarction. A meta-analysis. Circulation 1993; 88:2575–2581.

Sonnhag C, Kallryd A, Nylander E, Ryden L: Long-term efficacy of flecainide in paroxysmal atrial fibrillation. Acta Med Scand 1988; 224:563–569.

Sorota S, Siegal MS, Hoffman BF: The isoproterenol-induced chloride current and cardiac resting potential. J Mol Cell Cardiol 1991; 23:1191–1198.

Spach MS, Dolber PC: Relating extracellular potentials and their derivatives to anisotropic propagation at a microscopic level in human cardiac muscle. Evidence for electrical uncoupling of side-to-side fiber connections with increasing age. Circ Res 1986; 58:356–371.

Spach MS, Miller WT III, Geselowitz DB, Barr RC, Kootsey JM, Johnson EA: The discontinuous nature of propagation in normal canine cardiac muscle. Evidence for recurrent discontinuities of intracellular resistance that affect the membrane currents. Circ Res 1981; 48:39–54.

Spach MS, Miller WT III, Dolber PC, Kootsey JM, Sommer JR, Mosher CE Jr: The functional role of structural complexities in the propagation of depolarization in the atrium of the dog. Cardiac conduction disturbances due to discontinuities of effective axial resistivity. Circ Res 1982; 50:175–191.

Spach MS, Dolber PC, Heidlage JF, Kootsey JM, Johnson EA: Propagating depolarization in anisotropic human and canine cardiac muscle: Apparent directional differences in membrane capacitance. A simplified model for selective directional effects of modifying the sodium conductance on V_{max} τ foot, and the propagation safety factor. Circ Res 1987; 60:206–219.

Spach MS, Dolber PC, Heidlage JF: Influence of the passive anisotropic properties on directional differences in propagation following modification of the sodium conductance in human atrial muscle. A model of reentry based on anisotropic discontinuous propagation. Circ Res 1988; 62:811–832.

Spinelli W, Hoffman BF: Mechanisms of termination of reentrant atrial arrhythmias by class I and class III antiarrhythmic agents. Circ Res 1989; 65: 1565–1579.

Spinelli W, Parsons RW, Colatsky TJ: Effects of WAY-123,398, a new Class III antiarrhythmic agent, on cardiac refractoriness and ventricular fibrillation threshold in anesthetized dogs: A comparison with UK-68798, E-4031, and d1-sotalol. J Cardiovasc Pharmacol 1992; 20:913–922.

Strasberg B, Kusniec J, Lewin RF, Sclarovsky S, Arditti A, Agmon J: An unusual ventricular tachycardia responsive to verapamil. Am Heart J 1986; 111: 190–192.

Strauss HC: Antiarrhythmic implications from the CAST Trial: Impetus for new directions. In Spooner PM, Brown AM, Catterall WA, Kaczorowski GJ, Strauss HC (eds): Ion Channels in the Cardiovascular System. Function and Dysfunction. Armonk, NY: Futura Publishing Co, 1994, pp. 3–14.

Strauss HC, Bigger JT Jr, Hoffman BF: Electrophysiological and beta-receptor blocking effects of MJ 1999 on dog and rabbit cardiac tissue. Circ Res 1970; 26:661–678.

Stuhmer W: Structure-function studies of voltage-gated ion channels. Annu Rev Biophys Biophys Chem 1991; 20:65–78.

Stuhmer W, Ruppersburg JP, Schroter KH, Sakmann B, Stocker M, Giese KP, et al: Molecular basis of functional diversity of voltage-gated potassium channels in mammalian brain. EMBO J 1989; 8:3235–3244.

Sung RJ, Shen EN, Morady F, Scheinman MM, Hess D, Botvinick EH: Electrophysiologic mechanism of exercise-induced sustained ventricular tachycardia. Am J Cardiol 1983; 51:525–530.

Surawicz B: Ventricular fibrillation (Review). J Am Coll Cardiol 1985; 5(suppl 6):43B–54B.

Sutko JL, Ito K, Kenyon JL: Ryanodine: A modifier of sarcoplasmic reticulum calcium release in striated muscle. Fed Proc 1985; 44:2984–2988.

Suttorp MJ, Kingma HJ, Lie-A-Huen L, Mast EG: Intravenous flecainide versus verapamil for acute conversion of paroxysmal atrial fibrillation or flutter to sinus rhythm. Am J Cardiol 1989; 63:693–696.

Suttorp MJ, Kingma HJ, Jessurun ER, Lie-A-Huen L, van Hemel NM, Lie KI: The value of class 1C antiarrhythmic drugs for acute conversion of paroxysmal atrial fibrillation or flutter to sinus rhythm. J Am Coll Cardiol 1990; 16:1722–1727.

Tacker WA Jr, Niebauer MJ, Babbs CF, Combs WJ, et al: The effect of new antiarrhythmic drugs on defibrillation threshold. Crit Care Med 1980; 8: 177–180.

Tada M, Kirchberger MA, Repke DI, Katz AM: The stimulation of calcium transport in cardiac sarcoplasmic reticulum by adenosine 3':5'-monophosphate-dependent protein kinase. J Biol Chem 1974; 249:6174–6180.

Takei M, Furukawa Y, Narita M, Murakami M, Ren L-M, Karasawa Y, et al: Sympathetic nerve stimulation activates both β_1- and β_2-adrenoceptors of SA and AV nodes in anesthetized dog hearts. Jpn J Pharmacol 1992a; 59: 23–30.

Takei M, Furukawa Y, Narita M, Ren L-M, Shiba S: Cardiac electrical responses to catecholamines are differentially mediated by β_2-adrenoceptors in anesthetized dogs. Eur J Pharmacol 1992b; 219:15–21.

Tamkun MM, Knoth KM, Walbridge JA, Kroemer H, Roden DM, Glover DM: Molecular cloning and characterization of two voltage-gated K^+ channel cDNAs from human ventricle. FASEB J 1991; 5:331–337.

Taylor JW, Bidard J-N, Lazdunski M: The characterization of high-affinity binding sites in rat brain for the mast cell-degranulating peptide from bee venom using the purified monoiodinated peptide. J Biol Chem 1984; 259: 13957–13967.

Tempel BL, Papazian DM, Schwarz TL, Jan YN, Jan LY: Sequence of a probable channel component encoded at Shaker locus of *Drosophila*. Science 1987; 237:770–775.

Thandroyen FT, McCarthy J, Burton KP, Opie LH: Ryanodine and caffeine prevent ventricular arrhythmias during acute myocardial ischemia and reperfusion in rat heart. Circ Res 1988; 62:306–314.

Thompson KA, Roden DM, Wood AJJ, Siddoway LA, Barbey JT, Woosley RL: Suppression of ventricular arrhythmias in man by dextro-propranolol independent of beta-adrenergic receptor blockade. J Clin Invest 1990; 85: 836–842.

Thompson PD, Melmon KL, Richards JA, Cohn K, Steinbrunn W, Cudihee R, et al: Lidocaine pharmacokinetics in advanced heart failure, liver disease and renal failure in man. Ann Intern Med 1973; 78:499.

Touboul P, Attalah G, Gressade A, Michelson G, Chatelain MT, Delahaye JP: Effets electrophysiologiques des agents antiarrhythmiques chez l'homme. Tentative de classification. Archives des Maladies du Coeur 1979; 72:72–78.

Touboul P, Saoudi N, Atallah G, Kirkorian G: Catheter ablation for atrial flutter: Current concepts and results. J Cardiovasc Electrophysiol 1992; 3: 641–652.

Trappe HJ, Klein H, Lichtlen P: Sotalol in patients with life-threatening ventricular tachyarrhythmias. Cardiovasc Drugs Ther 1990; 4:1425–1432.

Trautwein W: Mechanisms of tachyarrhythmias and extrasystoles. In Sandoe E, Flensted-Jensen E, Olesen KH (eds): Symposium on Cardiac Arrhythmias. Sodertalje, Sweden: AB Astra, 1970, pp. 53–66.

Tseng G-N: Cell swelling increases the membrane conductance of canine ventricular myocytes. Evidence for a cardiac volume-sensitive chloride channel. Am J Physiol 1992; 262:C1056–1088.

Tseng G-N, Wit AL: Characteristics of a transient inward current that causes delayed afterdepolarizations in atrial cells of the canine coronary sinus. J Mol Cell Cardiol 1987; 19:1105–1119.

Tseng G-N, Boyden PA: Multiple types of Ca^{2+} currents in single canine Purkinje cells. Circ Res 1989; 65:1735–1750.

Tseng G-N, Hoffman BF: Two components of transient outward current in canine ventricular myocytes. Circ Res 1989; 64:633–647.

Tseng-Crank J, Yao J, Berman MF, Tseng GN: Functional role of the N-terminal cytoplasmic domain of a mammalian A-type K channel. J Gen Physiol 1993; 102:1057–1083.

Turgeon J, Murray KT, Roden DM: Effects of drug metabolism, metabolites and stereoselectivity on antiarrhythmic drug action. J Cardiovasc Electrophysiol 1990; 1:238–260.

Twidale N, Heddle WF, Tonkin AM: Procainamide administration during electrophysiology study—Utility as a provocative test for intermittent atrioventricular block. PACE 1988; 11:1388–1397.

Ursell PC, Gardner PI, Albala A, Fenoglio JJ Jr, Wit AL: Structural and electro-physiological changes in the epicardial border zone of myocardial infarcts during infarct healing. Circ Res 1985; 56:436–452.

Usui M, Inoue H, Saihars S, Sugimoto T: Antifibrillatory effects of Class III antiarrhythmic drugs: Comparative study with flecainide. J Cardiovasc Pharmacol 1993; 21:376–383.

Valdivia HH, Kirby MS, Lederer WJ, Coronado R: Scorpion toxins targeted against the sarcoplasmic reticulum Ca^{2+}-release channel of skeletal and cardiac muscle. Proc Natl Acad Sci USA 1992; 89:12185–12189.

Valentine PA, Frew JL, Mashford ML, Sloman JG: Lidocaine in the prevention of sudden death in the pre-hospital phase of acute infarction. N Engl J Med 1974; 291:1327–1331.

van Capelle FJL, Durrer D: Computer simulation of arrhythmias in a network of coupled excitable elements. Circ Res 1980; 47:454–466.

Vanoli E, DeFerrari GM, Stramba-Badiale M, Hull SS Jr, Foreman RD, Schwartz PJ: Vagal stimulation and prevention of sudden death in con-scious dogs with a healed myocardial infarction. Circ Res 1991; 68: 1471–1481.

Varnauskas E: Long-term results of prospective randomized study of coronary artery bypass surgery in stable angina pectoris. Lancet 1982; ii:1173–1180.

Vassalle M: Cardiac pacemaker potentials at different extra- and intracellular K concentrations. Am J Physiol 1965; 208:770–775.

Vassalle M: Electrogenic suppression of automaticity in sheep and dog Pur-kinje fibers. Circ Res 1970; 27:361–377.

Vassalle M: The relationship among cardiac pacemakers. Overdrive suppres-sion. Circ Res 1977; 41:269–277.

Vassalle M, Mugelli A: An oscillatory current in sheep cardiac Purkinje fibers. Circ Res 1981; 48:618–631.

Vaughan Williams EM: Classification of antiarrhythmic drugs. In Sandoe E, Flensted-Jensen E, Olesen K (eds): Cardiac Arrhythmias. Sodertaljie, Swe-den: AB Astra, 1971, pp. 449–472.

Vaughan Williams EM: A classification of antiarrhythmic actions reassessed after a decade of new drugs. J Clin Pharmacol 1984; 24:129–147.

Vaughan Williams EM: Significance of classifying antiarrhythmic actions since the Cardiac Arrhythmia Suppression Trial. J Clin Pharmacol 1991; 31: 123–135.

Verrier RL: Neurochemical approaches to the prevention of ventricular fibril-lation. Fed Proc 1986; 45:2191–2195.

Vetter VL, Josephson ME, Horowitz LN: Idiopathic recurrent sustained ven-tricular tachycardia in children and adolescents. Am J Cardiol 1981; 47: 315–322.

Visentin S, Wu S-N, Belardinelli L: Adenosine-induced changes in atrial action potential: Contribution of Ca and K currents. Am J Physiol 1990; 258: H1070–H1078.

Vlay SC: Catecholamine-sensitive ventricular tachycardia. Am Heart J 1987; 114:455–461.

Vos MA, Gorgels APM, Leunissen-Beekman JDM, Brugada P, Wellens HJJ:

The effect of an entrainment protocol on ouabain-induced ventricular tachycardia. PACE 1989; 12:1485–1493.

Vos MA, Gorgels APM, Leunissen-Beckman JDM, Brugada P, Wellens HJJ: Flunarizine allows differentiation between mechanisms of arrhythmias in the intact heart. Circulation 1990; 81:343–349.

Waldecker B, Coromilas J, Saltman AE, Dillon SM, Wit AL: Overdrive stimulation of functional reentrant circuits causing ventricular tachycardia in the infarcted canine heart. Resetting and entrainment. Circulation 1993; 87: 1286–1305.

Waldo AL: Mechanisms of atrial fibrillation, atrial flutter, and ectopic atrial tachycardia. A brief review. Circulation 1987; 75:III-37–III-40.

Waldo AL: Atrial flutter. In Podrid PJ, Kowey PR (eds): Arrhythmia: A Clinical Approach. Baltimore, MD: Williams & Wilkins. In press.

Waldo AL, MacLean WAH: Diagnosis and Treatment of Arrhythmias Following Open Heart Surgery: Emphasis on the Use of Epicardial Wire Electrodes. Mt Kisco, NY: Futura Publishing Co, 1980.

Waldo AL, Henthorn RW: Use of transient entrainment during ventricular tachycardia to localize a critical area in the reentry circuit for ablation. PACE 1989; 12:231–244.

Waldo AL, Wit AL: Mechanisms of cardiac arrhythmias. Lancet 1993; 341: 1189–1193.

Waldo AL, Wit AL: Mechanisms of Cardiac Arrhythmias and Conduction Disturbances. In Schlant RC, Alexander RW (eds): Hurst's The Heart. Eighth edition. New York, NY: McGraw Hill, 1994, pp. 659–704.

Waldo AL, MacLean WAH, Karp RB, Kouchoukos NT, James TN: Continuous rapid atrial pacing to control recurrent or sustained supraventricular tachycardias following open heart surgery. Circulation 1976; 54:245–250.

Waldo AL, MacLean WAH, Karp RB, Kouchoukos NT, James TN: Entrainment and interruption of atrial flutter with atrial pacing: Studies in man following open heart surgery. Circulation 1977; 56:737–745.

Waldo AL, Plumb VJ, Arciniegas JG, MacLean WAH, Cooper TB, Priest MF, et al: Transient entrainment and interruption of the atrioventricular bypass pathway type of paroxysmal atrial tachycardia. A model for understanding and identifying reentrant arrhythmias. Circulation 1983; 67:73–83.

Waldo AL, Henthorn RW, Plumb VJ, MacLean WAH: Demonstration of the mechanism of transient entrainment and interruption of ventricular tachycardia with rapid atrial pacing. J Am Coll Cardiol 1984; 3:422–430.

Waldo AL, Olshansky B, Okumura K, Henthorn RW: Current perspective on entrainment of tachyarrhythmias. In Brugada P, Wellens HJJ (eds): Cardiac Arrhythmias: Where to Go From Here? Mt. Kisco, NY: Futura Publishing Co, 1987, pp. 171–189.

Waldo AL, Akhtar M, Benditt DG, Brugada P, Camm AJ, Gallagher JJ, et al: Appropriate electrophysiologic study and treatment of patients with the Wolff-Parkinson-White Syndrome. J Am Coll Cardiol 1988; 11:1124–1129; PACE 1988; 11:536–543.

Walsh KB, Kass RB: Regulation of a heart potassium channel by protein kinase A and C. Science 1988; 242:67–69.

Wang GK, Brodwick MS, Eaton DC, Strichartz GR: Inhibition of sodium currents by local anesthetics in chloramine-T-treated squid axons. The role of channel activation. J Gen Physiol 1987; 89:645–667.

Wang J, Bourne GW, Wang Z, Villemaire C, Talajic M, Nattel S: Comparative mechanisms of antiarrhythmic drug action in experimental atrial fibrillation: Importance of use-dependent effects on refractoriness. Circulation 1933a; 88:1030–1044.

Wang Z, Fermini B, Nattel S: Delayed rectifier outward current and repolarization in human atrial myocytes. Circ Res 1993b; 73:276–285.

Ward DE, Camm AJ: Drug studies. In Ward DE, Camm AJ (eds): Clinical Electrophysiology of the Heart. London: E Arnold, 1987, pp. 271–298.

Ward DE, Garratt CJ: The substrate for atrioventricular "nodal" reentrant tachycardia: Is there a "third pathway"? J Cardiovasc Electrophysiol 1993; 4:62–67.

Ward DE, Nathan AW, Camm AJ: Fascicular tachycardia sensitive to calcium antagonists. Eur Heart J 1984; 5:896–905.

Wasserstrom JA, Ferrier GR: Voltage dependence of digitalis afterpotentials, aftercontractions, and inotropy. Am J Physiol 1981; 241:H646–H653.

Wasserstrom JA, Schwartz DJ, Fozzard HA: Catecholamine effects on intracellular sodium activity and tension in dog heart. Am J Physiol 1982; 243: H670–H675.

Watson RM, Josephson ME: Atrial flutter. I. Electrophysiologic substrates and modes of initiation and termination. Am J Cardiol 1980; 45:732–741.

Weidmann S: The effect of the cardiac membrane potential on the rapid availability of the sodium-carrying system. J Physiol (Lond) 1955; 127:213–224.

Weidmann S: Elektrophysiologie Der Herzmuskelfaser. Medizinischer Verlag Hans Huber, Bern Und Stuttgart, 1956.

Weismüller P, Mutter K, Kochs M, Richter P, Wiecha J, Grossmann G, et al: Wertigkeit von EKG-Morphologie und Zykluslänge von Salven im Langzeit-EKG bei Patienten mit Kammertachykardien. Z Kardiol 1992; 81:137. Abstract.

Wellens HJJ, Durrer D: Effect of digitalis on atrioventricular conduction and circus movement tachycardia in patients with Wolff-Parkinson-White syndrome. Circulation 1973; 47:1229–1233.

Wellens HJJ, Bär, FW, Gorgels AP, Vanagt EJ: Use of ajmaline in patients with the Wolff-Parkinson-White syndrome to disclose a short refractory period of the accessory pathway. Am J Cardiol 1980a; 45:130–133.

Wellens HJJ, Farré J, Bär FWHM: The Wolff-Parkinson-White syndrome. In Mandel WJ (ed): Cardiac Arrhythmias: Their Mechanism, Diagnosis and Management. Philadelphia, PA: JB Lippincott Co, 1980b, pp. 342–365.

Wellens HJJ, Brugada P, Roy D, Weiss J, Bär FW: Effect of isoproterenol on the antegrade refractory period of the accessory pathway in patients with the Wolff-Parkinson-White syndrome. Am J Cardiol 1982a; 50:180–184.

Wellens HJJ, Braat S, Brugada P, Gorgels AP, Bär FW: Use of procainamide in patients with the Wolff-Parkinson-White syndrome to disclose a short refractory period of the accessory pathway. Am J Cardiol 1982b; 50: 1087–1089.

Wellens HJJ, Brugada P, Stevenson WG: Programmed electrical stimulation of the heart in patients with life-threatening ventricular arrhythmias: What is the significance of induced arrhythmias and what is the correct protocol? Circulation 1985; 72:1–7.

Wells JL Jr, Karp RB, Kouchoukos NT, MacLean WAH, James TN, Waldo AL: Characterization of atrial fibrillation in man: Studies following open heart surgery. PACE 1978; 1:426–438.

Wells JL Jr, MacLean WAH, James TN, Waldo AL: Characterization of atrial flutter. Studies in man after open heart surgery using fixed atrial electrodes. Circulation 1979; 60:665.

Wesley RC Jr, Farkhani F, Morgan D, Zimmerman D: Ibutilide: Enhanced defibrillation via plateau sodium current activation. Am J Physiol 1993; 264: H1269–H1274.

Wharton J, Gulbenkina S: Peptides in the mammalian cardiovascular system. Experientia 1987; 43:821–832.

Wible FB, Wang Z, Fermini B, Faust F, Nattel S, Brown AM: Identity of a novel delayed rectifier current from human heart with a cloned K^+ channel current. Circ Res 1993; 73:210–214.

Wijffels M, Kirchhof C, Frederiks J, Boersma L, Allessie M: Atrial fibrillation begets atrial fibrillation. Circulation 1993; 88:I-18. Abstract.

Williams DO, Scherlag BJ, Hope RR, El-Sherif N, Lazzara R: The pathophysiology of malignant ventricular arrhythmias during acute myocardial ischemia. Circulation 1974; 50:1163–1172.

Wit AL, Cranefield PF: Triggered activity in cardiac muscle fibers of the simian mitral valve. Circ Res 1976; 38:85–98.

Wit AL, Cranefield PF: Triggered and automatic activity in the canine coronary sinus. Circ Res 1977; 41:435–445.

Wit AL, Cranefield PF: Reentrant excitation as a cause of cardiac arrhythmias. Am J Physiol 1978; 235:H1–H17.

Wit AL, Rosen MR: Cellular electrophysiology of cardiac arrhythmias. In Josephson ME, Wellens HJJ (eds): Tachycardias: Mechanisms, Diagnosis, Treatment. Philadelphia, PA: Lea & Febiger, 1984, pp. 1–17.

Wit AL, Rosen MR: Afterdepolarizations and triggered activity: Distinction from automaticity as an arrhythmogenic mechanism. In Fozzard HA, Haber E, Jennings RB, Katz AM, Morgan HE (eds): The Heart and Cardiovascular System. Scientific Foundations. New York, NY: Raven Press, Ltd, 1992, pp. 2113–2163.

Wit AL, Janse MJJ: The Ventricular Arrhythmias of Ischemia and Infarction. Electrophysiological Mechanisms. Mount Kisco, NY: Futura Publishing Co, 1993.

Wit AL, Hoffman BF, Cranefield PF: Slow conduction and reentry in the ventricular conducting system. I. Return extrasystole in canine Purkinje fibers. Circ Res 1972a; 30:1–10.

Wit AL, Cranefield PF, Hoffman BF: Slow conduction and reentry in the ventricular conducting system. II. Single and sustained circus movement in networks of canine and bovine Purkinje fibers. Circ Res 1972b; 30:11–22.

Wit AL, Fenoglio JJ Jr, Wagner BM, Bassett AL: Electrophysiological properties of cardiac muscle in the anterior mitral valve leaflet and the adjacent atrium in the dog. Possible implications for the genesis of atrial dysrhythmias. Circ Res 1973; 32:731–745.

Wit AL, Wiggins JR, Cranefield PF: Some effects of electrical stimulation on impulse initiation in cardiac fibers: Its relevance for the determination of the mechanisms of clinical cardiac arrhythmias. In Wellens HJJ, Lie KI, Janse MJ (eds): The Conduction System of the Heart. Philadelphia, PA: Lea & Febiger, 1976, pp. 163–181.

Wit AL, Cranefield PF, Gadsby DC: Electrogenic sodium extrusion can stop triggered activity in the canine coronary sinus. Circ Res 1981; 49:1029–1042.

Wit AL, Allessie MA, Bonke FIM, Lammers W, Smeets J, Fenoglio JJ Jr: Electrophysiological mapping to determine the mechanisms of experimental ventricular tachycardia initiated by premature impulses. Experimental approach and initial results demonstrating reentrant excitation. Am J Cardiol 1982; 49:166–185.

Wit AL, Dillon SM, Coromilas J, Saltman AE, Waldecker B: Anisotropic reentry in the epicardial border zone of myocardial infarcts. In Jalife J (ed): Mathematical Approaches to Cardiac Arrhythmias. Ann N Y Acad Sci 1990a; 591:86–108.

Wit AL, Tseng G-N, Henning B, Hanna MS: Arrhythmogenic effects of quinidine on catecholamine-induced delayed afterdepolarizations in canine atrial fibers. J Cardiovasc Elect 1990b; 1:15–30.

Woelfel A, Foster JR, McAllister RG Jr, Simpson RJ, Gettes LS: Efficacy of verapamil in exercise-induced ventricular tachycardia. Am J Cardiol 1985; 56:292–297.

Woods KL, Fletcher S, Roffe C, Haider Y: Intravenous magnesium sulphate in suspected acute myocardial infarction: Results of the second Leicester Intravenous Magnesium Intervention Trial (LIMIT-2). Lancet 1992; 339: 1553–1558.

Woosley RL, Roden DM: The importance of metabolites in antiarrhythmic therapy. Am J Cardiol 1983; 52:3C–7C.

Woosley RL, Drayer DE, Reidenberg MM, Nies AS, Carr K, Oates JA: Effect of acetylator phenotype on the rate at which procainamide induces antinuclear antibodies and the lupus syndrome. N Engl J Med 1978; 298:1157–1159.

Woosley RL, Siddoway LA, Duff HJ, Roden DM: Flecainide dose-response relations in stable ventricular arrhythmias. Am J Cardiol 1984; 53(supp): 59B–65B.

Woosley RL, Wood AJJ, Roden DM: Encainide. N Engl J Med 1988; 318: 1107–1115.

Woosley RL, Chen Y, Freiman JP, Gillis RA: Mechanism of cardiotoxic actions of terfenadine. JAMA 1993; 269:1532–1536.

Wu D, Kou H-C, Hung J-S: Exercise-triggered paroxysmal ventricular tachycardia. Ann Intern Med 1981; 95:410–414.

Yamashita T, Inoue H, Nozaki A, Sugimoto T: Role of anatomic architecture in sustained atrial reentry and double potentials. Am Heart J 1992; 124: 938–946.

Yanagihara K, Irisawa H: Potassium current during the pacemaker depolarization in rabbit sinoatrial node cell. Pflügers Arch 1980; 388:255–260.

Yatani A, Codina J, Brown AM, Birnbaumer L: Direct activation of mammalian atrial muscarinic potassium channels by GTP regulatory protein G_k. Science 1987; 235:207–211.

Yatani A, Okabe K, Codina J,Birnbaumer L, Brown AM: Heart rate regulation by G proteins acting on the cardiac pacemaker channel. Science 1990; 249: 1163–1166.

Yazawa K, Kameyama M: Mechanism of receptor-mediated modulation of the delayed outward potassium current in guinea pig ventricular myocytes. Am J Physiol 1990; 428:135–150.

Yeh JZ: Sodium inactivation mechanism modulates QX-314 block of sodium channels in squid axons. Biophys J 1978; 24:569–574.

Yusuf S, Peto R, Lewis J, Collins R, Sleight P: Beta blockade during and after myocardial infarction: An overview of the randomized trials. Prog Cardiovasc Dis 1985; 17:335–371.

Zaza A, Kline RP, Rosen MR: Effects of α-adrenergic stimulation on intracellular sodium activity and automaticity in canine Purkinje fibers. Circ Res 1990; 66:416–426.

Zeiler RH, Sequeria JM, Henkin R: Lysophospatidylcholine. Putative agent for maintained triggered activity in ischemic cardiac Purkinje fibers. J Am Coll Cardiol 1987; 9:252A.

Zipes DP: Electrophysiological mechanisms involved in ventricular fibrillation. Circulation 1975; 52(suppl II):120–130.

Zipes DP: A consideration of antiarrhythmic therapy. Circulation 1985; 72: 949–956.

Zipes DP: Antiarrhythmic uncoupling. PACE 1988a; 11:127–129.

Zipes DP: Proarrhythmic events. Am J Cardiol 1988b; 61:70A–76A.

Zipes DP: Cardiac electrophysiology: Promises and contributions. J Am Coll Cardiol 1989; 13:1329–1352.

Zipes DP: Specific arrhythmias: Diagnosis and treatment. In Braunwald E (ed): Heart Disease. A Textbook of Cardiovascular Medicine. Fourth edition. Philadelphia, PA: WB Saunders, 1992, pp. 667–725.

Zipes DP, Mendez C: Action of manganese ions and tetrodotoxin on atrioventricular nodal transmembrane potentials in isolated rabbit hearts. Circ Res 1973; 32:447–454.

Zipes DP, Foster PR, Troup PJ, Pedersen DH: Atrial induction of ventricular tachycardia: Reentry versus triggered automaticity. Am J Cardiol 1978; 44: 1–8.

Zuanetti G, Hoyt RH, Corr PB: Beta-adrenergic mediated influences on microscopic conduction in epicardial regions overlying infarcted myocardium. Circ Res 1990; 67:284–302.

Index

DATE DUE

AP 19 '97			